IMMUNOLOGICAL XENOGENIZATION
OF TUMOR CELLS

GANN Monograph on Cancer Research

The series of GANN Monograph on Cancer Research was initiated in 1966 by the late Dr. Tomizo Yoshida (1903–73) for the purpose of publishing proceedings of international conferences and symposia on cancer and allied research fields, and papers on specific subjects of importance in cancer research.

The decision to publish a monograph is made by the Editorial Board of the Japanese Cancer Association, with the final approval of the Board of Directors. It is hoped that the series will serve as an important source of information in cancer research.

Japanese Cancer Association

The publication of this monograph owes much to the financial support given by the late Professor Kazushige Higuchi of Jikei University.

JAPANESE CANCER ASSOCIATION

GANN Monograph on Cancer Research No. 23

IMMUNOLOGICAL XENOGENIZATION OF TUMOR CELLS

Edited by HIROSHI KOBAYASHI

JAPAN SCIENTIFIC SOCIETIES PRESS, Tokyo
UNIVERSITY PARK PRESS, Baltimore

Published jointly by

JAPAN SCIENTIFIC SOCIETIES PRESS

Tokyo

and

UNIVERSITY PARK PRESS

Baltimore

Library of Congress Cataloging in Publication Data
Main entry under title:

Immunological xenogenization of tumor cells.

(Gann monograph on cancer research; no. 23)
Papers presented at a workshop in Sapporo, Japan,
June 6–8, 1978, sponsored by International Cancer Research
Workshops, National Cancer Institute of the United States,
and the Japan Society for the Promotion of Science.
Bibliography: p.
1. Tumors—Immunological aspects—Congresses. 2.
Tumor antigens—Congresses.   3. Xenografts—
Congresses. I. Kobayashi, Hiroshi, 1927– II. Inter-
national Cancer Research Workshops.   III. United
States. National Cancer Institute.   IV. Nippon
Gakujutsu Shinkokai.   V. Series.
QR188.6.145   616.9′92′079   79-9414
ISBN 0-8391-1471-0

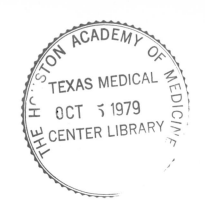
PREFACE

It is my great honor to be able to edit the monograph entitled "Immunological Xenogenization of Tumor Cells." This monograph documents the presentation given at the International Workshop of the same title held at the Park Hotel in Sapporo, Japan, on June 6–8, 1978. The workshop was sponsored by International Cancer Research Workshops (ICREW), the National Cancer Institute of the United States, and the Japan Society for the Promotion of Science.

The word "xenogenization" (i·bu·tsu·ka in Japanese) was first chosen to designate the spontaneous regression of tumors by artificial infection with nonlytic surface viruses by Kobayashi *et al.* in 1969. The regression of tumors is mainly based on the acquisition of virus-specific new antigen, which is foreign to the host. As is well known, an immunological characteristic of tumor cells is their low antigenicity, which is not easily recognized as foreign by the host. It is important, therefore, to explore how the antigenicity of tumor cells can be increased by biological and chemical modification, so that the modified tumor cells may be more effectively used in immunotherapy and immunodiagnosis. "Xenogenization" is now a general term used to describe all attempts at making a tumor cell antigenically foreign to the host (Greek: Xenos=foreign), for which either an *acquisition* of new foreign antigen (similar to the "heterogenization" of Dr. Svet-Moldavsky), or an *increase* in the antigenicity of formerly existing TSA, or both is required.

I would like to express my thanks to those from Sweden, the USSR, the United Kingdom, the United States, and Japan, who kindly participated in the workshop. I am sure that they have contributed greatly towards progress in cancer immunology in the new approach of how to create foreignness in tumor cells. I hope that the workshop and this monograph on xenogenization will be the first steps in solving the problem of weak antigenicity in tumor cells.

June 1978

Hiroshi KOBAYASHI

CONTENTS

viii

RECOGNITION OF CELL SURFACE ANTIGENS UNDERGOING XENOGENIZATION

XENOGENIZATION BY CELL HYBRIDIZATION

APPLICATION OF XENOGENIZATION TO HUMAN CANCER

XENOGENIZATION WITH VIRUS

GANN Monograph on Cancer Research 23, 1979

XENOGENIZATION BY VIRUSES: HOW COULD IT WORK?

J. LINDENMANN

*Institute of Medical Microbiology, Division of Experimental Microbiology, University of Zürich**

Although other mechanisms of virus-enhanced immunogenicity of cellular antigens are conceivable, such as activation of macrophages or interferon induction, this short review will focus on possible associations of viral epitopes with cellular epitopes. Such associations can occur at all levels of virus-cell interaction, but the following are the more obvious ones: Whereas mere adsorption of virus particles to cells is probably too superficial to have immunological consequences, those viruses which fuse their envelopes with the host cell cause a profound rearrangement of cellular and viral antigens within the plane of the cell membrane. At least in certain systems, the replicase offers a startling example of intimate collaboration between cellular and viral products: In the bacterial virus Q-beta the polymerase consists of virus-coded and host-coded polypeptides. In viruses where nucleoproteins are rapidly transported into and out of the nucleus, attachment to certain cellular transport elements must be postulated. The nascent viral proteins emerging from ribosomes will very soon assume their characteristic folding, resulting in the expression of viral epitopes still anchored to cellular material. In enveloped viruses, viral glycoproteins acquire, during their migration through the endoplasmic reticulum, carbohydrate epitopes patterned after the host, but now in conjunction with a viral carrier. The insertion of vast quantities of viral proteins in cell membranes concomitantly with elimination of cellular proteins must lead to considerable upheaval of membrane architecture, and, temporarily, to mosaic-like intercalation of viral and cellular patterns. After incorporation into the viral membrane glycolipids find themselves in entirely different protein surroundings, and this possibly affects their immunogenic behavior. In cytocidal as well as in noncytocidal virus-cell systems qualitatively similar relationships can be envisaged. Finally, many of the arguments presented above with viral structural epitopes in mind could also apply to non-structural, virus-coded antigens.

When considering the ways in which a virus-infected tumor cell might be a better immunogen than its non-infected counterpart, many possibilities come to mind (*1–5*). Thus, virus infection could lead to interferon production, which itself has an effect on expression of cell-surface antigens, on immune responsiveness, and on tumor cell growth potential. Alternatively, the virus-infected cell might exert a chemotactic attraction on macrophages, which in turn would result in an altered immunogenic behavior.

---

* CH-8006 Zürich, Switzerland.

The exciting discovery of an unexpectedly close interrelationship between viral anti-genic targets and cell-surface antigens, of which we will hear more in Dr. Zinkernagel's presentation, indicates that there may be a more specific element in the immunological consequences of virus-cell interactions.

Recognition of Self

Whereas the immune system has been regarded until recently as essentially geared to recognizing foreignness, there is now a tendency to assume that a weak interaction or "recognition" of self also exists. This in itself is apparently unable to trigger the immunological machinery. However, a second, possibly similarly weak, interaction may lead to the formation of cytotoxic cells. Alloantigens, the antigens by which members of the same species differ, may lead to strong interaction, and may by themselves trigger the immune response. If the structures involved in the weak self recognition are the very molecules on which the major histocompatibility complex harps its tune, then alloantigen recognition would involve a monovalent strong interaction, while at the same time abolishing the weak self interaction. The normal response against virus-infected cells would require a bivalent weak interaction. How is one now to regard those antigens that might conceivably serve as target in an antitumor response? It might be that these are, just as alloantigens, modifications of features normally per-ceived as "self"; this would also lead to an abolition of self interaction. But, in contrast to alloantigens, these more discrete modifications would themselves result in only weak interactions, and correspondingly to a recognition not above the level of self, and hence to a quiescent immune system.

Antitumor Response

Thus the problem in triggering the immune system in cases of an antitumor response is less one of recognizing the tumor epitope target, than one of allowing for a second, albeit weak interaction. Of course the two weak interactions visualized in such a scheme would have to fulfill certain criteria of spatial arrangement or surface distribu-tion of which we know at the moment very little. It is precisely this our ignorance which puts viruses in a particularly hopeful position, because we know that they interact in the proper manner with the normal "self" determinants. It is therefore tempting to assume that they interact similarly with the putative weak tumor-associated deter-minants.

Role of Viral Antigens

But do viruses alter the fabric of the cell surface in such a way that the immune system may be triggered? Although we still know very little at the molecular level, there are indications from morphology that this may indeed be the case. My collaborator Dr. Th. Bächi has studied the surface architecture of EL-4 tumor cells infected with Sendai virus. This is a system in which no infectious virions are formed, because cleavage of the F glycoprotein is not accomplished. Twenty-four hr after infection, viral antigens appear at the cell surface, as evidenced by cyto-hemadsorption. At the same

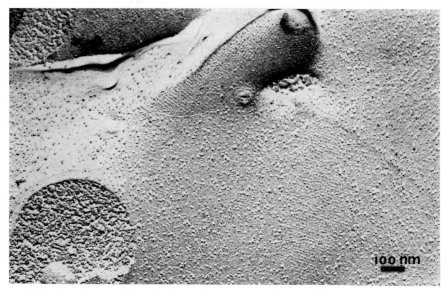

FIG. 1. Freeze-etching picture of EL-4 cell infected with Sendai virus, 24 hr after infection

Budding particle in the upper half of the picture. Note regular paracrystalline pattern on the budding particle and in the lower right-hand part of the fractured cell membrane (just left from the 100 nm bar). Normal intramembraneous particles with random distribution can be observed below the budding site. Picture by Dr. Th. Bächi.

time, freeze-etching reveals patches of paracrystalline arrangements of some finely granular material, smaller than the normal membrane particles, within the hydrophobic plane of cleavage (Fig. 1). Such arrays can also be seen on budding virus particles, but in pelleted virions prepared for electron microscopy by the same technique these structures are no longer visible. Thus they must represent a transient and labile stage in the course of virus-cell integration.

The paracrystalline aspect of these membrane changes suggests repetitive orderly presentation of epitopes, which may be sufficient to convert a T-dependent antigen into a T-independent one. It may also explain the strange observation that, whereas the immunogenicity of X-irradiated tumor cells as a rule is lost upon homogenization, that of the same cells, but virus-infected, is preserved (6).

CONCLUSION

In terms of more conventional immunology, it is known that most immunogens consist of a carrier moiety and a "haptenic" moiety, and that there is collaboration between T cells and B cells in recognition of the carrier and haptenic epitopes. Tolerance seems to be more generally engraved at the T cell than at the B cell level. Transfer of a haptenic epitope from a carrier with self characteristics to one of pronounced foreignness immediately results in a powerful immune response. In the course of virus replication numerous occasions for appositions of haptenic epitopes, for instance, host-determined patterns of sugar residues, on virus-coded polypeptides offer themselves.

There are even examples of enzymic machines composed of host-derived and virus-derived polypeptide chains working in unison. The problems with xenogenization by viruses are not due to the lack of possibilities, but to our lack of understanding which of the many possibilities, if any, could be harnessed for practical applications.

REFERENCES

1. Haller, O. and Lindenmann, J. Host-cell antigen potentiated by incomplete growth cycle of influenza virus. *J. Natl. Cancer Inst.*, **54**, 459–464 (1975).
2. Lindenmann, J. The use of viruses as immunological potentiators. *Ciba Found. Symp.*, **18**, 197–215 (1973).
3. Lindenmann, J. Viruses as immunological adjuvants in cancer. *Biochim. Biophys. Acta*, **355**, 49–75 (1974).
4. Lindenmann, J. Host antigens in enveloped RNA viruses. *In* "Virus Infection and the Cell Surface," ed. G. Poste and G. L. Nicolson, pp. 291–329 (1977). North-Holland Publ. Comp., Amsterdam, New York, Oxford.
5. Lindenmann, J. Strategies of active immunization applicable to cancer. Fogarty Int. Center Proc. No. 28. *In* "Modulation of Host Immune Resistance in the Prevention or Treatment of Induced Neoplasias," ed. M. A. Chirigos, pp. 187–190 (1977). Dept. of Health, Education and Welfare, U.S.A., Publ. No. (NIH) 77-893.
6. Wise, K. S. Vesicular stomatitis virus-infected L1210 murine leukemia cells: Increased immunogenicity and altered surface antigens. *J. Natl. Cancer Inst.*, **58**, 83–90 (1977).

VIRUS AUGMENTATION: INCREASED IMMUNOGENICITY OF TUMOR-ASSOCIATED TRANSPLANTATION ANTIGENS IN TUMOR CELL EXTRACTS AFTER INFECTION WITH SURFACE BUDDING VIRUSES

Charles W. Boone,[*1] Noritoshi Takeichi,[*1] Faye C. Austin,[*1]
Eiki Gotohda,[*1] Tsuneyuki Oikawa,[*1] and
Ronald Gillette[*2]

*Cell Biology Section, Laboratory of Viral Carcinogenesis,
National Cancer Institute, National Institutes
of Health[*1] and Cancer Center of Hawaii[*2]*

Eleven laboratories have now confirmed that immunogenicity of the tumor associated transplantation antigens (TATA) in tumor cell extracts or simple homogenates is increased by first infecting the tumor cells with a surface budding virus. The virus must infect the tumor cell to augment the TATA of that cell, a fact to be emphasized by using the term "vicinal adjuvanticity." Soluble extracts which retain virus-augmented TATA activity were prepared, indicating that the virus antigen and TATA may exist as a complex that lends itself to further purification.

It is important at the very outset to emphasize that there are two distinctly different groups of investigators who are interested in the use of viruses to augment the immunogenicity of tumor associated transplantation antigens TATA. One group deals exclusively with viable tumor cells and seeks to increase the immunogenicity of their TATA by productively infecting them with non-cytopathic viruses, usually oncornaviruses (*1, 12–14*). The other group deals exclusively with tumor cell extracts (or simple homogenates) and seeks to increase the TATA immunogenicity of the extracts by using tumor cells that have been lytically infected with a cytopathic surface-budding virus such as influenza virus or vesicular stomatitis virus (*2–6, 8–11, 15–19*). The interest of the former group appears to center around the use of the productively infected viable tumor cells as improved immunogens in immunotherapy. We belong to the latter group and, speaking at least for ourselves, are interested in attempting to purify from the lytically infected tumor cell extracts TATA of high specific activity which may then be of greater usefulness both in immunodiagnosis (as skin test antigens) and in immunotherapy (without the concern, justified or not, that customarily arises when the use of viable tumor cells or oncogenic viruses is considered).

We also wish to comment on the various definitions we observe being given to the term "xenogenization." As judged by its use in the session titles of this symposium

---

[*1] Bethesda, Maryland 20014,U.S.A. (武市紀年, 後藤田栄貴, 及川恒之).
[*2] Honolulu, Hawaii 96822, U.S.A.

(xenogenization with viruses, xenogenization with chemicals and enzymes, xenogenization by cell hybridization), "to xenogenize a cell" appears to mean simply to cause a foreign antigen to occur on the surface of that cell. This definition is immediately understandable and could be useful but other more inclusive and complicated definitions are also in current use (13), which tends to confuse the issue. It would be well if in the future every investigator who uses the term "xenogenization" were to carefully define it in each publication where it is used. In our case, for the present at least, we will continue to use the term "virus augmentation" or "virus augmented" to denote the increase in immunogenicity of a TATA produced by the insertion of a virus antigen into the cell membrane adjacent to that TATA.

Virus-augmented TATA in Crude Membrane Extracts of Tumor Cells

We will now quickly review the salient features of the phenomenon of virus-augmented TATA, and refer the reader to previous publications for details. In this work we have used an SV40-transformed BALB/3T3 tumor carried in BALB/c mice. TATA activity is routinely measured by the degree of resistance to tumor cell challenge conferred on animals 14 days after they have been immunized on days 0 and 3 with the material being tested. Homogenates and CM extracts of tumor cells infected with influenza virus or vesicular stomatitis virus possess increased TATA immunogenicity compared to extracts from non-infected cells, which have little or no TATA activity at all. Ultraviolet ray inactivation of the virus or Formalin fixation of the virus-infected material does not appreciably affect the augmented TATA immunogenicity (5). Immunization of mice with virus grown in eggs or in antigenically unrelated cells does not render the mice immune to tumor cell challenge. The tumor cells must be infected by the virus to at least the point of appearance of virus-coded antigens on the cell surface (16). Simply mixing virus with tumor cell homogenate or CM extract does not augment TATA immunogenicity (5).

Virus-augmented TATA in Soluble Extracts of Tumor Cells

We have found that soluble, as opposed to crude membrane, extracts of influenza virus-infected tumor cells still exhibit augmented TATA immunogenicity.* Table I compares the TATA immunogenicity of both CM and soluble extracts from influenza virus-infected and non-infected tumor cells. Tumor cell homogenates of hypotonically swollen cells ruptured in a Dounce apparatus were centrifuged at 1,500 rpm for 5 min to sediment nuclei. The supernatant was collected and subjected to a second centrifugation at high speed ($100,000 \times g$), after which the supernatant and resuspended pellet material were designated "soluble extract" and "CM," respectively, and were used to immunize mice according to the protocol given in Table I. Note that soluble extracts from influenza virus-infected tumor cells were more immunogenic than soluble extracts from non-infected cells. This result is an important advance toward the goal of obtaining purified virus-augmented transplantation resistant antigen (TRA) of high potency.

---

* Austin, F. C. Isolation of Virus-Augmented Tumor Antigens. Ph. D. dissertation, George Washington University, (1978).

TABLE I. Preparation of Soluble Virus-augmented Tumor Antigens by High-speed
Centrifugation $(100,000 \times g)$ of Nucleus-free Dounce Homogenates

| Group | Immunogen[a] | Results of tumor challenge | | p[b] |
		Tumor incidence (%)	Mean tumor wt(g)$\pm$SE	
1	10^6 X-ray inactivated tumor cells	0/20 (0)	—	
2	Tumor cell homogenate	8/13 (62)	0.39 ± 0.18	<0.01
3	Influenza virus-augmented tumor cell homogenate	3/13 (23)	0.45 ± 0.11	<0.005
4	Tumor cell crude membranes	17/20 (85)	0.67 ± 0.13	<0.05
5	Virus augmented tumor cell crude membranes	4/20 (20)	0.09 ± 0.06	<0.0005
6	Soluble extract from tumor cell homogenate	13/20 (65)	0.67 ± 0.14	<0.05
7	Soluble extract from virus-augmented tumor cell homogenate	4/14 (29)	0.36 ± 0.25	<0.025
8	Phosphate-buffered saline	17/20 (85)	1.03 ± 0.13	

[a] Mice were immunized with 10^6 X-irradiated tumor cells or 500 μg of antigen, s.c., on days 0 and 3.

[b] Comparison of mean tumor weight with that of control phosphate buffered saline (PBS) group by Student t-test. Comparisons of tumor weights from virus-augmented antigen groups with those of corresponding non-augmented groups shows significant difference in tumor size of Group 4 *vs* 5.

Basic Facts Regarding Virus Augmentation of TATA Immunogenicity

Following are some basic facts regarding virus augmentation of TATA that have been independently established in three or more laboratories.

1) The phenomenon of virus augmentation of TATA immunogencity in tumor cell extracts (or simple homogenates) is well established

Eleven different laboratories (*2, 3, 5, 6, 8, 10, 14, 16–19*) using six different viruses (influenza virus, Newcastle disease virus, Sendai virus, Semliki Forest virus, vesicular stomatitis virus, and vaccinia virus) and nine separate tumor systems, have reported the fact that the TATA immunogenicity of simple homogenates ro extracts of virus-infected tumor cells is greater than that of similar preparations of non-infected cells.

2) Virus augmentation of TATA works through the immune system

The following evidence from three different laboratories indicates that the immune system is involved in the virus augmentation effect. Priming mice with virus alone enhances (*15, 17*) or diminishes (*3, 5*) the augmented immunogenicity of virus-infected tumor cell homogenates. Homogenates of virus-infected tumor cells to which antiviral antibody has been added do not show augmented TATA immunogenicity (*15, 17*). Finally, mice made tolerant to influenza virus can no longer show augmented immunity when immunized with virus-infected tumor cell homogenate (*5*).

3) The immunogenicity of virus-augmented tumor cell homogenates is usually less than that of an equivalent number of X-ray inactivated whole cells

While the TATA immunogenicity of tumor cell homogenates and extracts is markedly improved after virus infection, it still is usually somewhat less than that of X-ray inactivated cells. One of our present goals is to purify the TATA-virus combination to a specific activity higher than that of X-ray inactivated cells.

4) The virus components must be on (or in) the plasma membrane of the same tumor cell that bears the TATA

This important fact, which has been shown in three different laboratories (*5, 15, 17*) deserves emphasis. Simply mixing virus with tumor cell homogenate does not augment TATA immunogenicity. The virus must infect the tumor cell whose TATA it augments, at least to the stage where virus-coded proteins appear within the plasma membrane. It appears that the viral antigen must be less than approximately a micrometer or two away from the TATA. A name we prefer which emphasizes this vicinity effect is "vicinal adjuvanticity," a term inspired by Dr. Lindenmann's term, "viral adjuvanticity." Thus, a virus-coded protein, a chemical adduct, or immunologically foreign membrane proteins produced by enzymic alteration or fusion with a foreign cell, may all act as vicinal adjuvants to the TATA. An interesting example of vicinal adjuvanticity in an unrelated system has been reported by Crum and McGregor (*7*) as follows: When a soluble tumor antigen from a chemically induced rat hepatoma (D37 tumor) was adsorbed to living BCG organisms and the antigen-BCG complex injected into syngeneic rats, resistance to challenge with D37 tumor cells was induced. However, no antitumor resistance occurred when the rats were immunized with the soluble tumor antigen alone.

Immunological Mechanism of the Virus Augmentation of TATA Effect

Some investigators have speculated that the virus augmentation of TATA may operate through a mechanism similar to that of the hapten-carrier effect familiar to humoral immunologists, where a determinant on the carrier gives a signal to a contacting helper T cell which in some way results in a nearby B cell responding more intensely to the adjacent hapten. By analogy, the vicinal virus antigen could convey a signal to a contacting helper T cell that would result in a nearby killer T cell precursor being induced to respond more intensely to the adjacent TATA. Of course other cellular immune interactions are possible. For instance, the vicinal viral antigen could separately call forth a local concentration of cellular and humoral immune mediators, such as macrophages and lymphocyte chemotactic factors, that would nonspecifically enhance the immune response to the TATA.

The fact that we were able to obtain virus augmented TATA in soluble form opens up new possibilities for elucidating the virus augmentation effect. At the moment we are attempting to determine if the solubilized TATA and virus antigen are bound together as a complex. If they are, the way will be open not only to purify the complex further, but also to analyze the virus augmentation of TRA phenomenon by *in vitro* methods.

REFERENCES

1. Al-ghazzouli, I. K., Donahoe, R. M., Huang, K-Y., Sass, B., Peters, R. L., and Kelloff,

G. J. Immunity to virus-free syngeneic tumor cell transplantation in the BALB/c mouse after immunization with homologous tumor cells infected with Type C virus. *J. Immunol.*, **117**, 2239–2248 (1976).

2. Ansel, S. Incorporation de L'antigene tumoral de transplantation specifique du SV40 (TSTA-SV40) dans le virus de la stomatite vesiculeuse cultive en cellules de hamster transformees par le SV40. *Int. J. Cancer*, **13**, 773–784 (1974).

3. Beverley, P.C.L., Lowenthal, R. M., and Tyrrell, D.A.J. Immune responses in mice to tumor challenge after immunization with Newcastle disease virus-infected or X-irradiated tumor cells or cell fractions. *Int. J. Cancer*, **11**, 212–223 (1973).

4. Boone, C. W. Augmented immunogenicity of tumor cell homogenates produced by infection with influenza virus. *Natl. Cancer Inst. Monogr.*, **35**, 301–307 (1972).

5. Boone, C. W., Paranjpe, M., Orme, T., and Gillette, R. Virus augmented tumor transplantation antigens. Evidence for a helper antigen mechanism. *Int. J. Cancer*, **13**, 543–551 (1974).

6. Cassel, W. A., Murray, D. R., Torbin, A. H., Olkowski, Z. L., and Moore, M. E. Viral oncolysate in the management of malignant melanoma. I. Preparation of the oncolysate and measurement of immunologic responses.

7. Crum, E. D. and McGregor, D. D. Induction of tumor resistance with BCG-associated tumor antigen. *Int. J. Cancer*, **20**, 805–812 (1977).

8. Eaton, M. and Almquist, S. J. Antibody response of syngeneic mice to membrane antigens from NDV-infected lymphoma. *Proc. Roy. Soc. Lond. (Biol)*, **148**, 1090–1094 (1975).

9. Gillette, R. and Boone, C. W. Augmented immunogenicity of tumor cell membranes produced by surface budding viruses: Parameters of optimal immunization. *Int. J. Cancer*, **18**, 216–222 (1976).

10. Griffith, I. P., Crook, N. F., and White, D. O. Protection of mice against cancer by immunization with membranes but not purified virions from virus infected cancer cells. *Br. J. Cancer*, **31**, 603–613 (1975).

11. Hakkinen, I. and Halonen, P. Induction of tumor immunity in mice with antigens prepared from influenza and vesicular stomatitis virus grown in suspension culture of Ehrlich ascites cells. *J. Natl. Cancer Inst.*, **45**, 1161–1167 (1971).

12. Kobayashi, H., Gotohda, E., Hosokawa, M., and Kodama, T. Inhibition of metastases in rats immunized with xenogenized autologous tumor cells after excision of primary tumor. *J. Natl. Cancer Inst.*, **54**, 997–999 (1975).

13. Kobayashi, H., Kodama, T., and Gotohda, E. "Xenogenization of Tumor Cells," Hokkaido University Medical Library Series 9, Hokkaido University Press (1977).

14. Kuzumaki, N., Fenyo, E. M., Giovanella, B. C., and Klein, G. Augmented immunogenicity of low antigenic rat tumors after superinfection with endogenous murine c-type virus in nude mice. *Int. J. Cancer*, (1978), in press.

15. Lindenmann, J. Viruses as immunological adjuvants in cancer. *Biochim. Biophys. Acta*, **335**, 49–76 (1974).

16. Lindenmann, J. Strategies of active immunization applicable to cancer. Fogarty Int. Center Proc. No. 28. *In* "Modulation of Host Immune Resistance in the Prevention or Treatment of Induced Neoplasias," ed. M. A. Chirigos, pp. 187–190 (1977). Dept. of Health, Education and Welfare, U.S.A., Publ. No. (NIH) 77-893.

17. Rukavishnikova, G. E. and Alekseyeva, A. K. Some immunological mechanisms of the influenza virus antitumor effect. *Acta Virol.*, **20**, 387–394 (1976).

18. Wallack, M. K., Steplewski, H., Koprowski, H., Rosata, E., George, J., Hulihan, B., and Johnson, J. A. A new approach in specific, active immunotherapy. *Cancer*, **39**, 560–564 (1977).

19. Wise, K. Vesicular stomatitis virus-infected L1210 murine leukemia cells: Increased immunogenicity and altered surface antigens. *J. Natl. Cancer Inst.*, **53**, 83–90 (1977).

ARTIFICAL HETEROGENIZATION OF TUMORS: GENERAL OUTLINE AND NEW APPROACHES

George SVET-MOLDAVSKY

Department of Neoplastic Diseases, Mt. Sinai School of Medicine*

    Artificial heterogenization of tumors is based on the artificial induction of new antigens in the tumor cells followed by the exposure of these antigens to actively or passively administered lymphoid cells or antibodies. Our general idea is to make tumor cells more heterogeneous in respect to other structures of the organism. To modify and augment the antigenicity of tumor cells, two approaches are suggested: Application of 1) chemical compounds; of 2) living biological oncotropic agents (viruses, bacteria, *Rickettsia*, and protists). Both approaches are now practiced. Quite a new approach was proposed by G. Klein to modifying the immunogenicity of tumor cells by using a somatic hybridization of tumor cells with other species cells.

    Current status of the problem and future possibilities are analyzed in the present paper, along with new experiments concerning the intensification of the effect of artificial heterogenization and the data on viral oncotropism obtained during the treatment of incurable cancer patients.

It is well known now that tumor antigens, especially of "spontaneous" tumors, are of very low activity. This is why the possibility of immunization and immunological treatment in respect to natural tumor antigens is very slight.

That stimulated us to seek another approach to the problem of immunological prophilaxis and therapy of tumors—artificial heterogenization. As it was formulated 14 years ago: "The general idea is to make the tumors more heterologous," more foreign to other structures of the organism. Artificial heterogenization of tumors is "based on artificial induction of new antigens in the tumor cells followed by the exposure of these antigens to actively acquired or passively administered lymphoid cells or antibodies" (*22, 65, 66*).

To modify and augment the antigenicity of tumor cells we suggest two approaches. The first is the application of chemical compounds and the second is the use of living tumorotropic agents (viruses, bacteria, *Rickettsiae*, and protists). Both approaches to artificial heterogenization of tumors are now practiced: Chemical and virus heterogenization.

A new and different approach to this problem was proposed by Klein (*34, 35*), *i.e.*, the heterogenization of tumor cells by fusion with allogeneic or xenogeneic cells. The different avenues of heterogenization are shown in Table I.

---

* New York, N.Y. 10029, U.S.A. on leave of absence from the Cancer Research Center, Moscow, U.S.S.R.

TABLE I.   Artificial Heterogenization of Tumors (=Xenogenization)

To make tumor cells (or part of them) more heterologous, more foreign to other structures of organisms by means of:

    I.   Compounds (for coupling)
   II.   Compounds (for induction)
  III.   Bacteria and bacterial products
  IV.   Bacterial enzymes
   V.   Fusion with allo-and xenogeneic cells
  VI.   Viral and virus-induced antigens

On new or modified antigenic determinants the immunological effect is produced which must work against the total population of tumor cells including newly appearing tumor cells. It is best to induce new antigenic determinants in as many tumor cells as possible.

Agents Used for Artificial Heterogenization

The lines of chemical, viral, and bacterial heterogenization were developed practically simultaneously. Now the fusion with allogenic and xenogenic cells is also added in this direction. Table II shows the agents that were used in different attempts to heterogenize tumor cells. Presented in Table III are the new methods proposed by us for heterogenization. Actovaccine means the vaccines prepared from macrophage-processed tumor or viral antigens (*15*). The processing with macrophages increases their immunogenicity. Interferons and hormones can change immunogenicity of tumor cells.

TABLE II.   Agents Used for Artificial Heterogenization of Tumors

Agents	References
I. Compounds (Coupling)	
N-Acetylgalactosaminuronic acid-(Vi-Antigen)	Hamburg, V. P., Svet-Moldavsky, G. J. (1964, 1965) (*22, 66*)
Bis-diazobenzidine	Czajkowski, N. P. *et al.* (1966) (*16, 17*)
Dinitrochlorobenzene	Klein, E.D.M. (1968) (*32, 33*)
Concanavalin A ; 2,4-dinitro phenylaminocaproate	Martin, W. *et al.* (1971) (*43*)
Iodoacetate	Affel, C. *et al.* (1966) (cited in *43*)
Iodoacetate	Wang, M., Halliday, W. (1967) (*72*)
L-Phenylalanine mustard	Arai, K. *et al.* (1973) (*2*)
II. Compounds (Induction)	
Bromodeoxyuridine	Silagi, S. *et al.* (1972) (*53*)
Compounds used for chemotherapy	Bonmassar, E. *et al.* (1970) (*9*)
	Nicolin, A. *et al.* (1972) (*48*)
III. Bacteria and their products	
Salmonella	Hamburg, V. P., Svet-Moldavsky, G. J. (1964, 1965) (*22, 66*)
O-Antigen, lipopolysacharides	Hamburg, V. P., Svet-Moldavsky, G. J. (1964, 1965) (*22, 66*)
Staphylococci and their antigenes	Hamburg, V. P., Svet-Moldavsky, G. J. (1964, 1965) (*22, 66*)
Live BCG	Zbar, B. (1970) (*75*)
Methanol extraction residue (M.E.R.)	Weiss. D. (1972) (*73*)

Continued...

TABLE II. Continued.

Agents	References
IV. Bacterial enzymes	
Neuraminidase	Bekesi, G. *et al.* (1971) (*7*)
V. Allogeneic and xenogeneic cells fused with tumor cells	Harris, H. *et al.* (1969) (*28*)
	Klein, G. *et al.* (1972) (*34*)
	Klein, G., Klein, E. (1977) (*35*)
VI. Viruses	
Rabbit virus III	Pearce, L. and Rivers, T. M. (1927) (cited in *65*)
Lymphogranuloma inguinale[a]	Hamburg, V. P., Svet-Moldavsky, G. J.
Vaccinia[a]	(1964) (*22, 62*)
Influenza[a]	
Poliomyelitis[a]	
Polyoma	Hamburg, V. P., Svet-Moldavsky, G. J. (1964) (*22, 62*)
	Sjogren (1964)
Herpes simplex	Hamburg, V. P., Svet-Moldavsky, G. J. (1964) (*22, 24*)
SV40	
Mouse leukemia virus (Rauscher)	Stück, B. *et al.* (1964) (*57*)
Parainfluenza sendai	Svet-Moldavsky G. J., Hamburg, V. P. (1965) (*62*)
Adenovirus	Hamburg, V. P. *et al.* (1966) (*23, 26*)
Influenza virus	Eaton *et al.* (1969) (*20*)
	Lindenmann, J. (1966) (*40, 41*)
	Boone, C. W. (1972) (*10–12*)
Mouse leukemia virus (Friend)	Kobayashi, H. *el at.* (1969) (*36, 37*)
Newcastle disease virus	Eaton. M. *et al.* (1967) (*19*)
Vesicular stomatitis virus	Defendi, V. *et al.* (1967) (*18*)
Rabies virus	Wiktor, T. *et al.* (1968) (*74*)
Mouse leukemia virus (Rauscher)	Otten, J. *et al.* (1971) (*49*)
	Barbieri, D. *et al.* (1971) (*4*)
	Baryshnikov, A. *et al.* (1973) (*5*)
Endogeneous C-virus	Silagi, S. *et al.* (1972) (*53*)
	Kuzumaki, N. *et al.* (1976) (*39*)
	Greenberger, J., Aaranson, S. (1973) (*21*)

[a] Tested with negative results.

TABLE III. Agents and Methods Proposed to Be Used for Artificial
Heterogenization of Tumors

Agents
1. Hormones
2. Interferons
3. Tumor antigens processed by macrophages (Actovaccines)
4. Different kinds of intracellular
Protists
Rickettsiae
5. Many other viruses such as Yaba virus. Cytomegaloviruses, *etc.*

Terminology

The definition of artificial heterogenization as a general approach of making tumor cells more foreign to the recognizing systems of organisms was proposed by Svet-Moldavsky and Hamburg in 1964–1965, (*22, 65, 66*). I do not see any scientific reason for changing the term heterogenization to xenogenization. The reason that the "hetero-transplantation" has changed now to "xenotransplantation" is not an argument.

It is impossible to postulate that induction of a new viral antigen or lectin-linked or other haptenic group makes tumor cells allogeneic or xenogeneic, but it makes them definitely foreign, *i.e.*, heterologous. The definition which Kobayashi gave that xenogenization is heterogenization without previous immunization also cannot be accepted. Our definition of heterogenization (see above) covers the heterogenization with simultaneous immunization, pre- and post-immunization. The heterogenization "without preimmunization" according to Kobayashi is heterogenization with simultaneous immunization. What is crucial is the fact that precisely on determinants artificially induced in the tumor cells by compounds or biological agents the immunological effect is produced, and this effect is working against modified and unmodified newly appeared tumor cells.

Now Kobayashi writes that "xenogenization in a strict sense differs from hetero-genization in that with xenogenization the regression of tumor cells is produced after infection with a virus." This was included in our definition of heterogenization. More-over, it was realized in our experiments in suppression of chemical and viral carcino-genesis by artificial heterogenization. We wrote in 1964 that "for artificial heterogeniza-tion of tumors, compounds or biological agents are administered to the tumors—affected organism which selectively accumulates or multiplies in the tumors." For regression of tumors, the heterogenization was proposed.

It should be emphasized that the definition of heterogenization as a general prin-ciple should not be mixed with the concrete experiments on heterogenization performed in our laboratory.

To investigate the possibility of artificial induction of new antigenic determinants in tumor cells and thereby using them for immunization, we began to study such compounds as Vi-antigen: N-acetylgalactosaminuronic acid, different bacterial anti-gens, and the different viruses. To check the possibility of inducing specific virus transplantation antigens in tumor cells, we of course used preimmunization of animals, and *vice versa* for suppressing of chemical and viral (induced by unrelated virus) car-cinogenesis we used postimmunization or immunization in latent period (*22–27*), some-times simultaneous immunization, *etc.*

To add the adjective "immunological" to the word heterogenization or xenogeni-zation is unnecessary because the word heterogenization (as well as xenogenization) includes the idea of "immunological response."

Natural Heterogenization

But it is important to speak about artificial or natural virus heterogenization of cells. Natural heterogenization of cells was defined by our laboratory in 1957 (*62–64*). It has been known since the late twenties, the time of Philibert (*51*) and Rivers (*52*) that the primary reaction of the cell to the reproduction of the virus consists in proliferation and destruction. I suggested that the most general type of primary cell reaction to the virus is heterogenization of the cells with regard to other structures of the organism. The primary idea was very simple: In unicellular organisms changes of antigenic structure (virus-infected) sometimes interferes with the normal relations inside the population. What will happen in the case of multicellular organisms? The changes in virus-infected cells may bring about a generalization of the pathological process which develops as a reaction of the organism to virus-infected cells. Subsequent study of the virus-induced autoimmune diseases fully confirmed these early ideas.

Symptoms of virus diseases were often mixed with hereditary signs. It is possible to postulate that the viruses can imitate the work of almost all genes. This general statement has become more and more evident.

Autoimmune diseases can appear in three cases (see review (64)). 1) If the function of lymphoid tissue is impaired, the recognizing function or effector ones; 2) If the antigenic properties of some other tissues or cells change, in particular, if new antigens appear; and 3) If the barriers are damaged which preserve (save) the cells "unknown" to an immunocompetent system.

Viruses might be the cause of each of the above mentioned disturbances. Viruses can change the antigenic properties of different tissues, to heterogenize various tissues of the organism. On the other hand, many viruses can strongly impair the work of immunocompetent systems, inducing, in particular, immunosuppression. There is a close connection between immunosuppressive and heterogenizing activity of the virus.

Some years ago, I thought that in some cases the virus immunosuppression is connected with the heterogenization of definite cells of the immunocompetent system: immune response is a result of cooperative work of several types of lymphoid cells. It is quite possible that the induction of virus coded or virus-induced antigens in one of these groups of cells leads to disturbance and, in particular, to the suppression of their functions, and especially the cell-to-cell cooperation.

It is preferable to speak on heterogenization, both natural and artificial, in respect to other structures of organisms because not only T cells and B cells, macrophages, and different types of antibodies play a role but many other still undetermined types of cells. A good example is the discovery of "natural killers." What is the best way of heterogenization in relation to these cells?

In 1967–1970 it was shown in this laboratory that interferon induces a strong cytotoxicity of normal lymphoid cells against syngeneic and allogeneic tumor targets *in vivo* and *in vitro* (14, 67).

Now Herberman and his colleagues (29) have confirmed this effect and show that it depends on the activation of natural killer cells. Now I think that what is most important in the antitumor defense are the early events of interaction of tumor cells with surrounding stromal ones and that the artificial heterogenization of tumors is necessary to make in the respect of the stromal fibroblast-like cells which make up the microenvironments.

Types of Artificial Heterogenization of Tumors

There are three basic types of artificial heterogenization in two main avenues (see Table IV).

The first is when heterogenized is only a "vaccine." Immune response work against new antigenic determinant of this vaccine which can be made by one of the above mentioned methods with the intention that this immunity will be strong enough to prevent the appearance of metastases. Two of these avenues particularly belong to the "virus-assisted immunotherapy" developed by Lindenmann (40, 41), Boone (10–12), and Eaton (19, 20).

Logically before the application of this method it is necessary to eliminate surgically or chemotherapeutically large masses of tumor tissue.

Until recently the best results were obtained by the authors who injected heterogenizing agents directly into the growing tumor nodes. This was work of Klein by using direct application of DNCB to tumor nodes (32, 33). Zbar by direct application of BCG (75) and Weiss by direct application of M.E.R. into tumor nodes (73). There is no convincing evidence that in these particular cases, heterogenization mechanisms are working, but many features of the phenomenon show that it is quite so. Such methods are possible to use only in very special cases when the tumor nodes are avail-

TABLE IV. Two Main Avenues of Tumor Heterogenization

1.   Heterogenized (by compounds, viruses or cell fusion) is the "vaccine" from tumor cells and their parts (for example, membranes) such a "vaccine" is used for immunization.
2.   The growing tumor is heterogenized *in vivo* (by various agents)
a) By direct application to the tumor nodesor.
b) By injection of heterogenizing agent into the bloodstream.

TABLE V. Attempts of Treatment of Incurable Patients with Adenovirus Type 16

No.	Patients	Diagnosis	Injected virus (TCID$_{50}$)	Study during life-time — Virus isolation	Study during life-time — Antibody to the virus
1.	SH	Metastases of testis teratoblastoma in the lungs, mediastinum, and retroperitoneal lymph nodes. Stage IV	4×10^9 i.v. 1×10^9 p.o.	Virus not isolated from blood	0–64 Day 5
2.	M	Melanoma of crus skin with metastases in the lungs, mediastinum, inguinal area, and pleura. Stage IV	3×10^9 i.v.	—	0–64 Day 11 0–64 Day 30
3.	B	Stomach cancer, metastases in the liver and peritoneum ascitis. Stage IV	3×10^9 i.v.	—	0–16 Day 8
4.	S	Stomach cancer, metastases in paraaortal, subclavicuar lymph nodes, lung, and bone marrow. Stage IV	3×10^9 i.v.	Virus not isolated from either blood or biopsies.	0–256 Day 8

Side reactions temperature rose to 38–39° in 2 patients on the day of injections.
There was no beneficial effect of the treatment.

able for direct injection of the heterogenization agent. This means that the most important aspect of this problem is to achieve a maximal accumulation of either the compounds or the organisms in the desired disseminated tumor nodes *via* the bloodstream.

Starting from the classical work of Levaditi, Nicolau, and Schoen (cited in Ref. *65*), the selective accumulation of different viruses in the tumor nodes (vaccinia, ectromelia rabies, lymphogranuloma inguinale, arthropode-borne encephalities, *etc.*) was well established. The basis for such a high accumulation of viruses in tumors is their selective multiplication. The oncotropic properties of some viruses were established in cancer patients by pioneers of virotherapy of cancer (Moore (*46–47*), Koprowski (cited in Ref. *74*), Huebner (*31*) and some others).

Here I will present some data on oncotropism of adenovirus 16 obtained in the course of the phase I study of adenovirus therapy of cancer (*68*). Attempts to treat the incurable patients with widely disseminated cancers by means of heterogenization were made on 8 patients. Five of them received intravenously and three local plus intravenous injections of the -10^9 $TCID_{50}$ of adenovirus-16. After inoculation of the virus containing fluid, minor immediate and delayed reactions were observed. No beneficial

TABLE VI. Postmorten Isolation of Virus from the Following Materials

1. Lung tissue, lung tissue pneumonic foci, tumor nodes in lungs (with lysis), tumor nodes in lungs (without lysis)
2. Pleura with metastasis, broncho-pulmonary lymph nodes with metastasis, trachea, paratracheal lymph nodes, para-aortal lymph node with metastasis
3. Mediastinum with metastases, subclavicular lymph node, retroperitoneal lymph nodes with matastasis
4. Heart, liver, tumor nodes in the liver, kidneys, kidneys with metastasis, normal stomach tissue, primary stomach tumor, large and small intestine, tumor nodes in the intestine, peritoneum with tumor, omentum with tumor, spleen, pancreas, pancreas with metastasis, urinary bladder tumor (metastases)
5. Adrenal gland, adrenal gland with metastasis thyroid gland, brain, cerebellum
6. Testicle, ovary, uterus (fibrous node), subcutaneous metastasis, inguinal lymph nodes with metastasis, ascitic fluid

TABLE VII. Postmortem Isolation of the Virus from Incurable
Patients Who Underwent Virotherapy

No.	Patients	Diagnosis	Life-time after injections (days)	Time of taking material after death (hr)	Study of autopsy material
1.	SH	Metastases of testis, teratoblastoma in the lungs, mediastinum, and retroperitoneal lymph nodes	17	4	Adenovirus-16 isolated from lung metastasis
2.	M	Melanoma of crus skin with metastases in the lungs, mediastinum, inguinal area, and pleura	35	6	Adenovirus-16 isolated from pleural and bronchopulmonal metastases
3.	B	Stomach cancer metastases in the liver and peritoneum ascites	52	60	Adenovirus-16 not isolated
4.	S	Stomach cancer metastases in para-aortal, subclavicular-lymph nodes, lung, and bone marrow	100	84	Adenovirus-5 isolated from lung metastases

effect was noticed. Adenovirus type 16 neutralizing antibodies were lacking in all the patients before inoculation but were detected after it (Table V).

Isolation of the virus was done posthumously from organs and tumor nodes of 4 patients (Table VI). It was isolated in 2 of 4 cases from living metastases (Table VII). It is interesting that we failed to isolate it from normal living tissue, from other tissues, and from tumor nodes in other tissues. In one case adenovirus type 5 that was not the injected type was recovered from the tumor tissue.

This is part of a larger work but I use it now as an illustration of adenovirus-16 oncotropism.

New Approaches

There are three basic problems of artificial heterogenization (Table VIII). For the increase of accumulation of the viruses in the tumor nodes we use previous loading of RES (the size of viruses is near the particles of the loading agents and previous loading markedly intensified the accumulation in 10–100 times of the vaccinia virus in the tumors). At the same time it markedly intensified the activity of leukemia viruses (*13*). The loading of RES is one of the possible approaches of increasing the primary accumulation of virus particles in the tumor nodes.

Immunosuppressive properties of the viruses are well known and it is possible to minimize these effects by choosing the best virus, and by the future development of the idea of selective protection of bone marrow and immunocompetent systems by agents linked to the carrier particles (*50*).

For selective protection in the course of cancer chemotherapy we are studying such an approach at the clinical level (*50*). For the heterogenization with compounds this method can also be used, but for viral heterogenization, it is first necessary to make experimental steps.

And finally, there is the problem of increasing the pathological reaction to the virus heterogenized cells. In this respect, the factor of great importance is the body temperature. For about 20 years the attention of the investigations have been concerned with the problem of the temperature and cell-virus interaction (see classical work of Lwoff (*42*) and many others) and brilliant achievements with temperature-sensitive virus mutants. However, there is quite another aspect of the problem—the temperature and virus infection at the level of organism.

Referring to my experiments performed commencing in 1949 (*58–61, 71*) to study the range of temperature of virus reproduction and range of temperature of development of pathological conditions, special systems were used: Reptiles, reptile embryos, newborn mice, and rabbits maintained a long period at a lowered body temperature. The infections with influenza, rabies, and vaccinia viruses were studied in these sys-

TABLE VIII.   Three Main Problems of Tumor Heterogenization
by Viruses Injected *in vivo*

1.	Maximal accumulation of injected virus particles in the tumor nodes
2.	Minimizing the immunosuppressive effect of the virus
3.	Increased response of different structures of the organism on heterogenized tumor cells (and on the remaining unheterogenized ones, also)

TABLE IX. Use of the RES-loading by Colloidal Gold and Hyperthermia for Enhancement of Artificial Heterogenization (Xenogenization) of Transplantable Syngeneic Sarcoma in C57BL/6J Mice by Means of Rauscher Leukemia Virus (RLV)

The treatment had begun after the appearance of the palpable tumor nodules (Exp 1).

Group	Tumors regressed	Average weight (g, M±m)	p
1. Tumor growth control	0/6	2.24±0.68	
2. Hyperthermia	0/3	0.46±0.38	>0.05
3. RLV	0/8	1.0 ±0.26	>0.05
4. RLV+Hyperthermia	0/8	1.9 ±0.37	>0.05
5. RES-loading	0/9	3.11±0.57	>0.05
6. RES-loading+RLV	0/7	1.8 ±0.43	>0.05
7. RES-loading+Hyperthermia	0/6	1.82±0.57	>0.05
8. RES-roading+RLV+Hyperthermia	4/8	0.8 ±0.26	<0.05

Nominator—the amount of mice with fully regressed tumors.
Denominator—the amount of mice in each group.

tems. It was shown that an increase in body temperature with certain limits may convert a latent infection into a clinically and pathologically manifested disease and, on the contrary, a decrease in body temperature of the host organism regularly makes a virus disease become dormant. For example a lowering of the body temperature in newborn mice and chick embryos below 30° resulted in symptomless replication of influenza virus, while at 36–37° the virus caused a lethal pneumonia. An increase of body temperature in snakes converted a symptomless infection with vaccinia virus into severe keratities (*58, 61, 71*).

In Table IX one of the heterogenization experiments is presented: Rauscher leukemia virus infection enhanced by previous loading of RES and hyperthermia in mice with growing (palpable) sarcomas. It is evident from this table that there is a marked effect of "enhanced" heterogenization treatment including full regression of some growing tumors.

Therefore, the combination of previous RES loading with hyperthermia must be considered to be a definite possibility in improving the positive effects of heterogenization therapy.

Acknowledgment

This work was supported by Grant #RD-19 from the American Cancer Society.

REFERENCES

1. Ancheva, M. N., Barchotkina, M. F., and Hamburg, V. P. Immunodepressive properties of the viruses. *Vopr. Virusol.*, No. 2, 132–138 (1975) (in Russian).
2. Arai, K., Wallance, H., and Blackmore, W. Immunotherapy of cancer with L phenylalanine mustard as a hapten. *Cancer Res.*, **33**, 1914–1920 (1973).
3. Bandlair, A. and Koszinowski, V. Increased cellular immunity against host cell antigens induced by vaccine virus. *Arch. Gesamt. Virusforsch.*, **45**, 122 (1974).
4. Barbieri, D., Balehradex, J., and Barski, G. Decrease in tumor-producing capacity of mouse cell lines following infection with mouse leukemia viruses. *Int. J. Cancer*, **7**, 364 (1971).

5. Baryshnikov, A. J., Buchman, V. M., and Svet-Moldavsky, G. J. Use of the loading of RES and hyperthermia for the increasement of virus heterogenization of tumors and direct viral oncolysis. *Vopr. Virusol.*, **16**, No. 1, 51–53 (1973) (in Russian, English Summary).

6. Basombrio, M. A. Rechazo de tumores no virales por infeccion con el virus de sarcomo murio. *Medicina (Buenos Aires)*, **37**, 127–132 (1977).

7. Bekesi, G., Arneanlt, St., and Holland, J. Increased immunogenicity of leukemia L-1210 cells after *Vibrio cholerae* neuraminadase treatment. *Proc. Am. Assoc. Cancer Res.*, **12**, 47 (1971).

8. Beverley, P., Lowenthal, R., and Tyrrell D. Immune response in mice to tumour challenge after immunization with Newcastle disease virus-infected or X-irradiated tumour cells or cell fractions. *Int. J. Cancer*, **11**, 212–223 (1973).

9. Bonmassar, E., Bonmassar, A., Vadlamudi, S., and Goldin, A. Immunological alteration of leukemic cells *in vivo* after treatment with antitumor drug. *Proc. Natl. Acad. Sci. U.S.*, **66**, 1089–1095 (1970).

10. Boone, C. Augmented immunogenicity of tumor cell homogenates produced by infection with influenza virus. *Natl. Cancer Inst. Monogr.*, **35**, 301–307 (1972).

11. Boone, C. and Blackman, K. Augmented immunogenicity of tumor cell homogenates infected with influenza virus. *Cancer Res.*, **32**, 1018–1022 (1972).

12. Boone, C., Paranjpe, M., Orme, T., and Gillette, R. Virus-augmented tumor transplantation antigens: Evidence for a helper antigen mechanism. *Int. J. Cancer*, **13**, 543–551 (1974).

13. Buchman, V. M., Radzichouskaya, R. M., Svet-Moldavsky, G. J., Kozlova, M. D., Mikaelian, S. E., and Levin, V. J. Loading of the reticuloendothelial system: Effect of the induction, development and chemotherapy of Rauscher virus leukemia. *Biomedicine* (Express) **19**, 335–339 (1973).

14. Chernyakhouskaya, J. Yr, Slavina, E. G., and Svet-Moldavsky, G. J. Antitumor effect of lymphoid cells activated by interferon. *Nature*, **228**, 71–72 (1978).

15. Chimishkyan, K. L. and Svet-Moldavsky, G. J. An approach to the development of actovaccines in the model of vaccinia virus. *Vopr. Virusol.*, **3**, 273–278, (1975) (in Russian).

16. Czajkowski, N., Rosenblatt, M., Cushing, F., Vasquez, J., and Woli, P. Production of active immunity to malignant neoplastic tissue. *Cancer*, **19**, 739 (1966).

17. Czajkowski, N., Rosenblatt, M., Wolf, P., and Vazquez, J. A new method of active immunization to autologous human tumor tissue. *Lancet*, **ii**, 905–907 (1967).

18. Defendi, V., Wiktor, T., and Koprowski, H. *In* "Cross-reacting Antigens and Neoantigens," ed. J. F. Trentin, p. 96 (1967). The Williams and Wilkins Co., Baltimore.

19. Eaton, M. and Levinthal, J. Contribution of antiviral immunity to oncolysis by Newcastle disease virus in murine lymphoma. *J. Natl. Cancer Inst.*, **39**, 1089–1097 (1967).

20. Eaton, M. and Scala, A. Further observation on the inhibitory effect of myxovirus on a transplantable murine leukemia. *Proc. Soc. Exp. Biol. Med.*, **132**, 20–23 (1969).

21. Greenberger, J. and Aaronson, S. *In vivo* inoculation RNA C-type virus inducing regression of experimental solid tumors. *J. Natl. Cancer Inst.*, **51**, 1935–1941 (1973).

22. Hamburg, V. and Svet-Moldavsky, G. Artificial heterogenization of tumors by means of herpes simplex and polyoma viruses. *Nature*, **203**, 772–773 (1964).

23. Hamburg, V. P., Liozner, A. L., and Svet-Moldavsky, G. J. Artificial induction of transplantation virus antigens in the chemical carcinogenesis. *Vopr. Oncol.* No. 8, 44–46 (1966) (in Russian, English Summary).

24. Hamburg, V. P. and Liozner, A. L. Growth stimulation and artificial heterogenization

of tumor cells by SV40 and adenovirus type 16. *Bull. Exp. Biol. Med.*, No. 10, 78–81, (1967) (in Russian, English Summary).

25. Hamburg, V. and Svet-Moldavsky, G. Suppression of viral and chemical carcinogenesis by means of artificial heterogenization. *Nature*, **215**, 230–232 (1967).

26. Hamburg, V. P. and Svet-Moldavsky, G. J. Further study of artificial heterogenization of tumors. Abstr. Meeting on tumor virology and immunology, Moscow. *Medicine*, 22–23 (1969).

27. Hamburg, V., Scherbakova, O., Trubcheninova, L., and Frolzova, A., Further study of artificial heterogenization of tumors in the course of chemical carcinogenesis. *Neoplasma*, **18**, 515–523 (1971).

28. Harris, H., Miller, O. I., Klein, G., Worst, P., and Tachibana, T. Suppression of malignancy of cell fusion. *Nature*, **223**, 363–366 (1969).

29. Herberman, R. Personal communication (1978).

30. Hosokawa, M., Sendo, F., Gotohda, E., and Kobayashi, H. Combination of immunotherapy and chemotherapy to experimental tumors in rats. *Gann*, **62**, 57 (1971).

31. Huebner, R., Smith, R., Row, W., Suskind, R., and Love, R. Experimantal approach to the virotherapy of cancer. *Science*, **1**, 124, 938 (1956).

32. Klein, E. Differential immunologic reactions in normal skin and epidermal neoplasms. *Fed. Proc.*, **26**, 430 (1967).

33. Klein, E. Tumors of the skin X. Immunotherapy of cutaneous and mucosal neoplasms. *N.Y. State J. Med.*, **68**, 900–911 (1968).

34. Klein, G. and Harris, H. Expession of polyoma-induced transplantation antigen in hybrid cell lines. *Nature New Biol.*, **237**, 163–164 (1912).

35. Klein, G. and Klein, E. Immune surveillance against virus-induced tumors and non-rejectability of spontaneous tumors: Contrasting consequences of host *versus* tumor evolution. *Proc. Natl, Acad. Sci. U.S.*, **74**, 2121–2125 (1977).

36. Kobayashi, H. An approach to the immunological regression of the tumor. *Acta Pathol. Jpn.*, **20**, 441 (1970).

37. Kobayashi, H., Sendo, F., and Shirai, T. Modification in growth of transplantable rat tumors exposed to Friend virus. *J. Natl. Cancer Inst.*, **42**, 413–419 (1969).

38. Kobayashi, H., Kodama, T., Shirai, T., Kaji, H., Hosokawa, M., Sendo, F., Saito, H., and Tateichi, N. Artificial regression of rat tumors infected with Friend virus (xenogenization), *Hokkaido J. Med. Sci.*, **44**, 133–135 (1969).

39. Kuzumaki, N., Fenyo, E. M., Ciovanella, B. C., and Klein, G. Increased immunogenicity of low antigenic rat tumor after super infection with endogenous murine C type virus in nude mice. *Int. J. Cancer*, **21**, 62–66 (1978).

40. Lindenmann, J. Immunity to transplantable tumors following viral oncolysis. I. Mechanisms of immunity to Ehrlich ascites tumor. *J. Immunol.*, **92**, 912–919 (1964).

41. Lindenmann, J. Viruses as immunological adjuvants in cancer. *Biochim. Biophys. Acta*, **355**, 49–75 (1974).

42. Lwoff, A. Factors influencing the evolution of viral diseases at the cellular level. *Bact. Rev.*, **23**, 109 (1959).

43. Martin, W. J., Wunderlich, J. R., and Fletcher, F. Enhanced immunogenicity of chemically coated syngeneic tumor cells. *Proc. Natl. Acad. Sci. U.S.*, **68**, 469–472 (1971).

44. Mitchison, N. Immunologic approach to cancer. *Transplant. Proc.*, **2**, 92–103 (1970).

45. Mizukami, T. and Takamura, Y. Beitrag zur immunologischen Krebstherapie-Versuche zur Midifikation der Tumorantigen Baschaffenheit. *Arch. Geschwulstforsch.*, **37**, 33–37 (1971).

46. Moore, A. Oncolytic properties of viruses. *Texas Rep. Biol. Med.*, **15**, 588–602 (1957).

47. Moore, A. The Oncolytic viruses. *Prog. Exp. Tumor Res.*, **1**, 411 (1960).

48. Nicolin, A., Vadlamudi, S., and Goldin, A. Antigenicity of L-1210 leukemic sublines induced by drugs. *Cancer Res.*, **32**, 653–657 (1972).

49. Otten, J., Tyndall, R., and Upton, A. Sarcoma rejection in mice born of mothers actively immunized against murine leukemia virus. *J. Natl. Cancer Inst.*, **43**, 499–508 (1969).

50. Pavlotsky, A. I., Novikova, L. A., Svet-Moldavsky, G. J., Toloknov, B. O., Buchman, V. M., and Radzikhovskaya, R. M. *Cancer Treat. Rep.*, **61**, 895–897 (1977).

51. Philibert, A. Virus cytotropes. *Ann. Med.*, **16**, 283–288 (1924).

52. Rivers, T. M. Some general aspects of pathological conditions caused by filterable viruses. *Am. J. Pathol.*, **4**, 91–96 (1928).

53. Silagi, S., Bejv, D., Wrathall, J., and Deharven, E. Tumorigenicity, immunogenicity, and virus production in mouse melanoma cells treated with 5-bromdeoxyuridine. *Proc. Natl. Acad. Sci. U.S.*, **69**, 3443–3446 (1972).

54. Sjogren, H. Studies on specific transplantation resistance to polyoma virus-induced tumors. II. Mechanism of resistance induced by polyoma virus injection. *J. Natl. Cancer Inst.*, **32**, 375–393 (1964).

55. Sjogren, H. and Hellstrom, J. Induction of polyoma specific transplantation of antigenicity in Moloney leukemia cells. *Exp. Cell Res.*, **40**, 208–211 (1965).

56. Smith, R., Huebner, R., Rowe, W., Schatten, W., and Thomas, L. Studies on the use of viruses in the treatment of carcinoma of the cervix. *Cancer*, **9**, 1211 (1956).

57. Stuck, B., Old, L., and Boyse, E. Antigenic conversion of established leukemias by an unrelated leukemogenic virus. *Nature*, **202**, 1016–1017 (1964).

58. Svet-Moldavsky, G. J. Experimental materials to the study of virus infection progress at the lowered body temperature. (thesis) Moscow (1952) (in Russian).

59. Svet-Moldavsky, G. J. On the temperature range limits at which virus reproduction and the development of a virus disease are possible. *In* "Problems of General Virology," Abstracts of the D. I. Ivanovsky Virology Institute Conference. Moscow 17 (1953) (in Russian).

60. Svet-Moldavsky, G. J. Viral infection and body temperature. Small pox-vaccinian keratitis in Natrix at various body temperatures. *Bull. Exp. Biol. Med.*, **4**, 64 (1955) (in Russian).

61. Svet-Moldavsky, G. J. Viral infection and body temperature. Influenza infection in newborn mice in case of durable cooling. *Bull. Exp. Biol. Med.*, **6**, 52–55 (1955) (in Russian).

62. Svet-Moldavsky, G. J. A symptomless viral infection as the main form of interaction between viruses and hosts. Materials of the conference of Tarasevitch State Control Institute. Moscow 15 (1957) (in Russian).

63. Svet-Moldavsky, G. J. Rous virus pathogenicity for mammals III. Sarcomas in rats, further study of cystic-hemorrhagic disease and attempts to isolate the infectious ribonucleic acid from Rous sarcoma (see: *Discussion*). *Acta Virol.*, **5**, 167–177 (1961).

64. Svet-Moldavsky, G. J. Viruses, autoimmune diseases and transplantation immunology in cellular basis of immunology. IV. All-Union Symposium on the problems of histophysiology of the connective tissue. *Novosib. Acad.*, **2**, 77–83, 1972 (in Russian).

65. Svet-Moldavsky, G. J. and Hamburg, V. Quantitative relationships in viral oncolysis and the possibility of artificial heterogenization of tumours. *Nature*, **202**, 303–304 (1964).

66. Svet-Moldavsky, G. J. and Hamburg, V. An approach to the immunological treatment of tumors by artificial heterogenization. Specific tumor antigens. *In* "Monograph Series," ed. R. J. Harris, p. 323 (1967). Munksgaard, Copenhagen.

67. Svet-Moldavsky, G. J. and Chernyakhovskaya, J. Yu. Interferon and the interaction of allogeneic normal and immune lymphocytes with L-cells. *Nature*, **215**, 1299–1300 (1967).

68. Svet-Moldavsky, G. J., Gibadullin, R. A., Froltzova, A. E., Hamburg, V. P., Perevod-chikova, N. Å., and Bychkov, M. B. Attempts to treat the incurable oncological patients with adenovirus type 16. *Vopr. Virusol.*, No. 6, 713–719 (1974).

69. Tennant, J. Immunogenetic approach to neoplasma. *Transplant. Proc.*, **2**, 104–116 (1970).

70. Tennant, J., Lambertenghi, G., Kingsley, S., and de Harven, E. Correlation between presence of leukemia virus in cultured cells and their immunogenicity in a leukemia isotransplant system. *J. Natl. Cancer Inst.*, **47**, 781–788 (1971).

71. Trubcheninova, L. P., Khutoryansky, A. A., Svet-Moldavsky, G. J., Kuznetsova, L. E., Sokolov, P. P., and Belianchykova, N. O. Body temperature and tumor virus infection. I. Tumorigenicity of Rous sarcoma virus for reptiles. *Neoplasma*, **24**, 3–19 (1977).

72. Wang, M. and Halliday, W. Immune response of mice to iodoaccetate-treated Ehrlich-ascites tumour cells. *Br. J. Cancer*, **21**, 346–353 (1967).

73. Weiss, D. W. Nonspecific stimulation and modulation of the immune response and of states of resistance by the methanol extraction residue fraction of tubercle bacilli. *Natl. Cancer Inst. Monogr.*, **32**, 157–172 (1972).

74. Wiktor, T., Kuwert, E., and Koprowski, H. Immune lysis of rabies virus infected cells. *J. Immunol.*, **101**, 1271, 1282 (1968).

75. Zbar, B. Tumor regression mediated by *Mycobacterium bovis* (strain BCG). *Natl. Cancer Inst. Monogr.*, **32**, 371–356 (1972).

IMMUNOGENICITY OF VIABLE XENOGENIZED TUMOR CELLS

Hiroshi KOBAYASHI*1 and Fujiro SENDO*2

*Laboratory of Pathology, Cancer Institute, Hokkaido University School
of Medicine*1 *and First Department of Pathology,
Yamagata University School of Medicine*2

In studies of tumor immunology, use of viable xenogenized tumor cells persistently infected with virus is advantageous, because they grow initially and regress in immunologically competent hosts, producing a strong immunity against identical types of tumor cells. This article describes the immunogenicity of viable tumor cells in rats after their infection with murine leukemia viruses, such as Friend and Gross. The immunogenicity produced in the host after regression of xenogenized tumor was very strong compared with conventional immunizations. This strong effect may be due to viable cell immunization, in which there is no danger of killing the host, if the host is normal or irradiated within 300 rad. In order to compare the strength of the immunogenicity of xenogenized and nonxenogenized tumor cells, they were first inactivated by X-irradiation, mitomycin C, glutaraldehyde, and formalin, after which the hosts were immunized and transplanted with a selected number of nonxenogenized tumor cells. Immunogenicity was better in xenogenized cell-immune rats, except for rats immunized with X-irradiated cells. Crude membrane obtained from xenogenized tumor cells also produced a much stronger immunizing effect than that from nonxenogenized tumor cells. Therefore, it was concluded that strong immunogenicity in viable xenogenized tumor cells may be produced by a qualitative increase in the immunogenicity of tumor-specific antigens (TSA), in addition to quantitative increase in the TSA due to viable cell immunization. Nevertheless, the immunogenicity produced by xenogenized tumor cells was still not satisfactory, and immunization with xenogenized tumor cells was combined with cyclophosphamide, resulting in a marked increase in the immunogenicity in the host. There has been no further progress in the experiments, but further increase in immunogenicity is planned by using viable xenogenized tumor cells.

Lindenmann, Boone, and others (*4–11, 13, 18, 40, 41, 61*) have noted that the immunogenicity of tumor-specific antigen increases after infection with oncolytic virus. Svet-Moldavsky and others (*12, 19, 21, 44, 46, 51–54*) have described how virus-specific new antigen can be produced on the surface of tumor cells infected

---

*1 Kita-15-jo, Nishi-7-chome, Kita-ku, Sapporo 060, Japan (小林　博).
*2 Nishinomae, Iida, Zao, Yamagata 990-23, Japan (仙道富士郎).

with virus and how these virus-infected tumor cells then become sensitive to immune attack by the host after previous immunization with virus. It could be said that Lindenmann and Boone have focused on increasing the immunogenicity of tumor-specific antigens (TSA) by infection with oncolytic virus, while Svet-Moldavsky has stressed producing new antigen on viable tumor cells. In comparing these results, we would like to emphasize that virus-specific new antigen produced by infection with nonlytic budding virus is foreign in the host; thus, the virus-infected cells immunologically regress by themselves without previous immunization, and that TSA is stable and highly antigenic in such viably growing virus-infected tumor cells.

Lethal Growth of Various Rat Tumors Artificially Infected with Friend Virus in Syngeneic Rats

"What is xenogenization of tumor cells?" Simply stated, xenogenization, in the strict sense of the word, is the phenomenon of immunological regression of tumors due to the acquisition of a new surface antigen which is foreign to the host (*26–28, 32, 48*). When rat tumors of various lines were artificially infected with murine leukemia viruses, such as Friend and Gross, they were not able to grow lethally in syngeneic rats and eventually they regressed in the host. We have already used more than ten thousand rats in our experiments, and we have succeeded in the regression of the growth of tumors in normal autochthonous and syngeneic hosts (Table I). For example, WST-5, a spontaneously developing fibrosarcoma artificially infected with Friend virus, is not able to kill the host and eventually regresses. There have been a few exceptional cases: Takeda sarcoma grew so rapidly when it was transplanted intraperitoneally that 6 out of 23 rats died of tumor. KNL-leukemia induced by N-nitrosobutylurea (NBU) also regressed when the leukemia cells were infected with the virus, but leukemias recurred 2–3 months after the regression. However, most rat tumors were not able to

TABLE I. Lethal Growth of Various Rat Tumors Artificially
Infected with Friend Virus in Syngeneic Rats

Tumors infected with virus		Lethal growth (%)
Spontaneous sarcoma:	WST-5	0/26 (0)
	Takeda	6/23 (26.1)
	KST-1	0/25 (0)
MCA sarcoma:	KMT-17	0/443 (0)
	KMT-19	0/80 (0)
	KMT-50	0/17 (0)
	AMC-60	0/10 (0)
4NQO lung cancer:	DLT	0/28 (0)
NBU breast cancer:	KBT-1	0/12 (0)
	KBT-2	0/8 (0)
DAB hepatoma:	AH 109	2/8 (25.0)
	KDH-8	0/58 (0)
NBU leukemia:	KNL-1	0/15 (0)[a]
Total		8/753 (1.1)

[a] Tumors recurred 2–3 months after the regression in all the cases.

kill the host, only 8 out of 753 rats, which is 1.1%, were killed by the tumor growth (Table I).

Regarding the mechanism of regression of rat tumors infected with murine leukemia viruses, we concluded that it was caused by a newly-acquired virus-specific antigen which was foreign in the host.

In order to maintain these virus-infected tumor cells, they were transplanted into immunologically tolerant rats, which had been infected with the virus at birth, or into immunologically suppressed rats which had been treated with chemical immunosuppressants or irradiation. The common method of infecting the tumors with viruses is to transplant tumors into syngeneic rats which have been infected with the virus at birth. While tumor cells and viruses are growing at the same time in the host, the tumor cells may be infected with the virus. Now we would like to move on to the main topic regarding the immunogenicity of virus-infected xenogenized tumor cells against the growth of transplanted noninfected tumor cells.

Immunogenicity of Viable Xenogenized (Friend Virus-infected) KMT-17 Tumor Cells in WKA Rats

Table II indicates the immunogenicity of viable xenogenized (Friend virus-infected) KMT-17 ascitic fibrosarcoma cells (10^7) in WKA rats compared to that of nonxenogenized tumor cells.

A characteristic of xenogenized tumor cells is that Friend virus-infected xenogenized tumor cells can be used as viable cell vaccine, because they regress after temporary growth in a normal host. In contrast, nonxenogenized, non-virus-infected tumor cells cannot be used, because they may grow and kill the host. Therefore, immunization resulting in the spontaneous regression of tumors is demonstrated only in xenogenized tumor cells persistently infected with Friend virus (Fig. 1, Table II). Only 1 of the 16 rats immunized with viable xenogenized tumor cells died from the growth of nonxenogenized KMT-17 tumor cells which were challenged 3 weeks later.

Next, in order to compare the strength of the immunogenicity of viable xenogenized and nonxenogenized tumor cells, viable xenogenized and nonxenogenized tumors were surgically removed on the 4th day after transplantation, and the intensity of the subsequent inhibition against tumor growth was compared (Fig. 1, Table II). There were no deaths before the challenge among the hosts immunized with xenogenized tumor

TABLE II. Immunogenicity of Viable Xenogenized (Friend Virus-infected) KMT-17 Tumor Cells (10^7) in WKA Rats[a]

Treatment of tumor	Lethal growth of KMT-17 in rats immunized with	
	Xenogenized KMT-17 tumor cells	Nonxenogenized KMT-17 tumor cells
Spontaneous regression	1/16	Not done
Surgery (4 th day)	6/16	7/16[b]–3/9

[a] Nonxenogenized tumor cells (1×10^6–10^7) were challenged on day 21 after treatment.

[b] Seven out of 16 rats immunized with nonxenogenized tumor died of recurrence and metastasis of the tumor before the challenge, and the remaining 9 rats were examined by immunogenicity test.

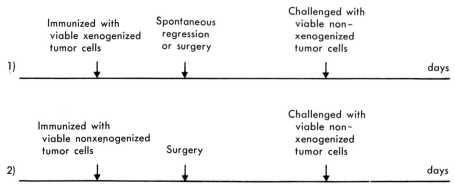

FIG. 1. Time schedule of the experiment in testing the immunogenicity of viable tumor cells

cells, and 6 out of 16 rats died of the challenged tumor. On the other hand, 7 out of 16 rats immunized with nonxenogenized tumor cells died of recurrence and metastasis of the tumor before the challenge, while 3 of the remaining 9 rats died of the challenged tumors. A definite conclusion cannot be made from such a small number of experiments, but our impression from data on the temporary growth of tumor is that the intensity of the antitumor effect produced in the remaining rats was slightly stronger in nonxenogenized tumor cells than in xenogenized tumor cells (unpublished data). This will be discussed again later.

Lethal Growth of Xenogenized (Friend Virus-infected) Tumor Cells (10^7) in Immunologically Suppressed Rats

Table III summarizes an experiment to determine the safety level when using viable xenogenized tumor cells, which, though they may be useful in immunizing the host, might grow and kill the host if immunologically suppressed. Two different types of tumors, a rapidly growing comparatively high antigenic KMT-17 sarcoma induced by 3-methylcholanthrene (MCA) and a slow growing low antigenic KDH-8 liver cell cancer induced by 4-dimethylaminoazobenzene (DAB), were infected with Friend virus and transplanted into rats X-irradiated with 200 to 600 rad. Xenogenized KMT-17 tumor regressed in all cases when the host was normal or irradiated within 300 rad. KDH-8 tumor regressed when the host was irradiated within 500 rad. We con-

TABLE III. Lethal Growth of Xenogenized (Friend Virus-infected) Tumor Cells (10^7) in Immunologically Suppressed Rats

Imm. suppressed by X-ray (rad)	Lethal growth of	
	Xenogenized KMT-17	Xenogenized KDH-8
None	0/5	0/4
200	0/5	—
300	0/5	0/4
400	4/5	0/4
500	9/9	0/4
600	10/10	2/4

clude that depending on the line of tumor, tumor cells will regress with no danger of killing the hosts if the hosts are normal or immunologically conditioned by 300 to 500 rad irradiation (unpublished data).

Immunogenicity of Irradiated Xenogenized and Nonxenogenized KMT-17 Tumor Cells

Xenogenized tumor cells may be useful as a viable cell vaccine to safely produce a strong immunity. In order to compare the qualitative strength of immunogenicity, xenogenized and nonxenogenized tumor cells were inactivated by irradiation (8,000–12,000 rad) (Table IV). We were surprised to observe an unexpectedly stronger antitumor immunity in the rats immunized with irradiated nonxenogenized tumor cells than with irradiated xenogenized tumor cells. Only 15 out of 46 or 32.6% of rats immunized with irradiated nonxenogenized tumor cells died of noninfected 10^5–10^7 KMT tumor cells. In contrast, 27 out of 50 or 54% of rats immunized with irradiated xenogenized tumor cells died. The difference is not large, but it is significant. Unfortunately, we cannot explain why the irradiated xenogenized tumor cells produced a slightly lower immunogenicity compared to the irradiated nonxenogenized tumor cells (unpublished data).

TABLE IV.   Immunogenicity of Xenogenized (Friend Virus-infected) KMT-17
Tumor Cells after Irradiation (8,000–12,000 rad) into Cells

Immunized with (10^7) irradiated	Lethal growth in rats, No. of tumor cells challenged			
	1×10^5	1×10^6	1×10^7	Total (%)
Nonxenogenized tumor cells	1/12	12/27	2/7	15/46 (32.6)
Xenogenized tumor cells	7/14	16/29	4/7	27/50 (54.0)
None	8/8	8/8	7/7	23/23 (100)

Immunogenicity of Xenogenized KMT-17 Tumor Cells after Treatment with Mitomycin C

Table V shows the levels of immunogenicity of xenogenized tumor cells treated with mitomycin C. Xenogenized tumor cells produced a stronger immunogenicity than did nonxenogenized tumor cells. However, the immunogenicity of tumor cells treated with mitomycin C was definitely lower than in previous experiments; 66% of rats were killed when challenged with only 10^5 cells (25).

TABLE V.   Immunogenicity of Xenogenized KMT-17 Tumor Cells
after Treatment with Mitomycin C[a]

Immunized with mitomycin C-treated	Lethal growth in rats No. of tumor cells challenged	
	1×10^5 (%)	1×10^6 (%)
Xenogenized tumor cells	12/18 (66.7)	8/8 (100)
Nonxenogenized tumor cells	18/18 (100)	8/8 (100)
None	10/10 (100)	8/8 (100)

[a] Treated with mitomycin C (20–40 μg) for 60 min with two immunizations being made.

Immunogenicity of Xenogenized KMT-17 Tumor Cells after Treatment with Glutaraldehyde

Table VI shows that xenogenized tumor cells treated with glutaraldehyde acquire a stronger immunogenicity than do nonxenogenized tumor cells. Although 35 out of 41 rats died of noninfected tumor, a much stronger inhibition against tumor growth was observed in xenogenized tumor cell-immune rats. However, the immunogenicity of glutaraldehyde-treated tumor cells is generally weak (*25*).

TABLE VI.   Immunogenicity of Xenogenized KMT-17 Tumor Cells
after Treatment with Glutaraldehyde[a]

Immunized with glutaraldehyde-treated	Lethal growth in rats No. of tumor cells challenged		
	1×10^5	1×10^6	Total (%)
Xenogenized tumor cells	20/23	15/18	35/41 (85.4)
Nonxenogenized tumor cells	23/23	18/18	41/41 (100)
None	23/23	18/18	41/41 (100)

[a] Treated with 0.25% glutaraldehyde with 2–3 immunizations being made.

Immunogenicity of Xenogenized KMT-17 Tumor Cells after Treatment with Formaldehyde

Table VII outlines a similar result, showing a much stronger immunogenicity in xenogenized tumor cells which were treated with formaldehyde (1.0%, 6 hr at 0°). However, the immunogenicity is generally weak (*25*).

TABLE VII.   Immunogenicity of Xenogenized KMT-17 Tumor Cells after
Treatment with Formaldehyde (1.0%, 6 hr at 0°)

Immunized with formaldehyde-treated	Lethal growth in rats No. of tumor cells challenged		
	5×10^4	5×10^5	Total (%)
Xenogenized tumor cells (2×)	3/5	4/5	7/10 (100)
Nonxenogenized tumor cells (2×)	5/5	5/5	10/10 (100)

Immunogenicity of Crude Membrane from Xenogenized KMT-17 Tumor Cells

A comparison of the immunogenicity of crude membranes obtained from xenogenized and nonxenogenized tumor cells was made (Table VIII). A much stronger immunogenicity was observed in rats immunized with the crude membrane obtained

TABLE VIII.   Immunogenicity of Crude Membrane from Xenogenized KMT-17 Tumor Cells

Immunized with crude membrane (10 mg) obtained from	Lethal growth in rats No. of tumor cells challenged		
	5×10^4	1×10^5	Total (%)
Xenogenized tumor cells (2×)	5/10	8/10	13/20 (65)
Nonxenogenized tumor cells (2×)	9/10	10/10	19/20 (95)

from xenogenized tumor cells. The difference was 65% in the one, as against 95% in the other (*25*).

Immunogenicity of Viable Xenogenized KMT-17 Tumor Cells Compared with That of X-irradiated Nonxenogenized Tumor Cells

As previously stated, irradiated nonxenogenized tumor cells produced a strong immunogenicity in the host. Therefore, we tried to compare the strength of immunogenicity of viable xenogenized tumor cells with that of irradiated nonxenogenized tumor cells.

Table IX indicates that the strength of one immunization with viable xenogenized tumor cells was stronger than that of 2–3 immunizations with irradiated nonxenogenized tumor cells. This is statistically significant (unpublished data).

TABLE IX. Immunogenicity of Viable Xenogenized KMT-17 Tumor Cells Compared with That of X-irradiated Nonxenogenized Tumor Cells

Immunized with	Lethal growth in rats No. of tumor cells challenged			
	10^5	10^6	10^7	Total (%)
Viable xenogenized tumor cells (one immunization)	0/2	2/9	5/19	7/30 (23.3)
Irradiated nonxenogenized tumor cells (2–3 immunizations)	1/2	9/21	12/19	22/42 (52.4)

Strength of Immunogenicity of Xenogenized KMT-17 Tumor Cells

Tables X and XI summarize the experiments regarding the strength of immunogenicity of xenogenized tumor cells.

Xenogenized tumor cells inactivated with mitomycin C, glutaraldehyde, or formalin, and crude membrane obtained from xenogenized tumor cells produce a much stronger immunogenicity than do nonxenogenized tumor cells, but in general they are weak. However, the immunogenicity of actively growing viable tumor cells is definitely stronger than that of inactivated tumor cells. The reason for the strong immunogenicity of viable tumor cells may be due to a quantitative increase in addition to a qualitative

TABLE X. Strength of Immunogenicity of Xenogenized KMT-17 Tumor Cells

Treatment		Xenogenized cells	Nonxenogenized cells
Actively growing viable cells:	Regression	‖‖	
	Surgery	‖‖	‖‖[a]
Viable cells:	X-ray	‖	‖‖
	Mitomycin C	+	−
Dead cells:	Glutaraldehyde	+	−
	Formalin	+	−
	Crude membrane	+	−

[a] Danger of metastasis and recurrence does not allow the use of surgery for ordinary immunization.

TABLE XI. Immunogenicity of Xenogenized FV-KMT-17 Tumor Cells
Compared with That of Nonxenogenized KMT-17 Tumor Cells

Immunization		LTD_{50}^a in immunized rats	Increase in LTD_{50}^a
with	times		
Viable			
FV-KMT-17	$1\times$	$10^{7.00}$	$1,000\times$
Irradiated			
FV-KMT-17	$2-3\times$	$10^{5.75}$	$56\times$
KMT-17	$2-3\times$	$10^{6.38}$	$240\times$
MMC-treated			
FV-KMT-17	$2\times$	$10^{4.75}$	$6\times$
KMT-17	$2\times$	$<10^{4.50}$	$<3\times$
GA-treated			
FV-KMT-17	$2-3\times$	$10^{4.65}$	$4.5\times$
KMT-17	$2-3\times$	$<10^{4.50}$	$<3\times$
Formalin-treated			
FV-KMT-17	$2-3\times$	$10^{4.70}$	$5\times$
KMT-17	$2-3\times$	$<10^{4.50}$	$<3\times$
Crude membrane			
FV-KMT-17	$2\times$	$10^{4.80}$	$5.5\times$
KMT-17	$2\times$	$<10^{4.50}$	$<3\times$
None		$10^{4.00}$	—

[a] LTD_{50}, 50%, lethal tumor dose. FV, xenogenized with Friend virus.

stability of TSA. For example, though the antigenicity of TSA is usually unstable and easily destroyed by treatment with chemicals and mechanical means, the TSA of viable tumor cells, particularly if infected with a virus, is very stable especially in the quality of the antigen. In addition, a large amount of TSA can be produced when the host is immunized with viable tumor cells. These allow the cells to grow for a certain period with no danger of killing the host. In contrast, there is danger of metastasis and recurrence when viable nonxenogenized tumor cells are used, even if they do produce stronger immunity in the host. Therefore, viable nonxenogenized tumor cells, naturally, cannot be used for ordinary immunization. We would like to emphasize from this table that the viable xenogenized tumor cells may be useful for the active immunization of tumor cells in the host.

We have been able, therefore, to conduct certain trials of immunotherapy by using viable xenogenized tumor cells. However, no such trials seem to have been effected previously.

Increase in the Immunogenicity of Xenogenized KMT-17 Tumor Cells When Combined with Cyclophosphamide (CY)

We have often been puzzled that the immunogenicity of viable xenogenized tumor cells is not so strong as might have been expected. Even after xenogenized tumor cells regressed following a temporary growth, the resistance against the challenge of tumor cells was still not satisfactory. Furthermore, as stated before, the immunogenicity of xenogenized tumor cells is weaker than that of nonxenogenized tumor cells when actively growing viable tumor cells and the irradiated viable tumor cells are used. Even when

TABLE XII. Increase in the Immunogenicity of Xenogenized KMT-17 Tumor
Cells by Combination with Cyclophosphamide (CY)

Immunization with FV-KMT-17[a]	CY (40 mg/kg) on day	Lethal growth in rats No. of tumor cells challenged		
		5×6^6	5×10^7	Total (%)
Yes	−3	2/13	5/7	7/20 (35.0)[b]
Yes	4, 8, 12, 18	22/29	18/20	40/49 (81.6)
Yes	No	7/13	7/8	14/21 (66.7)[b]
No	−3	4/4		4/4 (100)

[a] 1×10^7 of xenogenized (Friend virus-infected) KMT-17 cells were s.c. immunized on day 0, and
nonxenogenized tumor cells were challenged on day 21.
[b] Statistically significant, $\chi^2 (p < 0.05)$.

TABLE XIII. Effect of Cyclophosphamide Pretreatment on Immunogenicity
of Viable Xenogenized tumor Cells

Pretreated with CY	Immunized with	$LTD_{50}{}^a$ in immunized rat	Increase in $LTD_{50}{}^a$
Yes	FV-KMT-17	$10^{7.26}$	$1,800 \times$
No	FV-KMT-17	$10^{6.97}$	$930 \times$
Yes	None	10^4	—
No	None	10^4	—

[a] LTD_{50}, 50% lethal tumor dose.

repeated immunizations were made, a rather weaker immunogenicity was obtained
in the rats immunized with viable xenogenized tumor cells, compared to surgical
removal of the primary tumor and subsequent repeated immunization with viable nonxenogenized tumor cells, although in the latter there is a danger of killing the host
during the immunizations. Therefore, it was suspected that unknown factors produced
by viable xenogenized tumor cells might inhibit the production of a strong antitumor
immunity (unpublished data).

Tables XII and XIII are preliminary results indicating that immunogenicity of
viable xenogenized tumor cells may be enhanced by the previous administration of
cyclophosphamide (58). When cyclophosphamide was administered 3 days before the
immunization with xenogenized tumor cells, a strong immunogenicity was obtained.
Even when challenged with a large number of tumor cells, only 7 out of 20 rats were
killed, i.e., 35%. This shows a marked increase in the survival rate in comparison with
the immunogenicity of xenogenized tumor cells alone. However, no increase in the
survival rate was observed when cyclophosphamide was used on certain days after the
immunization. No inhibition of tumor growth was observed in rats treated with cyclophosphamide alone. From this preliminary experiment it can be suspected that unknown factors inhibiting the production of immunogenic activity may have appeared
when viable xenogenized tumor cells were used. It has not yet been determined what
factors caused the inhibition of xenogenized tumor cell-immunity. In any case, to
increase the immunogenicity of viable xenogenized tumor cells to higher levels and
to analyze the mechanism of inhibiting the production of viable xenogenized tumor
cell immunity must be the next step.

Thus, it is our intention to seek an application of stronger immunogenicity in the active immunotherapy of cancer by using viable xenogenized tumor cells.

REFERENCES

1. Barbieri, D., Belehradek, J., Jr., and Barski, G. Decrease in tumor-producing capacity of mouse cell lines following infection with mouse leukemia viruses. *Int. J. Cancer*, **7**, 364–371 (1971).
2. Basombrio, M. A. Antigenic conversion of established tumors with the Moloney sarcoma virus (MSV). *Proc. Am. Assoc. Cancer Res.*, **13**, 74 (1972).
3. Basombrio, M. A. Rejection of nonviral tumors after infection with murine sarcoma virus. *Medicina (Buenos Aires)*, **37**, 127–132 (1977).
4. Beverley, P.C.L., Lowenthal, R. M., and Tyrrell, D.A.J. Immune responses in mice to tumor challenge after immunization with Newcastle disease virus-infected or X-irradiated tumour cells or cell fractions. *Int. J. Cancer*, **11**, 212–223 (1973).
5. Boone, C. W. and Blackman, K. Augmented immunogenicity of tumor cell homogenates infected with influenza virus. *Cancer Res.*, **32**, 1018–1022 (1972).
6. Boone, C. W. and Blackman, K. Augmented immunogenicity of tumor cell homogenates produced by infection with influenza virus. *Natl. Cancer Inst. Monogr.*, **35**, 301–307 (1972).
7. Boone, C. W., Paranjpe, M., Orme, T., and Gillette, R. Virus-augmented tumor transplantation antigens: Evidence for a helper antigen mechanism. *Int. J. Cancer*, **13**, 543–551 (1974).
8. Cassel, W. A. and Garrett, R. E. Tumor immunity after viral oncolysis. *J. Bacteriol.*, **92**, 792 (1966).
9. Eaton, M. D., Levinthal, J. D., Scala, A. R., and Jewell, M. L. Immunity and antibody formation induced by intraperitoneal or subcutaneous injection of Krebs 2 ascites tumor cells treated with influenza virus. *J. Natl. Cancer Inst.*, **34**, 661–672 (1965).
10. Eaton, M. D., Levinthal, J. D., and Scala, A. R. Contribution of antiviral immunity to oncolysis by Newcastle disease virus in a murine lymphoma. *J. Natl. Cancer Inst.*, **39**, 1089–1097 (1967).
11. Eaton, M. D., Heller, J. A., and Scala, A. R. Enhancement of lymphoma cell immunogenicity by infection with non-oncogenic virus. *Cancer Res.*, **33**, 3293–3298 (1973).
12. Eiselein, J. and Biggs, M. W. Observations with a variant of lymphocytic choriomeningitis virus in mouse tumors. *Cancer Res.*, **30**, 1953–1957 (1970).
13. Gillette, R. W. and Boone, C. W. Augmented immunogenicity of tumor cell membranes produced by surface budding viruses: Parameters of optimal immunization. *Int. J. Cancer*, **18**, 216–222 (1976).
14. Gotohda, E., Sendo, F., Hosokawa, M., Kodama, T., and Kobayashi, H. Combination of active and passive immunization and chemotherapy to transplantation of methylcholanthrene-induced tumor in WKA rats. *Cancer Res.*, **34**, 1947–1951 (1974).
15. Gotohda, E., Sendo, F., Nakayama, M., Hosokawa, M., Kawamura, T., Kodama, T., and Kobayashi, H. Change of antigenic expression on rat tumor cells after their transplantation. *J. Natl. Cancer Inst.*, **55**, 1079–1083 (1975).
16. Gotohda, E., Moriuchi, T., Kawamura, T., Akiyama, J., Oikawa, T., Sendo, F., Hosokawa, M., Kodama, T., and Kobayashi, H. Stabilized expression of tumor-associated antigen on rat tumor cells by infection with Friend virus. Unpublished.
17. Greenberger, J. S. and Aaronson, S. A. *In vivo* inoculation of RNA C-type viruses

inducing regression of experimental solid tumors. *J. Natl. Cancer Inst.*, **51**, 1935–1938 (1973).

18. Häkkinen, I. and Halonen, P. Induction of tumor immunity in mice with antigens pre-pared from influenza and vesicular stomatitis virus grown in suspension culture of Ehrlich ascites cells. *J. Natl. Cancer Inst.*, **46**, 1161–1167 (1971).

19. Hamburg, V. P., Loizner, A. L., and Svet-Moldavsky, G. J. Artificial induction of transplantation viral antigens in the course of chemical carcinogenesis. *Nature*, **212**, 1495 (1966).

20. Holtermann, O. A. and Majde, J. A. An apparent histocompatibility between mice chronically infected with lymphocytic choriomeningitis virus and their uninfected syn-geneic counterparts. *Transplantation*, **11**, 20–29 (1971).

21. Hosokawa, M., Kodama, T., Sendo, F., Takeichi, N., and Kobayashi, H. Immunological characteristics of methylcholanthrene-induced tumors exposed to Friend virus. *J. Cancer Immunopathol.*, **3**, 42–46 (1967) (in Japanese).

22. Hosokawa, M., Sendo, F., Gotohda, E., and Kobayashi, H. Combination of immuno-therapy and chemotherapy to experimental tumors in rats. *Gann*, **62**, 57–60 (1971).

23. Hosokawa, M., Kasai, M., Yamaguchi, H., and Kobayashi, H. Increased immuno-sensitivity of xenogenized tumor cells to lymphocyte cytotoxicity. Unpublished.

24. Kaji, H., Sendo, F., Shirai, T., Saito, H. Kodama, T., and Kobayashi, H. Immuno-therapy of rat tumors with tumor cells artificially infected with mouse Friend virus. *Modern Med.*, **24**, 1329–1333 (1969) (in Japanese).

25. Katoh, H., Ikeda, K., Minami, A., Hosokawa, M., Kodama, T., and Kobayashi, H. Immunogenicity of inactivated xenogenized tumor cells. Unpublished.

26. Kobayashi, H., Sendo, F., Shirai, T., Kaji, H., Kodama, T., and Saito, H. Modification in growth of transplantable rat tumors exposed to Friend virus. *J. Natl. Cancer Inst.*, **42**, 413–419 (1969).

27. Kobayashi, H., Kodama, T., Shirai, T., Kaji, H., Hosokawa, M., Sendo, F., Saito, H., and Takeichi, N. Artificial regression of rat tumor infected with Friend virus (xenogeni-zation)—An effect produced by acquired antigen. *Hokkaido J. Med. Sci.*, **44**, 133–134 (1969).

28. Kobayashi, H. Growth of rat tumor cells infected with Friend virus: An approach to the immunological treatment of cancer. *In* "Immunity and Tolerance in Oncogenesis," ed. L. Severi, pp. 637–659 (1970). IV. Perugia Quadrenn. Int. Conf. on Cancer, 1969.

29. Kobayashi, H., Shirai, T., Takeichi, N., Hosokawa, M., Saito, H., Sendo, F., and Kodama, T. Antigenic variant (WFT-2N) of a transplantable rat tumor induced by Friend virus. *Eur. J. Clin. Biol. Res.*, **15**, 426–428 (1970).

30. Kobayashi, H., Sendo, F., Kaji, H., Shirai, T., Saito, H., Takeichi, N., Hosokawa, M., and Kodama, T. Inhibition of transplanted rat tumors by immunization with identical tumor cells infected with Friend virus. *J. Natl. Cancer Inst.*, **44**, 11–19 (1970).

31. Kobayashi, H., Gotohda, E., Hosokawa, M., and Kodama, T. Inhibition of metastasis in rats immunized with xenogenized autologous tumor cells after excision of the primary tumor. *J. Natl. Cancer Inst.*, **54**, 997–999 (1975).

32. Kobayashi, H., Kodama, T., and Gotohda, E. "Xenogenization of Tumor cells," Hok-kaido Univ. Med. Libr. Series, Vol. 9, Sapporo, pp. 1–24 (1977).

33. Kodama, T., Kobayashi, H., Saito, H., Shirai, T., and Matsumiya, H. Electron micro-scopic studies on cultured human cancer cells infected with Friend virus. *Gann*, **61**, 219–221 (1970).

34. Kodama, T., Gotohda, E., and Kobayashi, H. Immuno-electron microscopic studies on surface antigens of rat tumor cells infected with Friend virus. *Gann*, **64**, 475–479 (1973).

38   H. KOBAYASHI AND F. SENDO

35. Kodama, T., Gotohda, E., and Kobayashi, H. Morphological aspects of xenogenization of tumors by artificial infection with virus. *Gann Monogr. Cancer Res.*, **16**, 167–181 (1974).

36. Kodama, T., Gotohda, E., Takeichi, N., Kuzumaki, N., and Kobayashi, H. Histopathology of immunologic regression of tumor metastasis in the lymph nodes. *J. Natl. Cancer Inst.*, **52**, 931–939 (1974).

37. Kodama, T., Kato, H., Gotohda, E., Kobayashi, H., and Sendo, F. Regression of established tumors in rats by injection of diethylaminoethyl-dextran and Friend murine leukemia virus. *J. Natl. Cancer Inst.*, (1978) in press.

38. Kuzumaki, N. and Kobayashi, H. Reduced transplantability of syngeneic mouse tumors superinfected with membrane viruses in nu/nu mice. *Transplantation*, **22**, 545–550 (1976).

39. Kuzumaki, N., Fenyö, E. M., Giovanella, B. C., and Klein, G. Increased immunogenicity of low-antigenic rat tumors after superinfection with endogenous murine C-type virus in nude mice. *Int. J. Cancer*, **21**, 62–66 (1978).

40. Lindenmann, J. and Klein, P. A. Viral oncolysis: Increased immunogenicity of host cell antigen associated with influenza virus. *J. Exp. Med.*, **126**, 93–108 (1967).

41. Lindenmann, J. Viruses as immunological adjuvants in cancer. *Biochim. Biophys. Acta*, **355**, 49–75 (1974).

42. Moriuchi, T., Gotohda, E., Hosokawa, M., Kodama, T., and Kobayashi, H. Correlation between concanavalin A agglutinability and cytotoxic sensitivity to antiserum against tumor-associated antigen in rat fibrosarcoma cells. *J. Natl. Cancer Inst.*, **62**, 579–583 (1978).

43. Murray, D. R., Cassel, W. A., Torbin A. H., Olkowski, Z. L., and Morre, M. E. Viral oncolysate in the management of malignant melanoma. *Cancer*, **40**, 680–686 (1977).

44. Pasternak, G. and Pasternak, L. Demonstration of Graffi leukemia virus and virus-induced antigens in leukemic and nonleukemic tissues of mice. *J. Natl. Cancer Inst.*, **38**, 157–168 (1967).

45. Saito, H. Immunofluorescence studies on the transplantable rat tumor cells infected with Friend virus. *Gann*, **61**, 253–258 (1971).

46. Salaman, M. H., Turk, J. L., and Wedderburn, N. Foreign antigenicity in tissues of mice infected with a lymphomagenic virus. I. Antigenicity of spleen cells. *Transplantation*, **16**, 583–590 (1973).

47. Sauter, C., Gerber, A., Lindenmann, J., and Martz, G. Akute myeloische leukäemie: Behandlungsversuch mit einem an Myeloblasten adaptierten Myxovirus. *Schweiz. Med. Wochenschr.*, **102**, 285–290 (1972) (in German).

48. Sendo, F., Kaji, H., Saito, H., and Kobayashi, H. Antigenic modification of rat tumor cells artificially infected with Friend virus in the primary autochthonous host. *Gann*, **61**, 223–226 (1970).

49. Shirai, T., Kaji, H., Takeichi, N., Sendo, F., Saito, H., Hosokawa, M., and Kobayashi, H. Cell surface antigens detectable by cytotoxic test on Friend virus-induced and Friend virus-infected tumors in the rat. *J. Natl. Cancer Inst.*, **46**, 449–460 (1971).

50. Sinkovics, J. G., Plager, C., McMurtrey, M. J. Romero, J. J., and Romsdahl, M. M. Viral oncolysates for the immunotherapy of human tumors. *Proc. Am. Assoc. Cancer Res.*, **18**, 86 (1977).

51. Sjögren, H. O. and Hellström, I. Induction of polyoma-specific transplantation antigenicity in Moloney leukemia cells. *Exp. Cell. Res.*, **40**, 208–212 (1965).

52. Stück, B., Old, L. J., and Boyse, E. A. Antigenic conversion of established leukemias by an unrelated leukemogenic virus. *Nature*, **202**, 1016–1018 (1964).

53. Svet-Moldavsky, G. J. and Haumburg, V. P. Quantitative relationships in viral oncolysis

and the possibility of artificial heterogenization of tumors. *Nature*, **202**, 303–304 (1964).

54. Svet-Moldavsky, G. J. and Haumburg, V. P. An approach to the immunological treatment of tumors by artificial heterogenization. *UICC Monogr.*, **2**, 323–327 (1967).

55. Takeichi, N., Boone, C. W., Holden, H. T., and Herberman, R. B. Immunological study of two stocks of Moloney sarcoma virus producing regressor and progressor tumors in C57BL/6 mice. *Int. J. Cancer*, **21**, 78–84 (1978).

56. Takeichi, N., Austin, F. C., Oikawa, T., and Boone, C. W. Virus-augmentation of tumor-associated antigens. Comparison of influenza virus and murine sarcoma virus. *Cancer Res.*, **38**, 4580–4584 (1978).

57. Takeyama, H., Kawashima, K., Yamada, K., and Ito, Y. Induction of tumor resistance in mice by L1210 leukemia cells persistently infected with HVJ (Sendai virus). Unpublished.

58. Terashima, M., Mizushima, Y., Takeichi, N., Hosokawa, M., and Kobayashi, H. Immunogenicity of xenogenized tumor cells in rats pretreated with cyclophosphamide. Unpublished.

59. Wallack, M. K. and Steplewski, Z. Specific immunotherapy with vaccinia oncolysates. *Proc. Am. Assoc. Cancer Res.*, **18**, 18 (1977).

60. Wise, K. S. Vesicular stomatitis virus-infected L1210 murine leukemia cells: Increased immunogenicity and altered surface antigens. *J. Natl. Cancer Inst.*, **58**, 83–90 (1977).

61. Yamada, T. and Hatano, M. Lowered transplantability of cultured tumor cells by persistent infection with paramyxovirus (HVJ). *Gann*, **63**, 647–655 (1972).

GANN Monograph on Cancer Research 23, 1979

INCREASED IMMUNOGENICITY OF RAT TUMORS AFTER SUPERINFECTION WITH ENDOGENOUS MURINE C-TYPE VIRUS

Noboru Kuzumaki and George Klein

*Department of Tumor Biology, Karolinska Institutet**

Four chemical carcinogen-induced and two polyoma virus-induced rat tumors were repeatedly passaged through nude mice. A 3-methylcholanthrene (MC)-induced tumor in BDIX rats (MBDB) and a polyoma virus-induced tumor in Wistar/Fu rats (PW41) became infected with endogenous mouse virus (EMV), as judged by the expression of murine C-type virus-associated gp71, p30, and p12 antigens on their cell surface. Two ethylnitrosourea-induced tumors in BDIX rats (290T and GE3A) were exposed *in vitro* to the supernatant of EMV-infected PW41. Subsequently, 290T but not GE3A converted to murine gp71, p30, and p12 positivity. All these successfully infected rat tumors (EMV-MBDB, EMV-PW41, and EMV-290T) became less transplantable to, and more rejectable in otherwise susceptible syngeneic rats. To compare the immunogenicity of the virus-infected and noninfected tumors, syngeneic rats were immunized 3 times with irradiated cells, and challenged with the noninfected tumor. Wistar/Fu rats immunized with irradiated EMV-PW41 showed no improvement of PW41 rejection, compared to rats immunized with irradiated noninfected cells. On the other hand, BDIX rats immunized with EMV-MBDB or EMV-290T rejected MBDB or 290T, respectively, with no cross immunity, while the rats immunized with irradiated but noninfected tumors showed no significant rejection. These results indicate that EMV infection increased the immunogenicity of non-, or only low immunogenic rat tumors.

In contrast to the highly efficient surveillance against tumors induced by ubiquitous viruses in their natural host species, spontaneous tumors and a considerable proportion of the chemically-induced tumors evoke little or no rejection reaction (*4*). It is possible that a genetic deficiency of immune recognition is responsible for the outgrowth of many spontaneous or chemical tumors. If so, the preventive or immunotherapeutic effort will have to focus on the overcoming of unresponsiveness, rather than the correction of a presumptive immune breakdown. The nonrejectability of spontaneous or low antigenic chemical tumors may be overcome by target cell modification, *e.g.*, by chemical coupling, somatic cell hybridization or viral superinfection.

In the latter category, both lytic viruses (presented by Svet-Moldavsky, Lindenmann, and Boone at this workshop) and nonlytic oncogenic murine C-type viruses (presented by Kobayashi) were tested for their ability to increase the immunogenicity of nonrejectable tumors. The disadvantage of the former lies in the fact that a some-

---

* S-104 01 Stockholm 60, Sweden (葛巻　暹).

times striking oncolytic effect may be accompanied by cytotoxicity for the tumor-bearing animal. Viruses of the latter category are handicapped by their potential oncogenicity that limits the prospects of applicability to human tumors.

Endogenous C-type viruses found in natural species have so far not been found to induce tumors in the home or foreign species. Together with the ubiquitous occurrence of endogenous C-viral genomes in normal cells, this suggests that they may not carry any oncogenic information (3).

Nude mice have been broadly used for heterotransplantation of tumors. Since they contain endogenous, xenotropic mouse viruses (EMV) (8, 9), nude mouse passage is a convenient way to superinfect tumors of other species with EMV. Our experiments were designed to test whether EMV can increase the immunogenicity of low antigenic rat tumors.

Culture lines derived from two 3-methylcholanthrene (MC)-induced fibrosarcomas (MBDA and MBDB), two ethylnitrosourea-induced neurogenic tumors (290T and GE3A) in BDIX rats, and two polyoma virus-induced sarcomas (PW31 and PW41) in Wistar/Fu rats were inoculated subcutaneously and passaged 2 or 3 times through nude mice. Subsequently, the tumors were recultured and tested for sensitivity to anti-murine C-type viral gp71, p30, and p12 sera in a complement-dependent microcyto-toxicity assay (Table I). The original MBDB and PW41 tumors were not damaged by the anti-gp71, p30, and p12 sera, while nude mouse passaged MBDB and PW41 reacted with all three antisera, indicating successful superinfection with endogenous mouse virus (EMV). In contrast, nude mouse passaged MBDA, 290T, GE3A, and PW31 did not acquire any sensitivity to the reagents. We have therefore attempted to superinfect 290T and GE3A *in vitro* with the supernatant of nude mouse passaged, EMV-infected PW41 4 times weekly. Subsequently, 290T acquired sensitivity to anti-gp71, p30, and p12 sera (Table I), while the GE3A still failed to respond.

The three EMV-infected rat tumors (EMV-MBDB, EMV-290T, and EMV-PW41) were inoculated subcutaneously into untreated syngeneic rats in comparison with noninfected tumors (Table II). EMV-MBDB, EMV-290T, and EMV-PW41 showed a significantly reduced transplantability. EMV-MBDB and EMV-290T were

TABLE I. Expression of Mouse C-type Virus Components on Rat
Tumors after Superinfection with EMV

Rats	Tumors	Oncogenic agents	Method of superinfection	Expression of EMV after superinfection[a]		
				gp 71	p 30	p 12
BDIX	MBDA	MC	Nude mouse passage	−	−	−
	MBDB	MC	Nude mouse passage	+	+	+
	290T	ENU	Nude mouse passage	−	−	−
	GE3A	ENU	Nude mouse passage	−	−	−
W/Fu[b]	PW31	PV	Nude mouse passage	−	−	−
	PW41	PV	Nude mouse passage	+	+	+
BDIX	290T	ENU	*In vitro* superinfection[c]	+	+	+
	GE3A	ENU	*In vitro* superinfection	−	−	−

[a] None of the tumors expessed gp 71, p 30, and p 12 before superinfection.
[b] W/Fu, Wistar/Fu.
[c] With supernatant of EMV-infected PW41.

TABLE II. Reduced Transplantability of Rat Tumors Infected
with EMV in Untreated Syngeneic Rats

Tumors[a]	Dose	Incidence of lethal growths
MBDB	1×10^6	4/4
EMV-MBDB	1×10^6	0/4
290T	2×10^5	4/4
EMV-290T	2×10^5	0/4
PW41	5×10^5	6/6
EMV-PW41	5×10^5	2/7

[a] LD_{100} of MBDB, 290T, and PW41 in syngeneic rats was 1×10^5, 2×10^3, and 1×10^5, respectively (5).

rejected completely even at challenge doses that were 10 to 100 times above the LD_{100}.
Five out of 7 EMV-PW41 were also rejected by the hosts at a challenge dose exceeding
the LD_{100} 5 times. These results suggested that EMV-infected rat tumors were more
antigenic in syngeneic rats than noninfected tumors.

TABLE III. Growth Inhibition of Rat Tumors in Syngeneic Rats Immunized with
Irradiated Endogenous Mouse Virus-infected or Uninfected Tumors

Immunization[a]		Challenge[b]		
Tumors	Dose	Tumors	Dose	Lethal growths (MSD[c])
MBDB	1×10^6	MBDB	1×10^5	4/4 (72.0)
EMV-MBDB	1×10^6	MBDB	1×10^5	0/6
290T	5×10^6	MBDB	1×10^5	2/2 (57.5)
EMV-290T	1×10^6	MBDB	1×10^5	4/4 (62.0)
None		MBDB	1×10^5	4/4 (61.2)
MBDB	1×10^6	MBDB	1×10^6	4/4 (54.2)
EMV-MBDB	1×10^6	MBDB	1×10^6	0/4
None		MBDB	1×10^6	4/4 (57.5)
290T	5×10^6	290T	2×10^3	4/4 (67.5)
EMV-290T	5×10^6	290T	2×10^3	0/4
MBDB	1×10^6	290T	2×10^3	2/2 (59.5)
EMV-MBDB	1×10^6	290T	2×10^3	4/4 (56.5)
None		290T	2×10^3	4/4 (57.2)
290T	5×10^6	290T	2×10^4	5/5 (58.2)
EMV-290T	5×10^6	290T	2×10^4	4/6 (67.5)
None		290T	2×10^4	3/3 (52.3)
PW41	5×10^6	PW41	5×10^4	2/4 (67.5)
EMV-PW41	5×10^6	PW41	5×10^4	2/4 (63.0)
None		PW41	5×10^4	3/4 (48.6)
PW41	5×10^6	PW41	5×10^5	4/4 (54.5)
EMV-PW41	5×10^6	PW41	5×10^5	4/4 (61.0)
None		PW41	5×10^5	6/6 (37.6)

[a] Heavily irradiated (10,000 rad) cells were inoculated into syngeneic rats 3 times at weekly intervals.

[b] Challenge 8 days after final immunization. Hosts were irradiated 400 rads 24 hr before tumor
inoculation.

[c] Mean survival time in days (5).

In order to compare the immunogenicity of EMV-infected tumors with their noninfected counterparts, syngeneic rats were immunized with irradiated cells 3 times at weekly intervals. Seven days after the last immunization, the rats received 400 rad whole-body irradiation and, on the following day, they were challenged with different numbers of viable cells. BDIX rats immunized with irradiated noninfected MBDB failed to reject 10^5 of MBDB although their mean survival time increased in comparison with nonimmune rats. Rats immunized with irradiated EMV-MBDB completely rejected 10^5 and 10^6 viable cells (Table III). Similar results were obtained with 290T. All 4 BDIX rats immunized with EMV-290T rejected 2×10^3 290T cells that grew in all 4 controls. Two of 6 rats rejected 2×10^4 cells as well. BDIX rats immunized with irradiated EMV-MBDB did not reject 290T, and rats immunized with irradiated EMV-290T did not reject MBDB. These results show that superinfection with endogenous mouse virus could augment the low immunogenicity of the chemically-induced rat tumors tested, with maintained, noncross-reactive specificity. On the other hand, there was no difference between the Wistar/Fu rats immunized with irradiated PW41 compared to EMV-PW41. Neither group rejected 5×10^5 of PW41 cells although there was a clear retardation of mean survival time in both.

The present experiments show that low antigenic rat tumors can be infected with endogenous mouse C-type viruses that lack any known oncogenic activity, by nude mouse passage or *in vitro* exposure, with increased immunogenicity in transplantation and rejection tests, compared to the original tumors. In the mouse system, endogenous rat C-type viruses could infect mouse tumors, and the virus-infected tumors reduced their transplantability (7) as in murine sarcoma virus-infected mouse tumors (6). It has been shown that human tumors can also become infected with EMV in nude mice (1), thereafter they express mouse C-type virus-associated cellsurface antigens (2). This suggests that human tumors could be successfully xenogenized by nude mouse passage. Experiments to determine whether spontaneous rat tumors could also increase their immunogenicity after superinfection of endogenous mouse C-type viruses are now in progress.

REFERENCES

1. Achong, B. G., Trumper, P. A., and Giovanella, B. C. C-type virus particles in human tumors transplanted into nude mice. *Br. J. Cancer*, **34**, 203–206 (1976).

2. Kiessling, R., Haller, O., Fenyö, E. M., Steinitz, M., and Klein, G. Mouse natural killer (NK) cell activity against human cell lines is not influenced by superinfection of the target cell with xenotropic murine C-type virus. *Int. J. Cancer*, **21**, 460–465 (1978).

3. Klein, G. Mechanisms of carcinogeneis. *In* "Radiation Research, Biomedical, Chemical and Physical Perspectives," ed. O. F. Nygaard, H. I. Adler, and W. K. Sinclair, pp. 869–878 (1975). Academic Press, New York.

4. Klein, G. and Klein, E. Rejectability of virus-induced tumors and nonrejectability of spontaneous tumors: A lesson in contrasts, *Transplant. Proc.*, **9**, 1095–1104 (1977).

5. Kuzumaki, N., Fenyö, E. M., Giovanella, B. C., and Klein, G. Increased immunogenicity of low-antigenic rat tumors after superinfection with endogenous murine C-type virus in nude mice. *Int. J. Cancer*, **21**, 62–66 (1978).

6. Kuzumaki, N., Fenyö, E. M., Klein, E., and Klein, G. Protective effect of murine

sarcoma virus (MSV)-superinfected mouse tumor cells against the outgrowth of the corresponding noninfected tumor. *Transplantation*, **26**, 304–307 (1978).

7. Kuzumaki, N. and Kobayashi, H. Reduced transplantability of syngeneic mouse tumors superinfected with membrane viruses in nu/nu mice. *Transplantation*, **22**, 545–550 (1976).

8. Price, P. J., Arnstein, P., Suk, W. A., Vernon, M. L., and Huebner, R. J. Type-C RNA viruses of the NIH nude mouse. *J. Natl. Cancer Inst.*, **55**, 1231–1232 (1975).

9. Tralka, T. S., Rabson, A. S., and Hansen, C. T. C-type virus particles in a cell line from a lymphosarcoma of a nude mouse. *J. Natl. Cancer Inst.*, **55**, 197–198 (1975).

GANN Monograph on Cancer Research 23, 1979

STABILIZED EXPRESSION OF TUMOR-ASSOCIATED ANTIGEN IN XENOGENIZED TUMOR CELLS TO COMPLEMENT-DEPENDENT CYTOTOXICITY

Eiki Gotohda, Tetsuya Moriuchi, Takao Kodama, and
Hiroshi Kobayashi

Laboratory of Pathology, Cancer Institute,
*Hokkaido University School of Medicine**

The expression of cell surface antigens on a 3-methylcholanthrene (MCA)-induced rat transplantable tumor (KMT-17) or on the identical tumor artificially infected with Friend virus (FV-KMT-17) was studied by the complement-dependent cytotoxicity test. Both tumors killed syngeneic rats within 3 days if more than 10^8 cells were inoculated intraperitoneally (i.p.). The cytotoxicity test revealed that the sensitivity of KMT-17 to antiserum against histocompatibility antigen (R^w) was extremely stable and did not change after i.p. transplantation. However, cytotoxic sensitivity to antiserum against tumor-associated cell-surface antigen (TASA) decreased during the 3 days after transplantation; that of 1-day-old cells was the highest and that of 3-day-old cells the lowest. The sensitivity of 3-day-old cells was restored 1 day after transplantation into normal rats. With regard to the mechanism of the change in TASA expression, participation of host immunity was shown not to be involved. On the other hand, an inverse correlation was found between the density of tumor cells in the abdominal cavity and their sensitivity to anti-TASA serum. Therefore, the phenomenon of high cytotoxic sensitivity on the first day after transplantation dropping to sensitivity on the third day was not related only to days after transplantation. In addition, a newly-acquired antigen besides R^w and TASA appeared on the cell surface of KMT-17 after infection with Friend virus; the virus-associated cell-surface antigen (VASA). The sensitivities of FV-KMT-17 to antiserum against R^w or VASA were markedly stable and never changed regardless of the number of days after transplantation. However, most surprisingly, in contrast to the drop in anti-TASA sensitivity of the transplanted KMT-17 cells within 3 days as described above, the anti-TASA sensitivity of FV-KMT-17 cells did not drop, but remained stable at a high level after transplantation. This meant that the expression of TASA on the KMT-17 was stabilized by infection with Friend virus. Possible mechanisms concerning the change of TASA expression and significance of the stabilized expression of TASA in FV-KMT-17 will be discussed.

As already reported as "xenogenization" (7–9), chemical carcinogen-induced rat transplantable tumors which are infecetd with murine leukemia virus regress in syn-

* Kita-15-jo, Nishi-7-chome, Kita-ku, Sapporo 060, Japan (後藤田栄貴, 守内哲也, 小玉孝郎, 小林 博).

geneic hosts without any treatment. In a host which had rejected the virus-infected tumor, strong transplantation immunity against a virus-noninfected identical tumor was acquired. By comparing immunogenicity between a virus-infected and a noninfected tumor, the former was proved to possess much stronger immunogenicity than the latter. In order to know the mechanism of the above result, tumor-associated surface antigen (TASA), rat histocompatibility antigen (R^w), as well as virus-associated surface antigen (VASA) in virus-infected or noninfected identical tumors were examined quantitatively and qualitatively by a complement-dependent cytotoxicity test and an indirect membrane immunofluorescence test.

The tumor used in this experiment was induced by MCA in an inbred WKA rat and this tumor designated KMT-17, is a transplantable fibrosarcoma. This grows both intraperitoneally and subcutaneously but was usually maintained in an ascites form. One of the most remarkable characteristics of this tumor is its rapid growth. For example, an intraperitoneal inoculum of more than 10^8 cells kills normal rats within 3 days and the time needed for one cell cycle was estimated to be about 8 hr *in vivo*. On the other hand, Friend virus-infected KMT-17, designated FV-KMT-17, was obtained by artificial infection of KMT-17 with Friend virus in Friend-tolerant rats. When syngeneic WKA rats were inoculated subcutaneously (s.c.) with FV-KMT-17, the tumor grew initially and regressed completely within 2 weeks after inoculation.

Antiserum against the rat histocompatibility antigen of the WKA strain was obtained from Long-Evans rats that were given transplantations of WKA skin and immunization with spleen and lymph node cells from WKA rats. Antiserum against TASA was obtained from syngeneic rats immunized s.c. and i.p. with a large number of KMT-17 cells. No cytotoxicity was demonstrated with other tumor cell lines or normal spleen, lymph node or thymus cells from WKA rats. Antiserum against VASA was obtained in syngeneic WKA rats by s.c. and i.p. immunization with a Friend virus-induced rat tumor, WFT-13.

Antigenic Expression in KMT-17 Tumor

A WKA rat was given i.p. transplants of 10^8 KMT-17 cells every 3 days, then 1-, 2-, and 3-day-old KMT-17 tumors were prepared. Cytotoxic sensitivity of tumors from these 3 rats to antiserum against the histocompatibility antigen were examined. As shown in Fig. 1, 1-, 2-, and 3-day-old KMT-17 tumors showed almost identical sensitivity and they did not change with days after transplantation. On the other hand, Fig. 2 shows the cytotoxic sensitivity of KMT-17 tumors to antiserum against TASA; a 1-day-old tumor showed extremely high sensitivity but the sensitivity of 2-day-old KMT-17 decreased moderately. A 3-day-old tumor showed the lowest sensitivity. When a 3-day-old KMT-17 tumor was transplanted into other normal rats, the cytotoxic sensitivity was restored one day after the i.p. transplantation; thereafter it decreased daily as in the former rat. This means that the change of TASA expression by days after transplantation was reversible (3). Interestingly, the change of antigenic expression was restricted only to TASA and did not affect the histocompatibility antigen on the same cell surface. As one of the mechanisms for change of TASA expression by days after transplantation in the KMT-17 tumor, host immunity was considered to be an important factor. Then, the cytotoxic sensitivity of the KMT-17 tumor trans-

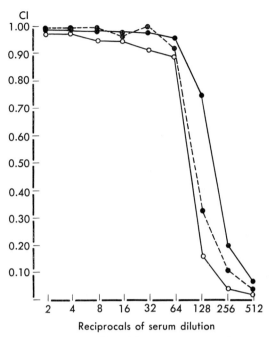

FIG. 1. Cytotoxic sensitivity of KMT-17 tumors to antiserum against histo-compatibility antigen by days after transplantation
●——● 1-day-old transplantation; ○——○ 2-day-old transplantation;
●－－－● 3-day-old transplantation.

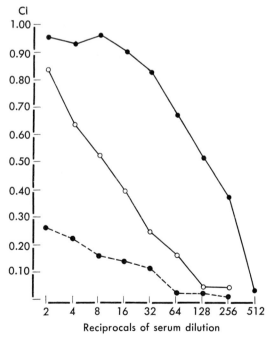

FIG. 2. Cytotoxic sensitivity of KMT-17 tumors to antiserum against TASA by days after transplantation
●——● 1-day-old transplantation; ○——○ 2-day-old transplantation;
●－－－● 3-day-old transplantation.

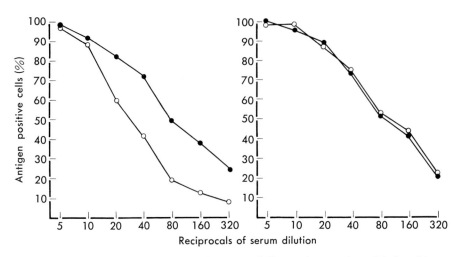

FIG. 3. Detection of TASA or histocompatibility antigen on 1- and 3-day-old KMT-17 tumors by the indirect membrane immunofluorescence test

    Left: Ratio of antigen-positive cells to antiserum against TASA. Right: That to antiserum against histocompatibility antigen. ●——● 1-day-old; ○——○ 3-day-old KMT-17 tumor.

planted in immunosuppressively irradiated rats was examined. Cytotoxic sensitivity of tumors transplanted into the irradiated rats also decreased daily like those of tumors transplanted into untreated rats. Therefore, host immunity such as immunoselection, the blocking factor, or TL-like antigenic modulation (*12*) does not participate in the change of TASA expression in a KMT-17 tumor (*3*).

    In order to know whether or not 3-day-old KMT-17 not sensitive to the antiserum and complement lost TASA on the cell surface, the ratio of TASA-possessing cells was checked in both 1- and 3-day-old KMT-17 tumors by indirect membrane immunofluorescence. Figure 3 shows that, at the highest concentration of antiserum, almost all cells in both tumors possessed distinct TASA. However, by diluting the antiserum the ratio in the 3-day-old tumor became gradually smaller than that in the 1-day-old tumor. On the other hand, the ratio of histocompatibility antigen-positive cells in 1- and 3-day-old KMT-17 tumors was almost identical at any dilution of antiserum.

    It has been suggested that the change was influenced by tumor cell density in the abdominal cavity since cytotoxic sensitivity was high when the tumor cells were less numerous in the abdominal cavity and, on the contrary, low when number of cells increased. Then, an experiment was designed to determine whether the sensitivity of KMT-17 to antiserum against TASA was influenced by the removal of tumor cells from the abdominal cavity or by transplantation with a large number of tumor cells. As a result, the change of TASA expression in KMT-17 was not due to days after transplantation but to the tumor cell density in the abdominal cavity of the rats (*3*).

Antigenic Expression in FV-KMT-17 Tumor

Friend virus-infected KMT-17, or a xenogenized tumor, grows lethally only in immunosuppressed or Friend virus-tolerant rats. However, when this is inoculated s.c. in syngeneic adult rats, it regresses by 2 weeks post-transplantation. The regression is due to newly-acquired VASA on the cell surface. As described previously, hosts which rejected the xenogenized tumor acquired strong transplantation resistance against a noninfected identical tumor (7). The main purpose in this experiment was to investigate whether this strong immunogenicity of the xenogenized tumor was induced by quantitative or qualitative changes in TASA after infection with Friend virus.

Cytotoxic sensitivity of FV-KMT-17 tumors to antisera against TASA and histocompatibility antigen was examined by days after transplantation in comparison with those of KMT-17 tumors. The KMT-17 tumor was not sensitive to anti-VASA serum but each of the FV-KMT-17 tumors was highly sensitive to the antiserum (4). Sensitivity of FV-KMT-17 tumors to antiserum against the histocompatibility antigen also did not change regardless of days after transplantation as those of the KMT-17 tumors. On the other hand, cytotoxic sensitivity of FV-KMT-17 tumors to anti-TASA serum did not change at all and were constantly high as shown in the righthand figure of Fig. 4. The sensitivity of KMT-17 tumors decreased by passaged days as mentioned previously (left figure). This means that the TASA expression which had changed in KMT-17 tumors was stabilized by infection with Friend virus. By the quantitative absorption test, there was no difference in the absorbing capacities of 1-day-old KMT-17 and FV-KMT-17 tumors (11).

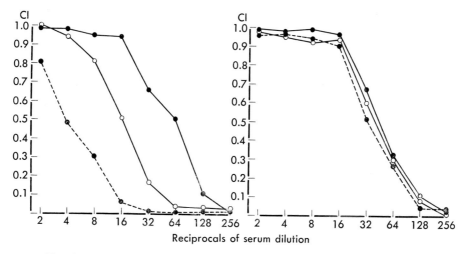

FIG. 4. Cytotoxic sensitivity of KMT-17 tumors (left) and FV-KMT-17 tumors (right) to antiserum against TASA by days after transplantation
●——● 1-day-old transplantation; ○——○ 2-day-old transplantation; ●---● 3-day-old transplantation.

Antigenic Expression and Antigen Movement on the Cell Membrane

Mechanisms of stabilization of TASA expression in FV-KMT-17 as well as

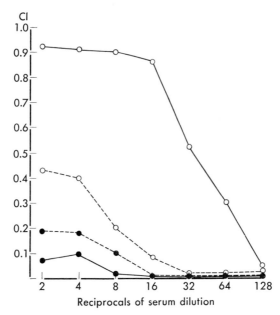

FIG. 5. Increased cytotoxic sensitivity of the 3-day-old KMT-17 tumor to antiserum against TASA by pretreatment with Con A at 37° for 15 min
●——● nontreated; ●- - -● treated with 13.0 μg/ml of Con A on ice; ○- - -○ treated with 1.3 μg/ml of Con A; ○——○ treated with 13.0 μg/ml of Con A.

change in KMT-17 are still not clear. However, if the cytotoxic sensitivity of tumors changes even though the content of TASA in them does not alter, changes or stabilization in TASA expression is probably due to complement activation. In fact, it is well known that antigens which are capped by antibody cannot activate a complement (2, 12). Therefore, the change in cytotoxic sensitivity followed by tumor growth *in vivo* seemed to depend on the modalities of existence of TASA on the cell surface. Therefore, an experiment was made to decide whether the decreased cytotoxic sensitivity of 3-day-old KMT-17 can be augmented by modification with some enzymes or lectins (5). Figure 5 shows the markedly increased cytotoxic sensitivity of a 3-day-old KMT-17 tumor to anti-TASA serum when it was treated with concanavalin A (Con A). In addition, it was also augmented by treatment with trypsin (5). Furthermore, the TASA expression correlated clearly with results detected by Con A-agglutinability; each of the FV-KMT-17 tumors showed similarly high agglutinability but the agglutinability of the 3-day-old KMT-17 was the lowest while that of the 1-day-old KMT-17 was as high as that of FV-KMT-17 tumors (11). By immunoferritin electron microscopic observations (10), TASA distribution was generally recognized as a cluster on the 1-day-old KMT-17 and on 1- and 3-day-old FV-KMT-17 cell surface but as a dispersed distribution on the 3-day-old KMT-17 cell surface. All of these results suggested that the expression of TASA in KMT-17 or xenogenized KMT-17 detected by complement-dependent cytotoxicity was regulated by antigen movement or lateral mobility of the antigen on the cell membrane (1, 13, 18). If the above speculation were correct, lateral mobility of TASA in KMT-17 may change as the tumor grows *in vivo*. On the contrary, it may be constantly high and stable if tumors are infected with the Friend virus. This will be supported by some reports (13, 14, 18) that cell agglutinability was augmented by infection with various types of viruses. Especially in the 3-day-old KMT-17 tumor, the lateral mobility might have been greatly decreased by unknown factors so that antigens on the cell membrane could not be concentrated enough to activate the complement even by sufficient antibodies. The expression of histocompatibility antigen which was always stable in both KMT-17 and FV-KMT-17 tumors might not be influenced even by the low lateral mobility because of a large amount of the antigen all over the cell membrane.

By malignant transformation, the content of the histocompatibility antigen was reduced in experimental (6, 17) as well as human tumors (16). Recently, interest has focused on the interrelationship between virus infection and the histocompatibility antigen (19), and H-2 and the virus antigen are likely to form hybrid antigens on the cell surface (15). We were also interested in whether the content of TASA and the histocompatibility antigen which already existed in KMT-17 was increased or decreased by the new acquisition of VASA in FV-KMT-17. Results obtained by the quantitative absorption test indicated that the content of either antigen in both tumors did not change (4). After all, changes brought about by Friend virus-infection on the cell membrane are qualitative rather than quantitative; one is an acquisition of distinct VASA and the other is the increased (or stabilized) lateral mobility of TASA by xenogenization.

Mechanisms for Augmented Immunogenicity of the Xenogenized Tumor

Transplantation resistance against the identical tumor was not augmented only by immunization with a mixture of Friend virus itself and the virus-noninfected tumor. Hence, the augmented immunogenicity of the xenogenized tumor is due to the participation of VASA which newly appeared on the cell surface after the virus infection. As already shown in this article, the content of TASA was proved to be unchanged in FV-KMT-17. It is therefore conceivable that VASA newly acquired on the cell surface might act as a helper antigen to recognize TASA easily or that there may exist a certain association between TASA and VASA on the Friend virus-infected cell membrane. Moreover, since not only TASA expression was stabilized at a high level but Con A-agglutinability was constantly high and stable in FV-KMT-17 tumors, it is also possible to think that the augmented immunogenicity of the xenogenized tumor was induced by high and stable lateral mobility of TASA on the cell membrane. As a certain amount of antigen concentration is required for activating the complement in the cytotoxicity test, an appropriate amount of antigen may be also demanded for recognition or killing in cell-mediated tumor immunity. It is possible to suppose that antigens which are freely mobile on the cell membrane can rapidly reach a certain degree of antigen concentration. As the content of TASA in both KMT-17 and FV-KMT-17 tumors was almost the same, the time required for the antigen to reach a certain concentration might have induced the difference in immunogenicity. However, further investigations are required to clarify the mechanism of the augmented immunogenicity of the xenogenized tumor.

REFERENCES

1. Boyle, M.D.P., Ohanian, S. H., and Borsos, T. Lysis of tumor cells by antibody and complement. III. Lack of correlation between antigen movement and cell lysis. *J. Immunol.*, **115**, 473–475 (1975).
2. Edidin, M. and Henney, C. S. The effect of capping H-2 antigens on the susceptibility of target cells to humoral and T cell-mediated lysis. *Nature New Biol.*, **246**, 47–49, (1973).
3. Gotohda, E., Sendo, F., Nakayama, M., Hosokawa, M., Kodama, T., and Kobayashi, H. Change of antigenic expression on rat tumor cells after their transplantation. *J. Natl. Cancer Inst.*, **55**, 1079–1083 (1975).
4. Gotohda, E., Moriuchi, T., Hosokawa, M., Kodama, T., and Kobayashi, H. Stabilized expression of tumor-associated surface antigen on rat tumor cells by infection with Friend virus. Unpublished.
5. Gotohda, E. Unpublished data.
6. Haywood, G. R. and McKhann, C. F. Antigenic specificities on murine sarcoma cells. Reciprocal relationship between normal transplantation antigens (H-2) and tumor-specific immunogenicity. *J. Exp. Med.*, **133**, 1171–1187 (1971).
7. Kobayashi, H., Sendo, F., Kaji, H., Hosokawa, M., and Kodama, T. Modification in growth of transplantable rat tumors exposed to Friend virus. *J. Natl. Cancer Inst.*, **42**, 413–419 (1969).
8. Kobayashi, H., Sendo, F., Shirai, T., Takeichi, N., Hosokawa, M., and Kodama, T. Inhibition of transplantable rat tumors by immunization with identical tumor cells infected with Friend virus. *J. Natl. Cancer Inst.*, **44**, 11–19 (1970).
9. Kobayashi, H., Kuzumaki, N., Gotohda, E., Takeichi, N., Hosokawa, M., and Kodama, T. Specific antigenicity of tumors and immunological tolerance in rat induced by Friend, Gross, and Rauscher viruses. *Cancer Res.*, **33**, 1589–1603 (1973).
10. Kodama, T., Gotohda, E., and Kobayashi, H. Immuno-electron microscopic studies of surface antigens of rat tumor cells infected with Friend virus. *Gann*, **64**, 475–479 (1973).
11. Moriuchi, T. Unpublished data.
12. Old, L. J., Stockert, E., Boyse, E. A., and Kom, J. H. Antigenic modulation. Loss of TL antigen from cells exposed to TL antibody. Study of the phenomenon *in vitro. J. Exp. Med.*, **127**, 523–539 (1968).
13. Poste, G. and Reeve, P. Agglutination of normal cells by plant lectins following with nononcogenic viruses. *Nature New Biol.*, **237**, 113–114 (1972).
14. Petria, S. D. and Raff, M. C. Ligand-induced redistribution of concanavalin A receptors on normal, trypsinized and transformed fibroblasts. *Nature New Biol.*, **244**, 275–278 (1973).
15. Schrader, J. W., Cunningham, B. A., and Edelman, G. M. Functional interactions of viral and histocompatibility antigens at tumor surfaces. *Proc. Natl. Acad. Sci. U.S.*, **72**, 5066–5070 (1975).
16. Siegler, H. F., Kremer, W. B., and Metzgar, R. S. HL-A antigenic loss in malignant transformation. *J. Natl. Cancer Inst.*, **46**, 577–584 (1972).
17. Ting, C. C. and Herberman, R. B. Inverse relationship of polyoma tumor specific cell surface antigen to H-2 histocompatibility antigens. *Nature New Biol.*, **232**, 118–120 (1971).
18. Zarling, J. M. and Tevethia, S. S. Expression of concanavalin A binding sites in rabbit kidney cells infected with vaccinia virus. *Virology*, **45**, 313–316 (1971).
19. Zinkernagel, R. M. and Doherty, P. C. H-2 compatibility requirement for T cell mediated

lysis of target cells infected with lymphocytic choriomeningitis virus. Different cytotoxic T cell specificities are associated with structures coded for in H-2K or H-2D. *J. Exp, Med.*, **141**, 1427–1436 (1975).

GANN Monograph on Cancer Research 23, 1979

LATERAL MOBILITY AND STABILIZED EXPRESSION OF TUMOR-ASSOCIATED SURFACE ANTIGEN IN XENOGENIZED TUMOR CELLS

Takao Kodama

Laboratory of Pathology, Cancer Institute,
Hokkaido University School of Medicine*

The distribution of tumor-associated surface antigen (TASA) was investigated by the immunoferritin method on the surface of 3-methylcholanthrene-induced transplantable KMT-17 and mouse Friend virus-infected KMT-17 (xenogenized KMT-17) tumor cells in WKA/Mk rats. The distribution of TASA on KMT-17 tumor cells was not stable and changed daily after intraperitoneal (i.p.) transplantation in the rat. Ferritin labeling of TASA of 1-day-old KMT-17 tumor cells clustered on the surface as discrete patches, while it was dispersed on the surface of 3-day-old cells. In contrast, however, the distribution of TASA on xenogenized KMT-17 tumor cells was stable. Ferritin labeling of TASA of both 1- and 3-day-old xenogenized KMT-17 tumor cells clustered on the surface. These results suggested that the lateral mobility of TASA after treatment with an antibody was changeable daily in KMT-17 tumor cells and was stable in xenogenized KMT-17 tumor cells after their i.p. transplantation. The findings of lateral mobility of KMT-17 and xenogenized KMT-17 tumor cells obtained from immunoelectron microscopy correlated well with complement-dependent cytotoxic sensitivity as well as agglutinability with concanavalin A (con A) and the appearance of microvilli on the cell surface. The results of these investigations are reviewed and discussed with reference to the relationship between the lateral mobility of TASA and the cytotoxic sensitivity of tumor cells.

Gotohda *et al.* (*2*) reported that the complement-dependent cytotoxicity test with antiserum against tumor-associated surface antigen (TASA) of 3-methylcholanthrene-induced transplantable KMT-17 tumor cells in WKA/Mk rats revealed a daily decrease in the cytotoxic sensitivity after transplantation. They also reported that the decrease in the cytotoxic sensitivity of KMT-17 disappeared after xenogenization of the tumor cells by infection with murine Friend leukemia virus (*3, 5*).

The present paper mainly deals with the investigation on the distributions of TASA on the surface membrane of KMT-17 and Friend virus-infected KMT-17 (xenogenized KMT-17) tumor cells by an immunoelectron microscopy. The results of these investigations are reviewed with reference to the relationship between the lateral mobility of TASA after treatment with antiserum, and the cytotoxic sensitivities of tumor cells.

---

* Kita-15-jo, Nishi-7-chome, Kita-ku, Sapporo 060, Japan (小玉孝郎).

Immunoelectron Microscopic Studies

Attempts were made to investigate the distribution of TASA on the surface of KMT-17 and xenogenized KMT-17 tumor cells by immunoelectron microscopy using an indirect method with ferritin-conjugated antibody (6). Antiserum against TASA (anti-TASA) was obtained from syngeneic WKA/Mk rats that resisted transplants of KMT-17 tumor in trocar dose after immunization by ligation and release methods.

a) KMT-17 tumor cells: After incubation with anti-TASA and ferritin-conjugated antibody at 20°, the label of ferritin granules was concentrated in relatively discrete patches on the 1-day-old KMT-17 cell surface. In contrast, on the surface of 3-day-old KMT-17 cells, the label was randomly and sparsely distributed over the whole cell surface. However, when 1-day-old and 3-day-old KMT-17 cells had been fixed previously with 1% glutaraldehyde, and then incubated with anti-TASA and ferritin-conjugated antibody, the label was distributed over the whole surface for both 1- and 3-day-old cells (Photos 1 and 2).

b) Xenogenized KMT-17 cells: After incubation at 20°, the label of ferritin granules was concentrated and clustered in discrete patches on both 1- and 3-day-old xenogenized KMT-17 cells. When 1- and 3-day-old xenogenized KMT-17 cells were fixed with 1% glutaraldehyde before incubation with anti-TASA and ferritin-conjugated antibody, the label was distributed over the whole surface of both cell groups as for pre-fixed KMT-17 cells (Photos 3 and 4).

From these above results, it may be suggested that the dissimilarity of ferritin labeling of TASA between 1- and 3-day-old KMT-17 cells might be due to the difference in the lateral mobility of TASA. The reason is that when tumor cells are previously fixed with glutaraldehyde and then incubated with ferritin-conjugated antibody, the labeling of TASA of KMT-17 as well as xenogenized KMT-17 tumor cells always shows a dispersed appearance similar to nonfixed 3-day-old KMT-17 tumor cells. Therefore, it can be said that TASA was originally distributed on the surface of KMT-17 and xenogenized KMT-17 tumor cells. Thus, lateral mobility of TASA with the treatment of antibody changed daily after the transplantation of KMT-17 tumor cells from high lateral mobility in 1-day-old cells to low lateral mobility in 3-day-old cells. On the other hand, the lateral mobility of TASA in xenogenized KMT-17 tumor cells might be high and stable after transplantation (7).

Scanning Electron Microscopic Studies

Morphological studies on the surface of KMT-17 and xenogenized KMT-17 tumor cells were performed by scanning electron microscopy. For scanning electron microscopy, tumor cells were fixed in 2.5% glutaraldehyde solution at 37° for 1 hr, rinsed once in Millonig buffer solution, and then post fixed in 2% OsO_4 solution at room temperature (10).

a) KMT-17 tumor cells: The results showed a different morphology of cell surface, especially in microvilli, between 1- and 3-day old KMT-17 tumor cells. The surface of 1-day-old cells was comparatively smooth, and microvilli were not in evidence. In contrast, the surface of 3-day-old cells was irregular and covered with an abundant number of microvilli (Photos 5 and 6).

b) Xenogenized KMT-17 tumor cells: The surface of xenogenized KMT-17 tumor cells did not show a daily change after the transplantation. The surface of both 1- and 3-day-old xenogenized KMT-17 tumor cells was comparatively smooth, and microvilli were not clear, like in the 1-day-old KMT-17 tumor cells (Photos 7 and 8).

The reason for the appearance of microvilli on the surface of 3-day-old KMT-17 tumor cells is still unknown, but it might be true that the appearance of microvilli reveals something of lateral mobility which in turn may possibly be related to TASA distribution on the tumor cell surface after treatment with an antibody.

Concanavalin A (Con A) Agglutinability of Tumor Cells

The agglutinability with Con A of KMT-17 and xenogenized KMT-17 tumor cells was investigated by means of scoring and turbidometric methods (*1, 8*). KMT-17 tumor cells showed a daily decrease in agglutinability with Con A after transplantation, from high agglutinability in 1-day-old cells to low agglutinability in 3-day-old cells. However, agglutinability of xenogenized KMT-17 tumor cells did not change after the transplantation, and was high and stable (Table I).

Thus, it can be seen that the lateral mobility of Con A receptors might decrease daily after transplantation in KMT-17 tumor cells, but might not change in xenogenized KMT-17 tumor cells (*4, 9*).

TABLE I. Summary of Results Obtained by Immunoferritin
Technique Incubated at 20°

Tumor cell	Findings of TASA	Con A agglut	Cytotoxic sensitive
KMT-17 (1)[a]	---- ----	⧺[b]	⧺
KMT-17 (3)	··········	+	+
FV-KMT-17[c] (1)	---⌒---	⧺	⧺
FV-KMT-17 (3)	---⌒---	⧺	⧺

[a] No. in parentheses; days after transplantation.
[b] Agglutinability and sensitivity; ⧺, high; +, low.
[c] FV-KMT-17, Friend virus infected KMT-17.

CONCLUSION

The results of lateral mobility of TASA obtained from the immunoelectron microscopy correlated well with the agglutinability with Con A as well as to the cytotoxicity test in KMT-17 and xenogenized KMT-17 tumor cells (Table I). The exact reason for the correlation between the lateral mobility of TASA and the cytotoxic sensitivity is still unknown. One possible explanation is that the antibody binding to TASA may depend on distribution of the antigen on the tumor cells. The apparent increase in the binding of the antibody may be due to an increase in the avidity of a low-affinity antibody for the TASA that are clustered into multivalent aggregates (*9*). Therefore, when the lateral mobility of TASA is high on the surface of tumor cells, cytotoxic sensitivity will increase. Thus, 1-day-old KMT-17 tumor cells as well as 1- and 3-day-old xenogenized KMT-17 tumor cells, which indicate high lateral mobility of TASA, showed a high cytotoxic sensitivity, and 3-day-old KMT-17 tumor cells, which indicate low lateral mobility of TASA, showed a low cytotoxic sensitivity. The meaning of the finding of microvilli on the surface of tumor cells was not clear. However, it might also be related to the lateral mobility of TASA on the surface of tumor cells. Further morphological studies will be conducted on the characteristics of xenogenization of tumor cells, with reference to the stabilized expression of TASA in tumor cells.

REFERENCES

1. Burger, M. M. and Goldberg, A. R. Identification on a tumor specific determinant on neoplastic cell surfaces. *Proc. Natl. Acad. Sci. U.S.*, **57**, 306–357 (1967).
2. Gotohda, E., Sendo, F., Nakayama, M., Hosokawa, M., Kawamura, T., Kodama, T., and Kobayashi, H. Change of antigenic expression on rat tumor cells after their transplantation. *J. Natl. Cancer Inst.*, **55**, 1079–1083 (1975).
3. Gotohda, E., Sendo, F., and Kawamura, T. Stabilization of the expression of tumor-specific antigen by xenogenization. *Proc. Jpn. Cancer Assoc., 34th Annu. Meet.*, p. 54 (1975).
4. Gotohda, E., Moriuchi, T., and Sendo, F. Enhancement of antigenic expression of rat tumor cells by trypsin and concanavalin A. *Proc. Jpn. Cancer Assoc., 35th Annu. Meet.*, p. 51 (1976).
5. Gotohda, E., Moriuchi, T., Kawamura, T., Akiyama, J., Oikawa, T., Sendo, F., Hosokawa, M., Kodama, T., and Kobayashi, H. Stabilized expression of tumor-associated antigen on rat tumor cells by infection with Friend virus. Unpublished.
6. Kodama, T., Kuzumaki, N., and Takeichi, N. Immunoelectron microscopic studies on cell surface antigens of Friend virus-induced tumor in the rat. *Gann*, **64**, 273–276 (1973).
7. Kodama, T., Moriuchi, T., and Gotohda, E. Immunoelectron microscopic studies on lateral mobility of membrane antigens of tumor cells. *Proc. Jpn. Cancer Assoc., 36th Annu. Meet.*, p. 88 (1977).
8. Maca, R. D. and Hoak, J. C. Improved method for quantitation of concanavalin A-induced agglutination. *J. Natl. Cancer Inst.*, **52**, 365–367 (1974).
9. Moriuchi, T., Gotohda, E., Kodama, T., Hosokawa, M., and Kobayashi, H. Correlation between concanavalin A agglutinability and cytotoxic sensitivity to antiserum against tumor-associated antigen in fibrosarcoma cells. *J. Natl. Cancer Inst.*, **62**, 579–583 (1979).
10. Tsutsui, K., Kumon, H., Ichikawa, H., and Tawara, J. Preparative method for suspended biological materials for SEM by using polycationic substance layer. *J. Electron Microsc.*, **25**, 163–168 (1976).

EXPLANATION OF PHOTOS

PHOTO 1. Ferritin labelings (arrow) of TASA on the surface of 1-day-old KMT-17 tumor cell clustered as discrete patches. ×100,000.

PHOTO 2. TASA on the surface of 3-day-old KMT-17 tumor cell dispersed. ×100,000.

PHOTO 3. TASA on the surface of 1-day-old xenogenized KMT-17 tumor cell clustered as discrete patches. ×100,000.

PHOTO 4. TASA on the surface of 3-day-old xenogenized KMT-17 tumor cells clustered. This was different from 3-day-old nonxenogenized KMT-17 tumor cells. ×100,000.

PHOTO 5. Scanning electron micrograph of 1-day-old KMT-17 tumor cells with relatively smooth surface. ×4,000.

PHOTO 6. Three-day-old KMT-17 tumor cells with a large number of microvilli. ×4,000.

PHOTO 7. One-day-old xenogenized KMT-17 tumor cells with relatively smooth surface. ×4,000.

PHOTO 8. Three-day-old xenogenized KMT-17 tumor cells relatively smooth surface differing from 3-day-old nonxenogenized KMT-17 tumor cells. ×4,000.

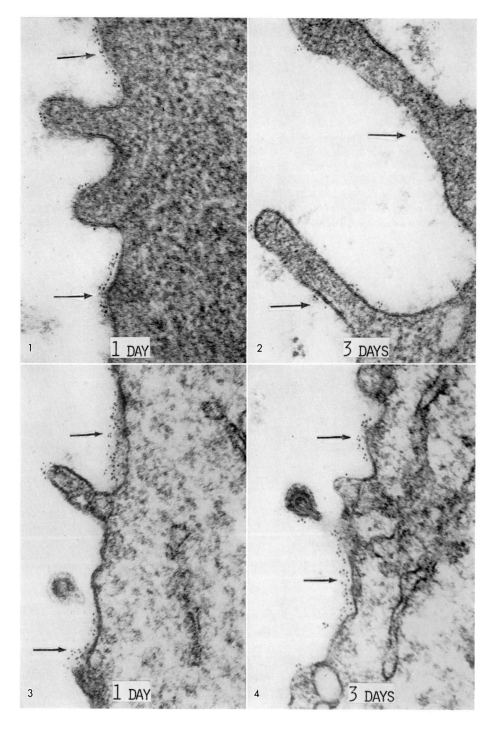

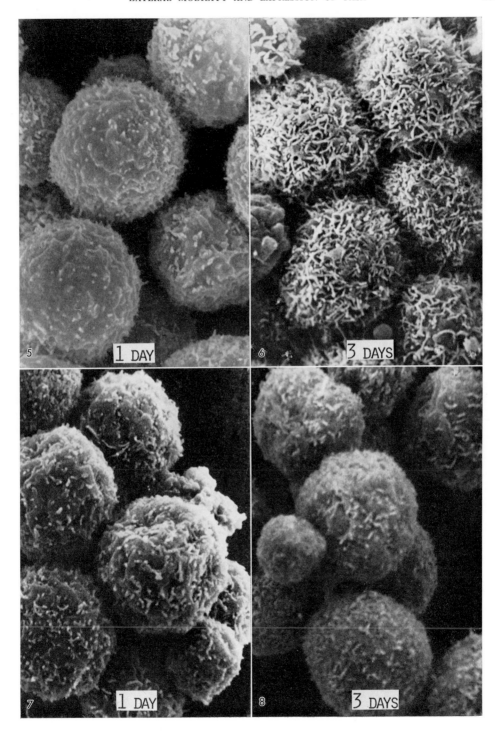

GANN Monograph on Cancer Research 23, 1979

ROLE OF VIRUS-ASSOCIATED ANTIGEN ON XENOGENIZED TUMOR CELL SURFACE IN PRODUCTION OF ANTIBODY AGAINST TUMOR-ASSOCIATED ANTIGEN

Tetsuya Moriuchi and Hiroshi Kobayashi

Laboratory of Pathology, Cancer Institute, Hokkaido University School of Medicine*

When rats are immunized with syngeneic tumor cells xenogenized by infection with murine leukemia virus, the rats recognize virus-associated antigen (VAA) in addition to tumor-associated antigen (TAA). In order to clarify the role of VAA in the production of anti-TAA antibody in immunization with xenogenized tumor cells, association between TAA and VAA on the cell surface was examined. Histocompatibility antigen was also examined for its relation to TAA. For the experiment, chemically-induced rat fibrosarcoma KMT-17 and Friend virus-infected KMT-17 (FV-KMT-17) were used.

FV-KMT-17 was incubated with antisera against TAA, VAA, or histocompatibility antigen, and the kinetics of antigenic modulation were determined. Modulation of TAA occurred rapidly, whereas the histocompatibility antigen was modulated very slowly. These results suggest that TAA and histocompatibility antigen have a different mobility on the cell surface. On the other hand, antigenic modulation of VAA was induced by a mechanism different from the other two kinds of antigens through the shedding of the antigen-antibody complex. Having attained modulation of TAA, inhibition of cytotoxic killing could be examined. FV-KMT-17 was incubated with antiserum against TAA, and antisera against either VAA or the histocompatibility antigen and complement were added. Inhibition of lysis was observed with antiserum against VAA but not with that against the histocompatibility antigen. These results suggest that there is an association between TAA and VAA but not between TAA and the histocompatibility antigen.

Antibody response against TAA was then examined. In the primary response, immunization with FV-KMT-17 and KMT-17 showed the same antibody level. In the secondary response, however, immunization with FV-KMT-17 produced a significantly higher antibody level than that with KMT-17.

Investigation of antitumor antibody response suggests that TAA and VAA may associate to form immunogenic units, with VAA functioning as a helper determinant.

Tumor cells possess a variety of surface antigens which may have different antigenic specificities, location, mobility, and role in tumor rejection. These antigens, particularly tumor-associated antigens (TAA), have been strongly implicated in host surveillance

---

* Kita-15-jo, Nishi-7-chome, Kita-ku, Sapporo 060, Japan (守内哲也, 小林　博).

against tumors. Cell-mediated immune reactions against TAA are widely considered to be of prime importance in the induction of resistance against transplanted tumors (3). In studies on allograft rejection, T cell killing plays a predominant role (1). However, in tumor immunology, the importance of non-T cell as well as the T cell, has been suggested (2). Although the antitumor antibody has been considered unimportant in the immunological control of chemically induced tumors, there are several recent studies which suggest that the antitumor antibody may play a more positive role in tumor rejection in combination with the non-T cell (ADCC) (4). Regarding cell-mediated response, enhancement of the immunogenicity of weak TAA using viruses (xenogenization) has previously been reported (5). In the present study, augumentation of humoral antibody response to virus-infected tumors was investigated. In order to clarify the role of virus-associated antigen (VAA) in the production of antitumor antibody, the relationship among TAA, VAA, and the histocompatibility antigen (R^w) was also studied.

Antigenic Modulation of VAA, TAA, and R^w on FV-KMT-17

We first examined the relationship among VAA, TAA, and R^w. In order to investigate the relationship by the complement-dependent cytotoxicity test, we examined whether antigenic modulation may be induced by specific antiserum. Figure 1 shows that preincubation of Friend virus-infected KMT-17 (FV-KMT-17) with rat antiserum to VAA at 37° led to "antigenic modulation" (7) of VAA on the cell surface as tested in the cytotoxicity test; *i.e.*, in the cytotoxicity test depending on the time of preincubation, the cell progressively lost its sensitivity to anti-VAA serum and guinea pig complement. Simultaneously, the fate of the cell-bound antibody during antigenic modulation was visualized by an indirect immunofluorescence technique. Following

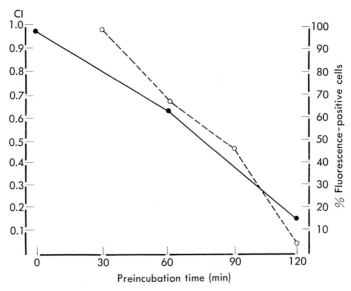

FIG. 1. Antigenic modulation of VAA on FV-KMT-17
● cytotoxic index; ○ % fluorescence-positive cells.

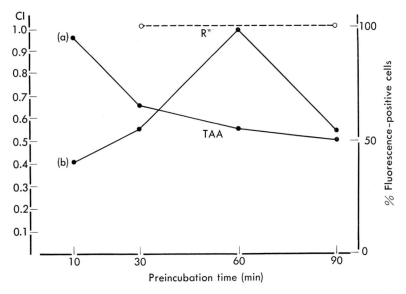

FIG. 2. Kinetics of antigenic modulation of TAA and R^w on FV-KMT-17
(a), FV-KMT-17+anti-TAA; (b), FV-KMT-17+anti-R^w
● cytotoxic index; ○ % fluorescence-positive cells.

modulation with anti-VAA at 37° for a particular length of time, FV-KMT-17 was incubated with goat anti-rat IgG/FITC antibody at 0° for 30 min and then examined by fluorescence microscopy. The percentage of fluorescence-positive cells during modulation decreased in parallel with the decrease in cytotoxicity of the complement. Capping and pinocytosis were not observed. Therefore, it can be suggested that VAA-anti-VAA complexes are shed from the cell surface.

Figure 2 shows the kinetics of antigenic modulation of TAA and R^w. FV-KMT-17 was preincubated with antisera at 37° and washed twice with cold minimum essential medium (MEM) and then incubated with the complement at 37° for 20 min. When incubated with anti-TAA, cytotoxic sensitivity to complement lysis became maximum

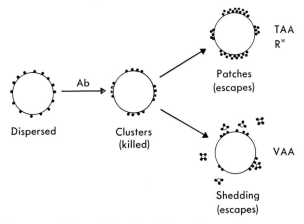

FIG. 3. Summary of data obtained by indirect immunofluorescence technique and cytotoxicity test in FV-KMT-17

at 10 min, whereas when incubated with anti-R^w cytotoxic sensitivity gradually increased, reaching the maximum sensitivity at 60 min and decreasing thereafter. Both antigens showed virtually 100% fluorescence-positive staining and small patches were observed over the entire cell surface. The different kinetics of modulation of both antigens indicate that TAA and R^w antigen have different mobilities, therefore it can be suggested that TAA and R^w are located on different molecules.

A summary of the data obtained by the indirect immunofluorescence technique and cytotoxicity test is shown in Fig. 3. Antigenic modulation of both TAA and R^w are due to patch formation which will inhibit complement activation by tightly packed immunoglobulin molecules, whereas antigenic modulation of VAA is due to the shedding of antigen-antibody complexes from the cell surface.

Relationship between TAA and VAA or R^w on the Cell Surface

On the basis of the experiments on antigenic modulation, the following experiments were carried out. In order to obtain antigenic modulation of TAA, FV-KMT-17 was incubated with anti-TAA at 37° for 90 min. Thereafter, either anti-VAA or anti-R^w and complement were added. As shown in Table I, when anti-VAA and complement were added, cytotoxic sensitivity of cells treated with anti-TAA was significantly lower than control cells treated with normal rat serum. In contrast, cell lysis by anti-R^w and complement was not inhibited by pretreatment with anti-TAA.

These results suggest that there is an association between TAA and VAA on the cell surface. On the other hand, it appears that TAA and R^w have no association. Figure 4 summarizes the results already described and the scheme of the hypothetical relationship between these antigens. According to this hypothesis, TAA, VAA, and R^w are present on separate molecules on the cell surface of FV-KMT-17; however, TAA and VAA are physically linked. In the presence of anti-TAA, TAA will redis-

TABLE I. Inhibition of Cytotoxicity by Preincubation with Anti-TAA in FV-KMT-17

		Preincubation with anti-TAA	
		(+)	(−)
Exp. 1	Anti-TAA+C	0.42	0.82
	Anti-VAA+C	0.35	0.63
Exp. 2	Anti-TAA+C	0.34	0.71
	Anti-VAA+C	0.31	0.52
	Anti-R^w+C	0.56	0.56

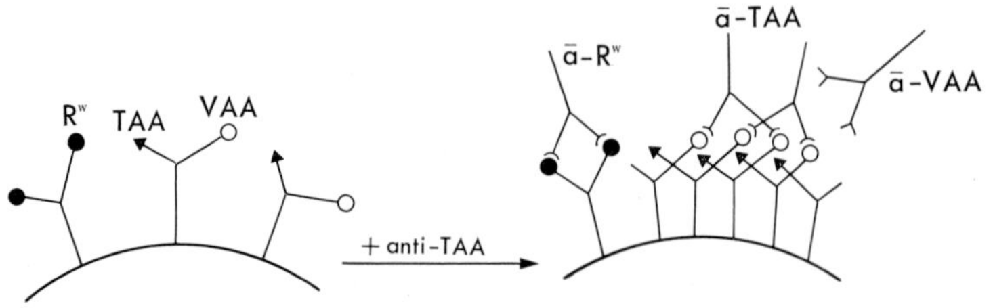

FIG. 4. Hypothetical relationship among TAA, VAA, and R^w on FV-KMT-17

tribute rapidly to form clusters and patches. At the same time, VAA will redistribute passively to form co-patches resulting in an escape from complement-dependent lysis. On the other hand, there is no association between TAA and R^w, therefore cytotoxic killing by anti-R^w will not be affected by anti-TAA.

Augumented Anti-TAA Antibody Response by Immunization with Xenogenized Tumor Cells

As the next step, we investigated whether there may be any effect of this association on anti-TAA antibody response. Figure 5 shows the primary antibody response following immunization against FV-KMT-17 and KMT-17. Each point on the curves represents the mean value for eight animals. Anti-TAA antibody was first detected on day 6, reached the peak titer on day 8, and decreased gradually thereafter. There was no apparent difference between FV-KMT-17 and KMT-17 with respect to the antibody level. Figure 6 shows the secondary antibody response following re-inoculation of the cells originally used for priming. Secondary immunizations were carried out subcutaneously. Antibody formation was significantly enhanced in the group given FV-KMT-17, compared with the group given KMT-17. In the FV-KMT-17 group, antibody formation reached a peak titer on day 5, whereas in the KMT-17 group it reached a peak titer on day 7. This result indicates that a rat primed with FV-KMT-17 developed an anti-TAA antibody at an accelerated rate after secondary immunization with FV-KMT-17. The same experiment was performed with rats receiving secondary immunization intraperitoneally. Figure 7 shows that the secondary anti-TAA antibody response was markedly enhanced by intraperitoneal immunization with FV-KMT-17.

On the assumption that VAA might be a carrier protein, rats were immunized with Friend virus-induced lymphoma WFT in an attempt to sensitize them to VAA. Four weeks later, they were immunized with FV-KMT-17, along with control rats which had not been primed with WFT. Table II shows that presensitization to VAA

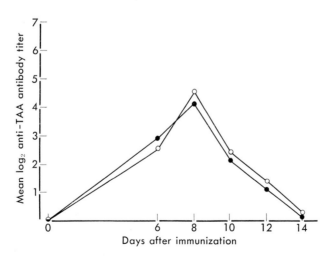

FIG. 5. Primary anti-TAA antibody response
○ FV-KMT-17; ● KMT-17.

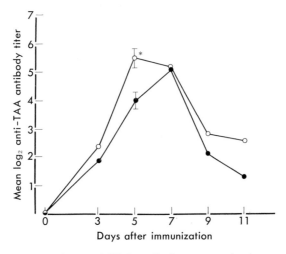

FIG. 6. Secondary anti-TAA antibody response (s.c.)
○ FV-KMT-17; ● KMT-17; * standard deviation. $p<0.01$.

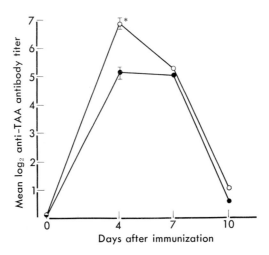

FIG. 7. Secondary anti-TAA antibody response (i.p.)
○ FV-KMT-17; ● KMT-17; * standard deviation. $p<0.01$.

TABLE II. Suppressed Anti-TAA Antibody Production by Preimmunization with WFT

Immunization protocol		Anti-TAA antibody ($\log_2$)	
		Day 7	Day 10
WFT	FV-KMT	1.00 ± 0.57^{a}	1.67 ± 0.61
	FV-KMT	3.67 ± 0.23	3.67 ± 0.23

[a] Mean±standard deviation. WFT, lymphoma induced in syngeneic rat by Friend virus.

significantly impaired the antibody response to TAA. This result indicates that VAA does not act as a carrier determinant.

Comparison of Amount of TAA between FV-KMT-17 and KMT-17

A quantitative absorption test was made to determine whether there was any quantitative difference between FV-KMT-17 and KMT-17 in TAA. As shown in Fig. 8, it is evident that there is no difference between FV-KMT-17 and KMT-17 in absorption activity to anti-TAA. Therefore it can be demonstrated that both tumor cells have the same amount of TAA on their cell surfaces.

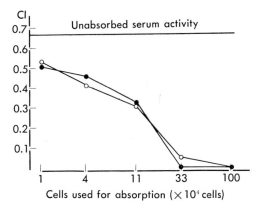

FIG. 8. Comparison of the absorbing activity of FV-KMT-17 and KMT-17 for the cytotoxicity of anti-KMT-17 antiserum against KMT-17

○ FV-KMT-17; ● KMT-17.

CONCLUSION

Two conclusions can be drawn from experiments with cell-surface antigens, if it can be shown that an increase in the response depends on association of two determinants on the same surface. One is that cell cooperation of the hapten-carrier type is probably operating. The other is that the two determinants are physically linked to an extent which enables them to be co-processed in the immune system (6). In our experiments, we demonstrated that VAA are not carrier determinants and that there is an association between TAA and VAA on the xenogenized cell surface. Therefore, it is suggested that VAA are physically linked with TAA on the cell surface to form a strong immunogenic unit and, in this case, VAA function as helper determinants for TAA in the antitumor antibody response.

REFERENCES

1. Cerottini, J. C., Nordin, A. A., and Brunner, K. T. *In vitro* cytotoxic activity of thymus cells sensitized to alloantigens. *Nature*, **227**, 72 (1972).
2. Greenberg, A. H. and Shen, L. A class of specific cytotoxic cells demonstrated *in vitro* by arming with antigen-antibody complexes. *Nature New Biol.*, **245**, 282 (1973).
3. Hellström, K. E. and Hellström, I. Lymphocyte-mediated cytotoxicity and blocking serum activity to tumor antigens. *Adv. Immunol.*, **18**, 209–277 (1974).

4. Hersey, P. New look at antiserum therapy of leukemia. *Nature New Biol.*, **244**, 22 (1973).
5. Kobayashi, H., Sendo, F., Kaji, H., Shirai, T., Saito, H., Takeichi, N., Hosokawa, M., and Kodama, T. Inhibition of transplanted rat tumors by immunization with identical tumor cells infected with Friend virus. *J. Natl. Cancer Inst.*, **44**, 11–19 (1970).
6. Lake, P. and Mitchison, N. A. Regulatory mechanisms in the immune response to cell-surface antigens. *Cold Spring Harbor Symp. Quant. Biol.*, **41**, 589–595 (1976).
7. Old, L. J., Stockert, E., Boyse, E. A., and Kim, J. H. Antigenic modulation. Loss of TL antigen from cells exposed to TL antibody. Study of the phenomenon *in vitro. J. Exp. Med.*, **127**, 523–539 (1968).

GANN Monograph on Cancer Research 23, 1979

INCREASED IMMUNOSENSITIVITY OF XENOGENIZED TUMOR CELLS TO LYMPHOCYTE CYTOTOXICITY

Masuo Hosokawa, Masaharu Kasai, Hideo Yamaguchi,
and Hiroshi Kobayashi

*Laboratory of Pathology, Cancer Institute,
Hokkaido University School of Medicine**

Immunosensitivity of xenogenized tumor cells to cell-mediated cytotoxicity was examined in comparison with that of nonxenogenized tumor cells. KMT-17, a transplantable fibrosarcoma induced by methyl-cholanthrene in WKA rats, was sensitive in a ^{51}Cr-release cytotoxicity test using spleen cells obtained from syngeneic WKA rats immunized with KMT-17 tumor cells. These hyperimmune spleen cells were also cytotoxic to xenogenized KMT-17 (Friend virus-infected (FV)-KMT-17 and Gross virus-infected (GV)-KMT-17) cells. No significant increase of immunosensitivity to hyperimmune spleen cells was observed in the xenogenized tumor cells. When effector spleen cells were obtained from WKA rats bearing KMT-17 tumors, significant cytolysis was observed in xenogenized KMT-17 cells but not in nonxenogenized KMT-17 cells. FV-KDH-8, a xenogenized transplantable liver carcinoma in WKA rats and antigenically unrelated to KMT-17, did not show cytolysis. Spleen cells obtained from WKA rats bearing KDH-8 were not cytotoxic against xenogenized KMT-17 cells. This indicated that the cytotoxicity of spleen cells from KMT-17-bearing rats to xenogenized tumor cells was tumor-specific and not caused by virus-related antigens on xenogenized tumor cells. In summary, an increase of immunosensitivity to cytotoxicity of spleen cells obtained from tumor-bearing animals was observed in xenogenized tumor cells. This result suggests that xenogenized tumor cells may be useful as highly sensitive target cells in the detection of a cell-mediated immune response to tumor cells in tumor-bearing hosts.

Since 1968, we have been experimenting with murine leukemia virus (MuLV)-infected tumor cells in rats for the study of tumor immunology. The most prominent characteristics of MuLV-infected tumor cells are that these tumor cells can grow only in syngeneic rats which are immunosuppressed or tolerant to MuLV, but cannot grow lethally in normal syngeneic rats. In rats that rejected the MuLV-infected tumor cells, a strong resistance against MuLV-noninfected identical tumors was observed. This phenomenon was referred to as xenogenization and the virus-infected tumor cells were termed "xenogenized tumor cells." Evidence regarding the immunogenicity of xenogenized tumor cells has been reported elsewhere (7–10).

Besides the above characteristics, rat tumor cells xenogenized by persistent infec-

---

* Kita-15-jo, Nishi-7-chome, Kita-ku, Sapporo 060, Japan (細川真澄男, 笠井正晴, 山口秀夫, 小林 博).

tion with MuLV retain their viability and shape, even after infection. Hence, xenogenized tumor cells can be used as target cells for cytotoxicity tests.

Cytotoxic sensitivity to humoral antibody against tumor-specific antigen has been stabilized and increased in xenogenized tumor cells (3, 4). Thus, it is important to evaluate the sensitivity of these cells to cell-mediated immunity against tumor-specific antigens.

A transplantable fibrosarcoma in an inbred WKA rat (KMT-17) and its xenogenized tumors infected either with Friend leukemia virus or Gross leukemia virus (FV-KMT-17 and GV-KMT-17) were used as target cells. *In vitro* cell-mediated cytotoxicity was performed by the ordinary ^{51}Cr-release technique, in which 5×10^4 ^{51}Cr-labeled target tumor cells with 3,000–5,000 cpm were incubated with effector lymphocytes in Eagle's minimum essential medium (MEM), containing 10% fetal calf serum (FCS), for 12 hr on a rocking platform.

Cytotoxic Sensitivity of Xenogenized Tumor Cells to Tumor-bearing Spleen Cells

It is well known that tumor-bearing hosts show a certain immune response against tumor cells (1, 12, 15). In our experiments, positive antitumor responses were detected by a radioisotopic footpad assay in rats which were subcutaneously transplanted with KMT-17 tumors. Using spleen cells from these tumor-bearing rats as effector cells, cytotoxic sensitivities were compared between xenogenized and nonxenogenized tumor cells. Figure 1 indicates the kinetics of the specific cytotoxicity of spleen cells from KMT-17-bearing rats, which were tested by the ^{51}Cr-release test. Slight cytotoxic activity against xenogenized tumor cells was observed in spleen cells obtained on day 8 after tumor transplantation, as indicated by the open circles. The activity increased until it reached 30% on day 12, after which it decreased on day 17 when the rats were dying of tumor growth. However, it is noteworthy that the cytotoxic activities were observable against xenogenized cells but not against nonxenogenized cells.

In order to confirm the above results regarding the different cytotoxic sensitivities

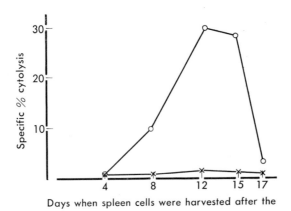

Days when spleen cells were harvested after the tumor transplantation

Fig. 1. Cytolysis of KMT-17 and FV-KMT-17 with spleen cells obtained from KMT-17-bearing rats measured by ^{51}Cr-release test
○ FV-KMT-17; × KMT-17.

TABLE I. Cytolysis of Xenogenized Tumor Cells with Spleen Cells
Obtained from KMT-17-bearing WKA Rats

Target cells	% cytolysis[a]±S.E. with spleen cells from		Specific % cytolysis[b]
	KMT-17-bearing rats[c]	Normal rats	
Xenogenized			
FV-KMT-17	30.2±5.1	5.0±1.0	25.2
GV-KMT-17	39.6±13.1	8.0±2.7	31.6
FV-KDH-8	−8.8±2.4	0.7±1.3	0
WLFT-6	6.8±2.5	9.0±1.9	0
Non-xenogenized			
KMT-17	1.7±0.8	5.8±1.4	0

[a] $\%\ \text{cytolysis} = \dfrac{\text{Release with spleen cells} - \text{spontaneous release}}{\text{Maximum release} - \text{spontaneous release}} \times 100.$

[b] Specific % cytolysis = difference in % cytolysis between tumor-bearring and normal spleen cells.

[c] Spleen cells were harvested 12 days after s.c. inoculation of 1×10^6 KMT-17 tumor cells.

between xenogenized and nonxenogenized tumor cells, ^{51}Cr-release tests were repeated with spleen cells obtained from WKA rats which were inoculated with KMT-17 tumors 12 days previously. Results of 13 different experiments are summarized in Table I. Positive specific cytolysis was observed in two lines of xenogenized tumor cells, FV-KMT-17 and GV-KMT-17, but not in nonxenogenized KMT-17 cells. Two lines of xenogenized tumors which antigenically differ from KMT-17 and possess Friend virus-specific antigens (FV-VSA), FV-KDH-8 and WLFT-6, showed no significant cytolysis with the KMT-17-bearing spleen cells. KDH-8 is a transplantable liver cell carcinoma in the WKA rat and WLFT-6 is a transplantable lymphoma induced by Friend lymphatic leukemia virus in the WKA rat. According to the above evidence, it cannot be said that lysis of xenogenized KMT-17 cells with KMT-17-bearing spleen cells is directly due to FV-VSA on xenogenized cells. Furthermore, any cross antigen between KMT-17 tumor-specific antigens (KMT-TSA) and FV-VSA cannot be detected by a humoral antibody tested by immunofluorescence tests or by complement-dependent cytotoxicity tests. The kinetics of cytotoxicity with tumor-bearing spleen cells (Fig. 1) suggests that the lysis of xenogenized tumor cells depends on spleen cells sensitized with KMT-17 cells.

TABLE II. Cytolysis of Xenogenized and Nonxenogenized Tumor Cells
with Spleen Cells Obtained from KDH-8-bearing WKA Rats

Target cells	% cytolysis[a] with spleen cells from		Specific % cytolysis[b]
	KDH-8-bearing rats[c]	Normal rats	
FV-KMT-17	9.2	14.3	0
FV-KDH-8	22.8	4.7	18.1
KDH-8	16.6	5.6	11.0

[a] $\%\ \text{cytolysis} = \dfrac{\text{Release with spleen cells} - \text{spontaneous release}}{\text{Maximum release} - \text{spontaneous release}} \times 100.$

[b] Specific % cytolysis = difference in % cytolysis between tumor-bearing and normal spleen cells.

[c] Spleen cells were harvested 35 days after s.c. inoculation of 1×10^6 KDH-8 tumor cells.

Thus, it was revealed that a significant increase of cytotoxic sensitivity was observable in xenogenized tumor cells to tumor-bearing spleen cells, compared with that in nonxenogenized tumor cells. As a corollary experiment, xenogenized FV-KMT-17 and FV-KDH-8 tumor cells were examined for their cytotoxic sensitivity to spleen cells obtained from syngeneic WKA rats which were bearing KDH-8. As indicated in Table II, FV-KMT-17 cells were not lysed by KDH-8-bearing spleen cells. On the other hand, FV-KDH-8 cells were lysed to a significant extent by these spleen cells (18.1% in specific % cytolysis). These results substantiate the fact that the cytotoxicity of tumor-bearing spleen cells is tumor specific. Cytolysis of xenogenized KDH-8 cells was slightly increased compared with that of nonxenogenized KDH-8 cells (11.0% in specific % cytolysis).

Amount of Tumor-specific Antigen (TSA) in Xenogenized Tumor Cells

A certain amount of KMT-TSA was investigated in xenogenized KMT-17 cells and compared with the amount in nonxenogenized KMT-17 cells. Capacity to absorb the anti-KMT-17 antibody was similar in xenogenized and non-xenogenized tumor cells (Fig. 2). This indicated that the amount of KMT-TSA did not increase in xenogenized tumor cells. This corresponded to previous results obtained from our laboratory (3, 4, 14). Thus, the increased cytotoxic sensitivity of xenogenized tumor cells is not due to an increase in the amount of TSA.

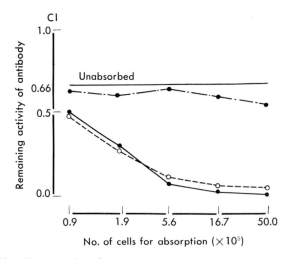

FIG. 2. Absorbing capacity of xenogenized and nonxenogenized tumor cells for anti-KMT-17 antibody
●——● KMT-17; ○---○ FV-KMT-17; ●—·—● thymus cells.

Cytotoxic Sensitivity of Xenogenized Tumor Cells to Immune Spleen Cells

Although cytotoxic sensitivity to tumor cells was detected in spleen cells from tumor-bearing rats, the rats could not reject their tumors and eventually they died from the tumor growth. On the other hand, WKA rats which were repeatedly immunized with KMT-17 cells eventually showed a strong resistance against KMT-17

TABLE III. Cytolysis of Xenogenized and Nonxenogenized Tumor Cells
with Spleen Cells Obtained from KMT-17 Immune WKA Rats

Target cells	% cytolysis[a]±S.E. with spleen cells from		Specific % cytolysis[b]
	Immune rats[c]	Normal rats	
Xenogenized			
FV-KMT-17	65.9±4.6	5.0±1.4	60.9
GV-KMT-17	53.3±2.2	8.0±2.7	45.3
Non-xenogenized			
KMT-17	59.4±5.6	5.8±1.4	53.6

[a] $\% \text{ cytolysis} = \dfrac{\text{Release with spleen cells} - \text{spontaneous release}}{\text{Maximum release} - \text{spontaneous release}} \times 100.$

[b] Specific % cytolysis=difference in % cytolysis between immune and normal spleen cells.

[c] Spleen cells were obtained from WKA rats repeatedly immunized with KMT-17 cells 5 days after a final booster with 1×10^8 cells.

and rejected 10^8 KMT-17 cells inoculated intraperitoneally (i.p.), which was 10^6 times more than the minimum number of cells (10^2) taken by normal nonimmunized rats. It was thought that immune spleen cells obtained from immunized rats might show different activity from those of tumor-bearing rats, thus, the cytotoxic activity of immune spleen cells was examined in xenogenized and nonxenogenized tumor cells.

As the results indicate in Table III, the immune spleen cells lysed xenogenized FV-KMT-17 and GV-KMT-17 cells as well as nonxenogenized KMT-17 cells. No difference in specific % cytolysis could be observed between xenogenized and non-xenogenized cells. Immune spleen cells showed higher cytotoxic activity to xenogenized tumor cells than tumor-bearing spleen cells (Table I). It was of interest to know whether the increased cytotoxic sensitivity of xenogenized cells would be observed at a lower target-effector (T/E) ratio. Table IV indicates the results of an experiment which was carried out at various T/E ratios. No difference in cytotoxic activity was observed even at T/E ratios of 1: 100 or 1: 200. As can be seen in Table IV at the T/E ratio of 1: 200, xenogenized FV-KMT-17 cells were lysed to 39.7% and nonxenogenized KMT-17 cells were lysed in 30.7%. Therefore, it is unlikely that these results, which differ from

TABLE IV. Immunosensitivity of Xenogenized and Nonxenogenized KMT-17
Cells to Spleen Cells Obtained from KMT-17 Immune WKA Rats

Target cells	T/E ratio	% cytolysis[a] with spleen cells		Specific % cytolysis[b]
		Immune rats[c]	Normal rats	
KMT-17	1: 100	28.7	7.9	20.8
	1: 200	36.9	6.2	30.7
	1: 400	46.3	10.1	36.2
FV-KMT-17	1: 100	31.7	12.3	19.4
	1: 200	49.5	9.8	39.7
	1: 400	54.9	10.4	44.5

[a] $\% \text{ cytolysis} = \dfrac{\text{Release with spleen cells} - \text{spontaneous release}}{\text{Maximum release} - \text{spontaneous release}} \times 100.$

[b] Specific % cytolysis=Difference in % cytolysis between immune and normal spleen cells.

[c] Spleen cells were obtained from WKA rats repeatedly immunized with KMT-17 cells 5 days after a final booster with 1×10^8 cells.

those of tumor-bearing spleen cells, are due to the strength of the killing activity of spleen cells. Thus, an increased cytotoxic sensitivity of xenogenized cells only to tumor-bearing spleen cells was observed. However, in the case of hyperimmune spleen cells no increase was observed.

Increased Immunosensitivity of Xenogenized Tumor Cells

The cytotoxic sensitivity of xenogenized tumor cells was first reported by Stück et al. in 1964 (17). EL4 leukemia cells were converted with Rauscher leukemia virus (RV) antigen and then the converted cells were lysed with anti-RV antibody with a complement. Hamburg and Svet-Moldavsky (5) reported that tumor cells could acquire viral antigen and be rejected in animals previously immunized with the virus. We also observed that the growth of methylcholanthrene-induced tumors infected with FV in mice was inhibited by preimmunization with FV-VSA (6) and that FV-infected rat tumor cells were sensitive to anti-FV-VSA antibody in complement-dependent cyto-toxicity tests (4, 16). There have been many reports showing that, after infection with a virus, the virus-related antigen is expressed on the surface of the infected cells and the virus-infected cells are destroyed by immunity to the virus-related antigen. How-ever, there are very few reports concerned with an increased immunosensitivity of virus-infected cells to immunity against tumor-specific antigen which originally existed on the tumor cells. An increased immunosensitivity of xenogenized tumor cells to anti-TSA antibody was first reported by Shirai et al. (16) in FV-infected DLT cells in the Donryu strain of rats. Using KMT-17 tumor cells, an increased cytotoxic sensitivity of xenogenized cells was also found by complement-dependent cytotoxicity tests with anti-KMT antibody (3, 4). The lateral mobility of antigen on the cell surface plays an important role in the sensitivity of xenogenized tumor cells in a complement-dependent cytotoxicity test (11). In addition, an association was found between VSA and TSA in the xenogenized tumor cells infected with FV (4, 13).

We have presented an evidence of the increased cytotoxic sensitivity of xeno-genized tumor cells to lymphocyte cytotoxicity in FV-infected and GV-infected KMT-

TABLE V. Specificity of Delayed Hypersensitivity in WKA Rats Bearing KMT-17 Tumor to DOC-extracts of Tumor Antigens Measured by Radioisotopic Footpad Assay

Rats	On day[a]	FCR[b]±S.D. (I/N[c]) with indicated antigen		
		DOC-KMT-17	DOC-KDH-8	DOC-WFT-2N
KMT-17-bearing	8	1.57±0.14[d] (1.30)	N.T.	N.T.
KMT-17-bearing	12	1.60±0.13[e] (1.32)	1.10±0.10 (0.91)	1.10±0.12 (1.10)
Normal	—	1.21±0.06[d,e]	1.20±0.17	1.00±0.16

[a] Days after the transplantation of 1×10^6 KMT-17 tumor cells.

[b] FCR, Foot count ratio$= \dfrac{\text{cpm with antigen}}{\text{cpm with saline}}$.

[c] I/N, $\dfrac{\text{FCR in tumor-bearing rats}}{\text{FCR in normal rats}}$.

[d] Statistically significant at $0.001 < p < 0.01$.

[e] Statistically significant at $p < 0.001$.

17 tumor cells in rats with KMT-17-bearing spleen cells. Cell-mediated immunity which was specific against KMT-TSA was found in KMT-17-bearing rats by radio-isotopic footpad assay which has been reported by Paranjpe and Boone (14). As indicated in Table V, in KMT-17-bearing rats, positive footpad reactions were observed only with deoxycholate extracts of KMT-17 cells (DOC-KMT-17), not with either DOC-KDH-8 or DOC-WFT-2N. WFT-2N is a lymphoma induced by Friend leukemia virus and possessing FV-VSA. These data suggest that tumor-bearing spleen cells are sensitized with KMT-17 tumor cells but not with FV-VSA.

Although no cytolysis has been observed in non-xenogenized KMT-17 cells in this work, it was revealed that tumor-bearing spleen cells could show a slight toxicity to nonxenogenized cells by Winn's assay (unpublished data). Thus, increased cytotoxic sensitivity in xenogenized cells could be considered due to KMT-TSA-sensitized lymphocytes. Similar evidence has been found by Takeichi et al. (18). They observed an increased cytotoxic sensitivity of Moloney sarcoma virus-infected E-4 cells in the BALB/c mouse by microcytotoxicity tests. In a chemical modification of tumor cells, Tsukagoshi and Hashimoto (19) reported that a nitromin-resistant line of Yoshida sarcoma showed a higher cytotoxic sensitivity to the lymphocyte than suggested by the original line.

Mechanisms of Increased Immunosensitivity

Further experiments should be carried out for the mechanisms of the increased cytotoxic sensitivity. Amount of TSA did not increase in xenogenized tumor cells as compared with their nonxenogenized counterparts. An association between TSA and VSA was suggested to explain the increase of cytotoxic sensitivity to the antibody (4). It is possible that VSA might act as a helper determinant of TSA-sensitized lymphocytes. Immunosuppressive cells could be involved in tumor-bearing spleen cells, since immune spleen cells lysed nonxenogenized cells as well as xenogenized cells. It is possible that suppressive cells do not work on xenogenized cells, because of the conformational changes of the surface antigens on xenogenized cells. It is also possible that populations of effector killer cells of tumor-bearing spleen cells differ from those of immune spleen cells.

CONCLUSION

The use of lymphocyte cytotoxicity to tumor cells *in vitro* is now available to detect the immune response to tumor cells in cancer patients and to analyse tumor immunity. However, for many reasons, *e.g.*, the low antigenicity of tumor cells and the immunosuppressive effect of serum factors and suppressor cells, the cytotoxicity of lymphocytes is not observed in all cases. The increase of cytotoxic sensitivity in xenogenized cells indicates that xenogenized cells may be useful for the detection of immune responses in tumor-bearing hosts. This idea has also been presented by Boone et al. (2) who have reported the usefulness of the crude membrane of xenogenized melanoma cells infected with vesicular stomatitis virus through skin tests in melanoma patients. It is important to consider the increase in immunosensitivity of tumor cells in studies on a weak and complicated immune surveillance against tumor cells.

REFERENCES

1. Baldwin, R. W., Embleton, M. J., and Robins, R. A. Cellular and humoral immunity to rat hepatoma-specific antigens correlated with tumor status. *Int. J. Cancer*, **11**, 1–10 (1973).

2. Boone, C. W., Takeichi, N., and Klein, E. Improved delayed hypersititivity skin test responses to malignant melanoma membranes isolated from cultured tumor cells infected with vesicular stomatitis virus. *Proc. Jpn. Cancer Assoc., 35th Annu. Meet.*, p. 64 (1976).

3. Gotohda, E., Moriuchi, T., Kodama, T., and Kobayashi, H. Stabilized expression of tumor-associated antigen in xenogenized tumor cells to complement-dependent cytotoxicity. This volume, 47–55 (1979).

4. Gotohda, E., Moriuchi, T., Kawamura, T., Akiyama, J., Oikawa, T., Sendo, F., Hosokawa, M., Kodama, T., and Kobayashi, H. Stabilized expression of tumor-associated antigen on rat tumor cells by infection with Friend virus. Submitted to *J. Natl. Cancer Inst.* (1978).

5. Hamburg, V. P. and Svet-Moldavsky, G. J. Artificial heterogenization of tumours by means of viral herpes simplex and polyoma viruses. *Nature*, **203**, 772–773 (1964).

6. Hosokawa, M., Kodama, T., Sendo, F., Takeichi, N., and Kobayashi, H. Immunological characteristics of methylcholanthrene-induced tumors exposed to Friend virus. *J. Cancer Immunopathol.*, **3**, 42–46 (1967) (in Japanese).

7. Kobayashi, H., Kodama, T., Shirai, T., Kaji, H., Hosokawa, M., Sendo, F., Saito, H., and Takeichi, N. Artificial regression of rat tumors infected with Friend virus (xenogenization). An effect produced by acquired antigen. *Hokkaido J. Med. Sci.*, **44**, 133–134 (1969).

8. Kobayashi, H. and Sendo, F. Immunogenicity of viable xenogenized tumor cells. This volume, 27–39 (1979).

9. Kobayashi, H., Sendo, F., Kaji, H., Shirai, T., Saito, H., Takeichi, N., Hosokawa, M., and Kodama, T. Inhibition of transformed rat tumors by immunization with identical tumor cells infected with Friend virus. *J. Natl. Cancer Inst.*, **44**, 11–19 (1970).

10. Kobayashi, H., Sendo, F., Shirai, T., Kaji, H., Kodama, T., and Saito, H. Modification in growth of transplantable rat tumors exposed to Friend virus. *J. Natl. Cancer Inst.*, **42**, 413–419 (1969).

11. Kodama, T. Lateral mobility and stabilized expression of tumor-associated surface antigen in xenogenized tumor cells. This volume, 57–63 (1979).

12. Lavrin, D. H., Herberman, R. B., Nunn, M., and Soares, N. *In vitro* cytotoxicity studies of Murine sarcoma virus-induced immunity in mice. *J. Natl. Cancer Inst.*, **513**, 1497–1508 (1973).

13. Moriuchi, T. and Kobayashi, H. Role of virus-associated antigen on xenogenized tumor cells surface in production of antibody against tumor-associated antigen. This volume, 65–72 (1979).

14. Paranjpe, M. S. and Boone, C. W. Delayed hypersensitivity to simian virus 40 tumor cells in BALB/c mice demonstrated by a radioisotopic footpad assay. *J. Natl. Cancer Inst.*, **48**, 563–566 (1972).

15. Paranjpe, M. S. and Boone, C. W. Kinetics of the anti-tumor delayed hypersensitivity response in mice with progressively growing tumors. Stimulation followed by specific suppression. *Int. J. Cancer*, **13**, 179–186 (1974).

16. Shirai, T., Kaji, H., Takeichi, N., Sendo, F., Saito, H., Hosokawa, M., and Kobayashi,

H. Cell surface antigens detectable by cytotoxic test on Friend virus induced and Friend virus-infected tumors in the rat. *J. Natl. Cancer Inst.*, **46**, 449–460 (1971).

17. Stück, B., Old, L. J., and Boyse, E. A. Antigenic conversion of established leukemias by a unrelated leukemogenic virus. *Nature*, **202**, 1016–1018 (1964).

18. Takeichi, N., Austin, F., Oikawa, T., and Boone, C. W. Virus-augmentation of tumor associated antigens. Comparison of influenza virus and murine sarcoma virus. *Cancer Res.*, **38**, 4580–4584 (1978).

19. Tsukagoshi, S. and Hashimoto, Y. Increased immunosensitivity in nitrogen mustard-resistant Yoshida sarcoma. *Cancer Res.*, **33**, 1038–1042 (1973).

INDUCTION OF IMMUNE RESISTANCE BY HVJ-INFECTED L1210 LEUKEMIA CELLS

Kohei Kawashima,[*1] Hideo Takeyama,[*1] Kazumasa Yamada,[*1]
and Yasuhiko Ito[*2]

First Department of Internal Medicine[*1] *and Germ-free Life Research
Institute,*[*2] *Nagoya University School of Medicine*

It is well known that tumor immunity can be augmented by virus-infected tumor cells. Tumor immunity was induced against syngeneic tumor cells by employing HVJ-pi-infected L1210 leukemia cells. The infectious, nononcogenic virus, a temperature-sensitive (ts) mutant of HVJ, showed little or no cytopathic effect and led to the establishment of carrier cultures in several cell lines. By the use of this characteristic quality, HVJ-pi-infected L1210 leukemia cell line (L1210/c-HVJ-pi) was established, almost all of which were positively stained with fluorescent HVJ antibody. They are viable and able to grow almost as well as un-infected L1210/c leukemia cells *in vitro*. Nude mice, deficient in T cells, succumbed to inoculation of L1210/c-HVJ-pi cells, as well as uninfected L1210/c cells. The leukemia cells in the ascites of the nude mice con-sisted of HVJ-pi-infected and -uninfected cells. However, viable L1210/c-HVJ-pi cells were not transplanted easily into the susceptible mice. As they were serially subcultured *in vitro*, a decreased rate of HVJ antigen positive cells was observed and reversely led to a step-by-step increase in leukemia death among the semisyngeneic mice inoculated with L1210/c-HVJ-pi cells of each culture generation. The strong inhibition of growth of 10^5 intact L1210/c cells was recognized in the semi-syngeneic or syngeneic mice previously immunized with 10^5 L1210/c-HVJ-pi cells. These immune mice became refractory to challenge with 10^7 intact L1210 cells after progressive monthly inoculation of L1210 cells. This finding was more prominent in hybrid than in DBA/2 syngeneic mice. In BDF_1 mice hyperimmunized with repeated L1210 cell challenge, the complement-dependent cytotoxic antibody against L1210 cells was demonstrated in 29 out of 30 mice. The activity of this antibody was not absorbed with normal mouse tissues and various tumor cells except P388 leukemia cells originating in DBA/2 mice.

Since the tumor-associated antigen on the surface of tumor cells is weakly immuno-genic, its activity is markedly reduced once the tumor cell is destroyed. Attempts have long been made to augment immunogenicity by means of modified preparations of virus-infected tumor cells (*1, 4, 7*). Boone *et al.* (*2*) have recently proposed a helper antigen mechanism in order to explain the virus-augmented tumor immunity. They have in-sisted on the importance of the juxtaposition within the structure of the plasma mem-brane between the relatively weak tumor-associated antigen and a strong virus-asso-

---

[*1],[*2] Tsurumai-cho 65, Showa-ku, Nagoya 466, Japan (川島康平, 竹山英夫, 山田一正, 伊藤康彦).

ciated antigen. In these studies, a cytopathic virus was usually employed to modify the tumor-associated antigen on the cell surface membrane.

However, of interest is that modification of the growth of the transplantable rat tumor exposed to Friend virus indicated the significance of using a noncytopathic virus which alters the surface of tumor cells and which is scarcely infectious to the host (*5*).

The infectious virus, HVJ-pi, obtained from baby hamster kidney cells persistently infected with HVJ was found to be temperature-sensitive as well as causing little or no cytopathic effect (*8*, *9*). Utilizing this characteristic, we established that HVJ-pi persistently infected L1210/c leukemia cells (L1210/c-HVJ-pi). In this work, we will describe some information regarding the growth of L1210/c-HVJ-pi cells, the change of their transplantability in semisyngeneic or syngeneic mice and tumor immunity against intact L1210 leukemia cells.

Growth of HVJ-pi-infected L1210/c Leukemia Cells

As shown in Fig. 1, HVJ-w infected L1210/c (L1210/c-HVJ-w) cells revealed no proliferation in the growth medium because of cytopathic effect of HVJ-w on L1210/c cells, but L1210/c-HVJ-pi grew almost equally as uninfected L1210/c cells in the growth medium at 35°. For viral infection, the leukemia cells were suspended approximately 10^7/ml in serum free medium and infected with egg-grown HVJ-pi or HVJ-w at multiplicity of infection (moi) 20–200/cell. After a virus adsorption period of one hour at 32°, the virus-infected cells were washed with phosphate-buffed saline (PBS) and resuspended in Eagle's minimum essential medium (MEM), followed by incubation at 32° for 24 hr.

L1210/c-HVJ-pi cells could be serially subcultured easily, resulting in the establishment of a carrier state in which almost all cells carried viral antigen of HVJ. Direct immunofluorescence study demonstrated the strong positive staining of L1210/c-HVJ-

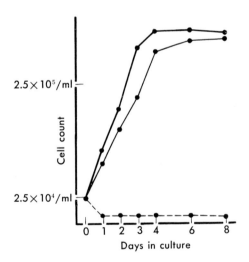

Fig. 1.   Growth rate of HVJ-infected L1210/c cells incubated at 35°
——— uninfected L1210/c;   ——— HVJ-pi-infected L1210/c (L1210/c-HVJ-pi);
– – – HVJ-w-infected L1210/c (L1210/c-HVJ-w).

pi cells with fluorescein-labeled rabbit antiviral envelope or antiviral nucleocapsid.

When 10^5 L1210/c-HVJ-w cells were inoculated intraperitoneally into semi-syngeneic or syngeneic mice, their growth was inhibited. This was expected because HVJ-w is cytopathic. However, despite the fact that viable L1210/c-HVJ-pi cells remained morphologically intact, they could not grow, particularly in semisyngeneic mice. Ninety percent of BDF_1 or CDF_1 mice survived over 40 days, whereas about 50% of DBA/2 mice died of leukemia although they had prolonged survivals. In case of athymic nude mice (BALB/c nu/nu), all mice which were inoculated with 10^5 L1210/c-HVJ-pi cells died of leukemia within 13 days. About 5 to 50% of cells in the ascites of dead nude mice revealed viral antigens with immunofluorescent antibody staining.

Change of Transplantability of HVJ-pi-infected L1210/c Leukemia Cells

Next, we investigated the tumorigenicity of L1210/c-HVJ-pi cells at several culture generations (Table I). Nearly all L1210/c-HVJ-pi cells incubated at 32° or 38° contained V (viral envelope) and S (viral nucleocapsid) antigens in their cytoplasm at the primary infection. HVJ-pi is temperature-sensitive and virus particles are released readily from L1210/c-HVJ-pi cells incubated at 32° but not that at 38°. The 10^5 L1210/c-HVJ-pi cells incubated at 32° were rejected in almost all BDF_1 mice which survived free of tumor for over 60 days. During incubation at 38° when the cells carried the viral antigen in their cytoplasm but did not produce virus particles, rejectability of L1210/c-HVJ-pi cells in BDF_1 mice decreased by 10 to 40%. As L1210/c-HVJ-pi cells were readily subcultured in the growth medium at 35°, the rate of viral antigen-positive cells and production of virus particles in the culture medium decraesed and, in the 10th subculture, the viral antigen-positive cells were below 5%. In proportion to the decreasing rate of viral antigen-positive cells, the survival rate of BDF_1 mice which received tumor cells of each subculture generation decreased significantly.

TABLE I. Relation between HVJ Antigen Expression and Tumorigenicity of L1210/c-HVJ-pi in BDF_1 Mice

| | HA in culture fluid (HAU/ 0.25 ml) | Fluorescent antibody staining (%) | | | No. of survivors/ No. of mice inoculated[c] |
| | | Cytoplasm | | Membrane | |
		V^a	S^b	V	
Primary infection[d]					
L1210/c-HVJ-pi at 32°	4	>99	>99	25–50	9/10–10/10
L1210/c-HVJ-pi at 38°	<1	>99	>99	0	3/10– 4/10
5 th subculture at 35°					
L1210/c-HVJ-pi	4	75–90	75–90	5–10	5/10– 6/10
10 th subculture at 35°					
L1210/c-HVJ-pi	<1	<5	<5	<1	0/10– 1/10

[a] Viral envelope antigen.

[b] Viral nucleocapsid antigen.

[c] 1×10^5 L1210/c-HVJ-pi were inoculated i.p. in BDF_1 mice.

  Mice surviving longer than 60 days after inoculation were considered as survivors.

[d] Incubation for 48 hr in the medium.

Antitumor Effect in Mice Immunized with L1210/c-HVJ-pi Cells

Resistance of the mice which survived for over 30 days after a single immunization with 10^5 HVJ-infected L1210/c cells or its homogenates was tested against intact L1210/c leukemia cells. (Table II) These survivors were challenged with a sample of 10^5 intact L1210/c cells. Ninety percent of BDF_1 mice immunized with 10^5 L1210/c-HVJ-pi cells were protected from this challenge, whereas the mice inoculated with L1210/c-HVJ-w cells or homogenates of 10^5 L1210/c-HVJ-pi cells were much less protected. Even in syngeneic DBA/2 mice, single preimmunization with 10^5 L1210/c-HVJ-pi

TABLE II.   Survival Rate of Mice Challenged L1210/c Cells after
Immunization of HVJ-infected L1210/c Cells

Method of Immunization[a]			Challenge of L1210	
Antigen for immunization	No. of cells inoculated (i.p.)	Strain	No. of cells (i.p.)	Survival rate[b]
L1210/c-HVJ-pi	1×10^5	BDF_1	1×10^5	9/10
L1210/c-HVJ-w	1×10^5	BDF_1	1×10^5	2/10
L1210/c-HVJ-pi	1×10^5 (sonicated)	BDF_1	1×10^5	2/10
L1210/c	1×10^5 (sonicated)	BDF_1	1×10^5	0/10
HVJ-pi	8HA/0.2 ml	BDF_1	1×10^5	0/10
Control (no immunization)		BDF_1	1×10^5	0/10
L1210/c-HVJ-pi	1×10^5	DBA/2	1×10^5	6/10
L1210/c-HVJ-w	1×10^5	DBA/2	1×10^5	1/10
Control (no immunization)		DBA/2	1×10^5	0/10

[a] Each group of mice was immunized with reference antigen 4 weeks before challenge with L1210/c cells.

[b] No. of mice surviving more than 60 days after challenge/No. of mice immunized.

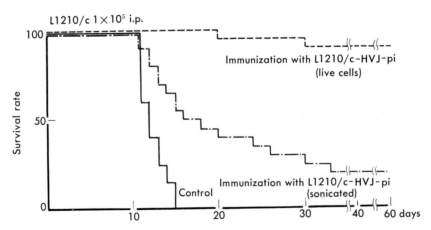

FIG. 2.   Survival rate of BDF_1 mice challenged with L1210/c cells after immunization with L1210/c-HVJ-pi

BDF_1 mice were immunized with either 1×10^5 L1210/c-HVJ-pi (live cells) or L1210/c-HVJ-pi (soniated) 4 weeks before challenge of 1×10^5 L1210/c cells.

cells induced about 60% protection. A single inoculation of HVJ-pi alone did not inhibit the growth of L1210/c leukemia cells inoculated subsequently.

Figure 2 shows an example of the survival curve of BDF_1 mice immunized with 10^5 L1210/c-HVJ-pi leukemia cells or its homogenates after challenge with 10^5 intact L1210/c cells. Ninety percent of the mice immunized with the cells survived more than 60 days after challenge without any evidence of leukemia, whereas only 20% of the mice immunized with the homogenate survived free of disease, although prolonged survival was obtained. These findings indicate that proliferative, viable L1210/c-HVJ-pi cells would be the effective immunogen for evoking tumor immunity.

The next problem was to discover how powerful was the tumor immunity. Figure 3 shows the refractoriness of semisyngeneic mice to challenge with varying dose of uninfected L1210/c cells after a single immunization with HVJ-pi infected L1210/c leukemia cells. Both BDF_1 and CDF_1 mice received a single inoculation of 10^5 L1210/c-HVJ-pi cells intraperitoneally. The mice were challenged 30 days later with 10^3 to 10^7 uninfected L1210/c cells. The immune hybrid mice resisted up to 10^6 intact L1210/c cells at the rate of more than 80%. This implies a remarkably increased immunogenicity of HVJ-pi infected L1210/c leukemia cells.

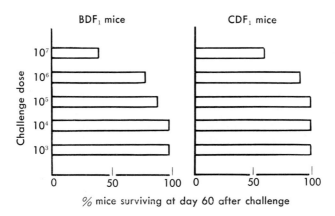

Fig. 3.   Strength of immunity in BDF_1 and CDF_1 mice induced by L1210/c-HVJ-pi

BDF_1 or CDF_1 mice was immunized with 10^5 of L1210/c-HVJ-pi i.p. Challenge of the immunized mice was made 30 days later by various dose of uninfected L1210/c cells i.p. Each group represents 10 mice.

Humoral Immunity in Immune BDF_1 Mice

I would like to consider another aspect in mice immunized with L1210/c-HVJ-pi cells; that is, the cytotoxic antibody in immune mice. It is important to note that there was a measurable humoral immunity in immune mice. In this experiment (Table III), 30 BDF_1 mice which survived free of tumor after a single inoculation of 10^5 L1210/c-HVJ-pi cells were challenged monthly with increasing dose of 10^5, 10^6, and 10^7 viable L1210/c cells. The cytotoxic activity against intact L1210 leukemia cells of sera from the immune mice was examined by a standard complement-dependent cytotoxicity test. Twenty-one of 30 immune mice were found to be high producers of the antibody

TABLE III. Cytotoxic Activity of BDF$_1$ Antisera for L1210 Leukemia Cells

Immune mouse No.	1) 1/Dilution of antisera[a]			2) 1/Dilution of antisera[b]			Results[c]
	16	32 (% cell lysis)	64	16	32 (% cell lysis)	64	
1	< 5	< 5		43	21	5	Low
2	>90	>90		>90	>90	>90	High
3	81	61		>90	>90	>90	High
4	>90	>90					High
5	>90	73					High
6	66	50	25	>90	>90	>90	High
7	53	47	30	>90	>90	>90	High
8	>90	>90	85				High
9	>10	<10	<10	<10	<10	<10	Low
10	>90	>90	83				High
11	<10	<10		>90	>90	>90	High
12	>90	>90	>90				High
13	27	20	<10	>90	>90	>90	High
14	25	10	<10	>90	>90	68	High
15	>90	>90	>90				High
16	>90	>90	>90				High
17	>90	>90	>90				High
18	84	82	57				High
19	>90	>90	>90				High
20	>90	>90	>90				High
21	>90	>90	>90				High
22	>90	>90	>90				High
23	21	<10	<10	12	<10	10	Low
24	>90	>90	>90				High
25	22	10	<10	13	<10	10	Low
26	32	12	11	23	49	17	Low
27	>90	69	67				High
28	28	19	18	28	30	18	Low
29	>90	>90	>90				High
30	78	50		>90	>90	>90	High
Normal BDF$_1$ mouse	<10	<10					
L1210-bearing BDF$_1$ mouse	<10	<10					

[a] BDF$_1$ mice were challenged monthly with 10^5, 10^6, and 10^7 L1210 leukemia cells after immunization with 10^5 L1210/c-HVJ-pi leukemia cells. These mice were bled within 2 months after the last challenge.

[b] These immune mice were further challenged with 10^7 L1210 leukemia cells and bled 1 month later.

[c] "High" means a high producer of the antibody with a titer of more than 32, "Low" with a titer of less than 16.

with a titer of more than 32. The other 9 were found to be low responders. The latter were further challenged with 10^7 uninfected L1210/c cells. One month later, the sera again were studied for cytotoxic activity. Finally, 24 of 30 mice were identified as high producers and 6 as low producers. Even low producers could reject a subsequent challenge dose of L1210/c cells, but most of them died with a tumor in an ascitic or solid form at the site of injection or somewhere in the body, although they usually had a much more prolonged survival than the control mice.

Now, I wish to discuss the specificity of this antisera against L1210 leukemia cells. We absorbed the immune sera with various tissues from normal BDF_1 or C3H/He mice, such as thymus, bone marrow, spleen, lymph nodes, and liver. As a result, remarkable, residual cytotoxic activity against intact L1210 leukemia cells was observed, suggesting that humoral immunity is not against some antigen present on the normal cell surface.

It has been reported by Chen et al. (3) at the Sloan-Kettering Institute that L1210 leukemia cells carry both murine leukemia virus and mammary tumor virus (MTV), as demonstrated by electron microscopy. Neither Passage A Gross virus-induced tumor, E♂G2, nor spontaneous mammary tumor in C3H/HeJ mice could remove cytotoxic activity against L1210 leukemia cells, while P388 leukemia cells originating in DBA/2 mouse could completely remove this activity as well as L1210 leukemia cells. This finding suggests that common leukemia-associated antigen, not murine leukemia virus (MuLV)-associated or MTV-associated, exists on the surface of both L1210 and P388 leukemia cells.

In accord with this finding, it is of interest that Leffell and Coggin (6) recently reported the presence of common transplantation antigens on methylcholanthrene-induced murine sarcomas.

CONCLUSION

The nononcogenic, infectious virus (HVJ-pi), a ts mutant of HVJ, known to be little or noncytopathic, led the culture line of L1210 leukemia cells to the establishment of a carrier state (L1210/c-HVJ-pi). These HVJ-pi infected L1210/c cells grew almost as well as uninfected L1210/c cells *in vitro*. Further, BALB/c nude mice succumbed to the inoculation of L1210/c-HVJ-pi cells. However, L1210/c-HVJ-pi cells were not easily transplanted into susceptible mice. As they were serially subcultured *in vitro*, the rate of HVJ-antigen-positive cells decreased. In accordance with the decreasing rate, the survival rate of the BDF_1 mice for over 60 days after inoculation decreased. In these surviving immune mice, strong, inhibition of growth of intact L1210/c leukemia cells was observed with a high production of cytotoxic antibody against L1210 cells. These findings suggest that HVJ-associated antigens at the cell membrane of tumor cells have augmented the immunogenicity of L1210 leukemia cells.

REFERENCES

1. Boone, C. and Blackman, K. Augmented immunogenicity of tumor cell homogenates infected with influenza virus. *Cancer Res.*, **32**, 1018–1022 (1972).
2. Boone, C. W., Paranjpe, M., Orme, T., and Gillette, R. Virus-augmented tumor transplantation antigens: Evidence for a helper antigen mechanism. *Int. J. Cancer*, **13**, 543–551 (1974).
3. Chen, P. L., Hutchison, D. J., Sarker, N. H., Kramarsky, B., and Moore, D. H. Identification of the virions in the *in vitro* L1210 (V) leukemia cell lines by morphological, virological and immunological techniques. *Cancer Res.*, **35**, 718–728 (1975).
4. Hakkinen, I. and Halonen, P. Induction of tumor immunity in mice with antigens pre-

pared from influenza and vesicular stomatitis virus grown in suspension culture of Ehrlich ascites cells. *J. Natl. Cancer Inst.*, **46**, 1161–1167 (1971).

5. Kobayashi, H., Sendo, F., Shirai, T., Kaji, H., Kodama, T., and Saito, H. Modification in growth of transplantable rat tumor exposed to Friend virus. *J. Natl. Cancer Inst.*, **42**, 413–419 (1969).
6. Leffell, M. S. and Coggin, J. H., Jr. Common transplantation antigens on methyl-cholanthrene-induced sarcomas detected by three assays of tumor rejection. *Cancer Res.*, **37**, 4112–4119 (1977).
7. Lindenmann, J. and Klein, P. A. Viral oncolysis: Increased immunogenicity of host cell antigen associated with influenza virus. *J. Exp. Med.*, **126**, 93–108 (1967).
8. Nagata, I., Kimura, Y., Ito, Y., and Tanaka, T. Temperature sensitive phenomenon of viral maturation observed in BHK cells persistently infected with HVJ. *Virology*, **49**, 453–461 (1972).
9. Nishiyama, Y., Ito, Y., Shimokata, K., Kimura, Y., and Nagata, I. Relationship between establishment of persistent infection of hemagglutinating virus of Japan and the properties of the virus. *J. Gen. Virol.*, **32**, 73–83 (1976).

DECREASED TRANSPLANTABILITY OF CULTURED TUMOR CELLS PERSISTENTLY INFECTED WITH NONONCOGENIC VIRUSES

Motoichi Hatano, Hisashi Ogura, Hiroshi Sato, and Junji Tanaka

Department of Virology, Cancer Research Institute, Kanazawa University[*]

Using two nononcogenic viruses (HVJ-Sendai virus and Rubella virus), the effect of persistent infection with these viruses on the antigenic conversion of cultured tumor cells was examined, in view of their low pathogenicities to normal cells. Cultured THEL and GENO cells formed a transplantable tumor in a hamster (noninbred or inbred GN strain) and caused animal death. The cells were easily infected persistently by both viruses, particularly with the temperature-sensitive (ts) variant, HVJ_{ts}, and Mav (Rubella virus), without the viral cytopathic effect (CPE) or a retarded cell growth in culture.

These virus carrier cells generally showed decreased transplantability even by transplantation with 10^6 cells per hamster, accompanied by an occasional loss of tumorigenicity. Immunological analysis using the macrophage migration inhibition test and cell-mediated cytotoxicity test revealed that the phenomena may be due to an increased induction of cellular immunity in a hamster transplanted with the carrier cells. In this analysis, the HVJ_{ts} genomes carried in the cells were found to play an important role in the antigenic conversion of the cell membrane, making for an enhancement of the cellular immune response *in vivo*.

In general tumor-specific antigenicity may be recognized from some difference in the immunological reactivity between tumor cells and their normal, origin cells. However, it is well known that tumor cells usually show a poor antigenicity *in vivo* or *in vitro*. Therefore, various trials to enhance the tumor-specific antigenicity have been described consisting of viral infection (*3–5, 7, 8*), treatment with chemicals (*2, 9*), cell-fusion techniques (*14*), *etc*. Previously we reported the lowered transplantability of hamster tumor cells persistently infected with Sendai virus (HVJ) (*15*). In connection with this problem, the induction of cellular immunity in hamsters transplanted with virus-carrier cells and the role of temperature-sensitive (ts) virus genomes carried in the cells were further examined here.

Establishment of Stable Carrier State

THEL (derived from noninbred hamster embryonic lung) (*15*) and GENO (derived from inbred hamster, GN strain and transformed *in vitro* by treatment with nitro-

---

[*] Takara-machi 13-1, Kanazawa 920, Japan (波多野基一, 小倉　寿, 佐藤　博, 田中淳之).

soguanidine) cells were cultured with Eagle's minimum essential medium (MEM) containing 10% calf serum. These two cell lines showed a high transplantability with subsequent animal death. Temperature-sensitive variants of HVJ or Rubella virus were extracted from the stable carrier cells, according to our previous procedures (*12, 13*). It should be noted here that the extracted HVJ_{ts} or Mav (Rubella$_{ts}$) could easily infect the cultured cells by the establishment of a carrier state. The stable persistent infection of the cells (*12, 13*) was confirmed by fluorescent antibody staining and the hemadsorption phenomenon of the cells as well as by recovery of a few infectious viruses from the cells, though the cells lacked viral cytopathic effect (CPE) and showed a non-retarded cell growth in culture.

Decreased Transplantability of HVJ_{ts} or Mav Carrier Tumor Cells

The results are shown in Table I. It is clear that these carrier cells generally decrease their transplantabilities and occasionally lose them. However, THEL-HVJ$_{ts}$ cells cultured at 37° or 39° (nonpermissive temperature for HVJ$_{ts}$ growth) regained transplantability as shown in the parent THEL cells. These recoveries in the tumorigenicity were complete after culture at 39° and partial at 37°, suggesting the important role of carried HVJ genomes in the present phenomena.

TABLE I. Tumorigenicity of HVJ$_{ts}$-or Rubella (Mav)-carrier Tumor Cells, THEL (Allogenic) and GENO (Syngeneic) Cells

Cells cultured at	Dose (cells/hamster)	Tumor incidence at (weeks)						Latent period (days)
		2	3	4	5	6	8	
THEL	35° (10⁴/n.i. G.H.)	9/14 (2.1 ±1.5)ᵃ		14/14 (13.5 ±7.8)		14/14 (30.6 ±10.4)	14/14 (43.5 ±10.2)	10–18
THEL-HVJ$_{ts}$ { 35°		0/14 (0)		2/14 (2.0)		6/14 (3.0 ±2.1)	6/14 (8.6 ±4.3)	28–42
37° (10⁴/n.i. G.H.) (1 day)		0/12 (0)		8/12 (5.6 ±4.3)				21–28
39° (5 day)		4/6 (1.5 ±0.9)		6/6 (15.8 ±4.7)				10–18
THEL-Mav	35° (10⁴/n.i. G.H.)	0/11 (0)	0/11 (0)	2/11 (1.0)	2/11 (2.3)	2/11 (3.0)	2/11 (5.8)	23–28
GENO	35° (10⁶/i. GN-H.)	3/3 (3.8 ±1.2)	3/3 (8.0 ±1.1)	3/3 (9.0 ±1.2)	3/3 (9.7 ±1.7)	3/3 (11.2 ±0.6)		7
GENO-HVJ$_{ts}$	35° (10⁶/i. GN-H.)	3/4 (1.5)	2/4 (1.0)	1/4 (1.0)	3/4 (1.0)	2/4 (1.0)	2/4 (1.5)	7
GENO-Mav	35° (10⁶/i. GN-H.)	0/8 (0)	1/8 (1.0)	1/8 (1.0)	1/8 (1.7)	1/8 (2.0)	1/8 (3.8)	21

ᵃ Mean diameter (mm) of tumor±S.D.
n.i. G.H., noninbred golden hamster; i. GN-H., inbred golden hamster, GN strain.

MMI Test in Hamsters Transplanted with Carrier Cells

Immunoreactivity of peritoneal exudate cells from the hamsters was assayed by the macrophage migration inhibition test (MMI) (*1, 10*) every week from 1 to 6 weeks after transplantation as shown in Fig. 1. These tests in the group transplanted with HVJ_{ts} carrier cells generally showed positive results against THEL-HVJ_{ts} cells in from 1 to 4 weeks. Then also proved significant against parent THEL cells at 3 and 4 weeks (Fig. 1, THEL-HVJ_{ts} bearer). During these positive periods (1–4 weeks) for the MMI test, usually no causative tumors occured, as seen in Table I.

On the other hand, tests in the group with parent THEL cells were positive against both the HVJ_{ts}-carrier and the parent THEL cells only 1 week after transplantation, but thereafter turned to negative levels with the tumor occurrences (Fig. 1, THEL bearer). Similar results to these in the MMI tests were also obtained by the cell-me-diated cytotoxicity test (*6*) of spleen cells from transplanted animals. Thus, it may be safely concluded that transplantation with HVJ_{ts}-carrier cells induced a more enhanced response of cellular immunity in animals for a longer period, though a detailed pattern against carrier or parent cell antigen differed even at the early stage.

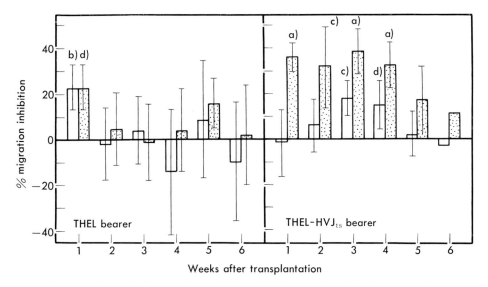

FIG. 1. Macrophage migration inhibition (MMI) test of peritoneal exudate cells from hamsters transplanted with THEL or THEL-HVJ_{ts} cells
THEL antigen; THEL-HVJ_{ts} antigen; transplanted dose was 10^4 cells per hamster. Significant at a) $p<0.005$; b) $p<0.025$; c) $p<0.01$; d) $p<0.05$.

Effect of Temperature Shift of Cell Culture on the Antigenicity of HVJ_{ts}-carrier Cells

Other evidence concerned the important role of HVJ_{ts} gene function and the con-sequent antigenic conversion of the cell membrane is shown in Table II. By the shift of the culture temperature to 37° from the usual 35°, the THEL-HVJ_{ts} cells slightly altered in antigenicity, as found by the MMI test, yet clear differences from the parent THEL cells still remained. However, when it was raised to 39° (completely non-per-

TABLE II. Effect of Temperature Shift of Cell Culture on the Antigenicity of HVJ_{ts}-carrier Cells Observed by the MMI Test

PE cells from hamsters transplantation with (cultured at)		Antigen cells (cultured at)		Migration inhibition (%)					
				Exp. 1	$p<$	Exp. 2	$p<$	Exp. 3	$p<$
THEL (35°)		THEL	(35°)	-3.4 ± 16.2	N.S.	0.1 ± 1.9	N.S.		
		THEL-HVJ$_{ts}$		-2.8 ± 5.2	N.S.	6.0 ± 19.0	N.S.		
THEL-HVJ$_{ts}$	(35°)	THEL	(35°)	12.2 ± 6.9	N.S.	10.0 ± 6.1	N.S.	-1.2 ± 3.0	N.S.
		THEL-HVJ$_{ts}$		51.9 ± 12.3	0.005	46.7 ± 4.3	0.005	51.4 ± 3.8	0.005
	(37°, 1 day)	THEL	(37°, 1 day)	13.2 ± 1.3	0.025	8.0 ± 5.3	0.025		
		THEL-HVJ$_{ts}$		45.5 ± 3.9	0.005	37.3 ± 5.9	0.005		
	(39°, 5 days)	THEL	(39°, 5 days)	-15.4 ± 8.2	N.S.				
		THEL-HVJ$_{ts}$		-9.4 ± 5.5	N.S.				

PE (peritoneal exudate) cells were obtained at 18 days after the transplantation with 1×10^4 cells/hamster. N.S., not significant, $p>0.05$.

missive temperature for HVJ_{ts} growth), HVJ_{ts}-carrier cells lost their HVJ_{ts}-specific antigenicity and became negative in the MMI test with an identical pattern to those of the parent THEL cells (Table II). Those carrier cells cultured at 39° recovered their transplantabilities (tumorigenicities) to the extent of those in the parent THEL cells, as seen in Table I. These data seemed to indicate a close correlation of the HVJ_{ts} gene function to the antigenicity of the cell membrane and subsequently to tumorigenicity.

DISCUSSION

In addition to the ts characteristics of HVJ or Mav, another problem possibly related to the tumorigenicity of the carrier cells should be noted here. Sato *et al.* (*11*) have reported the activation of latent oncorna virus by Rubella virus infection of BHK-21 cells. The culture fluid of our HVJ_{ts}- or Mav-carrier cells cultured at 32–35° was preliminarily observed to contain significant amounts of latent oncorna virus expressed by reverse transcriptase activity together with released HVJ_{ts} or Mav. An analysis of the possible interaction between this activated latent virus and carrying viruses is now in progress in relation to decreased tumorigenicity or immunological implications.

REFERENCES

1. Blasecki, J. and Tevethia, S. S. *In vitro* assay of cellular immunity to tumor-specific antigen(s) of virus-induced tumor by macrophage migration inhibition. *J. Immunol.*, **110**, 590–594 (1973).
2. Czajkowski, N. P., Rosenblatt, M., Cusing, R. R., Vasquez, J., and Wolf, P. Production of active immunity to malignant neoplastic tissue: Chemical coupling to an antigenic protein carrier. *Cancer*, **19**, 739–749 (1966).
3. Eaton, M. D., Heller, J. A., and Scala, A. R. Enhancement of lymphoma cell immunogenicity by infection with nononcogenic virus. *Cancer Res.*, **33**, 3293–3298 (1973).

4. Gillette, R. and Boone, C. W. Augmented immunogenicity of tumor cell membranes produced by surface budding viruses: Parameters of optimal immunization. *Int. J. Cancer*, **18**, 216–222 (1976).

5. Grifth, I. P., Crook, N. E., and White, D. O. Protection of mice against cancer by immunization with membranes, but not purified virions, from virus-infected cancer cells. *Br. J. Cancer*, **31**, 603–613 (1975).

6. Hashimoto, Y. and Sudo, H. Evaluation of cell damage in immune reactions by release of radioactivity from ³H-uridine labelled cells. *Gann*, **62**, 139–143 (1971).

7. Kobayashi, H., Sendo, F., Kaji, H., Shirai, T., Saito, H., Takeichi, N., Hosokawa, M., and Kodama, T. Inhibition of transplanted rat tumors by immunization with identical tumor cells infected with Friend virus. *J. Natl. Cancer Inst.*, **44**, 11–19 (1970).

8. Lindenmann, J. and Klein, P. A. Viral oncolysis: Increased immunogenicity of host cell antigen associated with influenza virus. *J. Exp. Med.*, **126**, 93–108 (1967).

9. Martin, W. J., Wunderlich, J. R., Fletcher, F., and Inman, J. K. Enhanced immunogenicity of chemically-coated syngenic tumor cells. *Proc. Natl. Acad. Sci. U.S.*, **68**, 469–472 (1971).

10. Rees, R. C., Potter, C. W., and Shelton, J. The specificity of cellular immune reactions to three DNA virus induced tumors, as measured by the macrophage migration inhibition test. *Eur. J. Cancer*, **11**, 79–86 (1975).

11. Sato, M., Yamada, T., Yamamoto, K., and Yamamoto, N. Evidence for hybrid formation between rubella virus and latent virus of BHK-21/WI-2 cells. *Virology*, **69**, 691–699 (1976).

12. Tanaka, J., Ogura, H., and Hatano, M. Cellular proteases increased in paramyxovirus (Sendai virus) carrier cells possibly responsible for enhanced formation of cowpox virus-specific cell surface antigen. *Arch. Virol.*, **53**, 87–99 (1977).

13. Tanaka, J., Morita, O., and Hatano, M. Factors involved in the expression of cowpox virus-specific antigen in Sendai virus carrier cells. *J. Gen. Virol.*, **33**, 87–97 (1976).

14. Watkins, J. F. and Chen, L. Immunization of mice against Ehrlich ascites tumor using a hamster/Ehrlich ascites tumor hybrid cell line. *Nature*, **223**, 1018–1022 (1969).

15. Yamada, T. and Hatano, M. Lowered transplantability of cultured tumor cells by persistent infection with paramyxovirus (HVJ). *Gann*, **63**, 647–655 (1972).

BREAKDOWN OF MuLV-INDUCED TOLERANCE AND SUBSEQUENT REGRESSION OF XENOGENIZED TUMORS

Noritoshi Takeichi and Hiroshi Kobayashi

*Department of Pathology, Cancer Institute Hokkaido University School of Medicine**

Immunological tolerance to murine leukemia virus (MuLV)-induced tumors in rats can be produced by a neonatal injection of MuLV. In this study, rats given neonatal injections of Gross virus (GV) or Friend virus (FV) always became tolerant to virus-specific transplantation antigens (VSTA) and eventually developed lymphoma. The tolerant rats did not show any cellular or humoral immune response to VSTA, even though these lymphomas are so highly antigenic that they will not grow in syngeneic nontolerant rats. To prevent development of primary lymphomas in the tolerant rats, attempts were made to break the tolerant state by adoptive transfer with syngeneic spleen and lymph node cells. The inoculation of immune lymphoid cells into FV-tolerant rats always brought about the runting syndrome, and the tolerant state was not broken in any survivors. In the runted rats, high-titered cytotoxic antibody to FV-lymphomas (WFT) was detected, and thymic atrophy and enlarged spleens with a depletion of lymphocytes were observed. It is suggested that the specific immune reaction of inoculated lymphoid cells against FV-infected cells of tolerant rats causes massive destruction of the lymphoid organs and results in a runting death.

On the other hand, immunological tolerance to GV-VSTA in rats given neonatal injection of GV was broken by adoptive transfer with lymphoid cells. When tolerance was abrogated, the rats produced cytotoxic antibody and resisted transplantation to GV-induced lymphomas (WGT); none developed primary thymomas. Immunotherapy of WGT and a GV-infected fibrosarcoma (a xenogenized tumor) growing in the tolerant rats was also successfully attained by inoculation of immune lymphoid cells. Immunological differences between GV-tolerance and FV-tolerance in the process of breakdown were significant.

Murine leukemia viruses (MuLV) are known to induce immunological suppression or tolerance in rodents during leukemogenesis. In high-leukemic AKR and C58 strains of mice, vertical transmission of Gross virus (GV) produces immunological tolerance to GV-induced cell surface antigens and induces leukemia in over 90% of the progeny (*3*). In our study, rats given neonatal injection of murine leukemia viruses such as Gross, Friend, or Rauscher virus always became tolerant to virus-induced cell surface antigens and eventually developed malignant lymphomas (*5, 6*). Tolerant rats do not

---

* Kita-15-jo, Nishi-7-chome, Kita-ku, Sapporo 060, Japan (武市紀年, 小林 博).

show any cellular or humoral immune response to virus-induced lymphomas, even though these lymphomas are so highly antigenic that they cannot grow in syngeneic normal adult rats. As previously reported (7, 14, 15), nonvirally-induced tumors which are generally of low antigenicity and rapid growing can be made highly antigenic by infection with MuLV. We termed this phenomenon "xenogenization of tumor cells," which is defined as immunological regression of xenogenized tumors in syngeneic normal rats owing to newly-acquired, virus-induced cell-surface antigens.

In spite of their high antigenicity, however, both the virus-induced lymphomas and virus-infected tumors (xenogenized tumors) will grow and kill rats made tolerant to virally-induced antigens. We have reported that the immunologically tolerant state in rats induced by GV or Friend virus (FV) can be broken down by the adoptive transfer of spleen and lymph node cells from syngeneic rats immunized with the virus-induced lymphomas (16, 17). The experimental results presented here attempt to describe a model for the immunotherapy of tumors growing in immunologically tolerant hosts by the breakdown of the tolerant state.

Induction of Tolerance to FV-induced Cell Surface Antigens

It has been reported that Friend (9), Moloney (10), and Gross (4) leukemia viruses can transcend species barriers and produce leukemias in rats by a neonatal injection of the virus. Rats given neonatal injection of high doses of FV grew up normally as FV-tolerant rats which were more susceptible to a subsequent challenge with FV-induced lymphomas (WFT) and were unable to produce circulating antibodies (18, 19). During the tolerant state, the rats developed a cell-mediated immunity against

TABLE I. Lethal growth of FV-induced Tumors Inoculated i.p. in FV-tolerant and Normal WKA/Mk rats

Tumor line	Friend virus-tolerant rats[a]		No. of lethal growths in normal rats/No. tested
	No. of lethal growths/No. tested	Mean survival days	
WFT-1	128/129	33.2	3/38
WFT-2	113/113	10.2	0/53
WFT-3	84/84	19.5	0/26
WFT-4	25/25	20.0	0/9
WFT-5	9/12	52.3[b]	
WFT-6	9/9	21.8	0/4
WFT-7	7/13	25.4	0/3
WFT-8	11/11	35.0	0/5
WFT-9	13/13	24.3[b]	0/4
WFT-10	2/2	36.0[b]	
WFT-11	2/2	28.5[b]	
WFT-12	2/2	21.0[b]	
WFT-13	19/19	18.2	0/26
Total	424/434 (97.7%)		3/168 (1.8%)

[a] Given injections of FV at birth.
[b] Inoculated s.c.

nonspecific antigens such as allogeneic skin grafts or chemicals for delayed-type hypersensitivity tests. However, FV-tolerant rats showed depression of antibody formation to sheep red blood cells and reduced γ-globulin concentrations. Values of α- and β-globulins were essentially within normal ranges. From these results, FV-tolerant rats were completely lacking in specific cellular and humoral immunity and nonspecifically depressed only in antibody production. All FV-tolerant rats developed primary lymphomas about 200 days after injection. The primary organ mostly involved was the spleen in the tolerant rats and the histological types of Friend lymphomas are mostly lymphoblastic and, in some cases, reticulocellular sarcomas. Transplantable WFT lines were so highly antigenic that they did not grow in normal syngeneic rats. They grew lethally in FV-tolerant rats or immunologically depressed rats (Table I).

Development of Runting Syndrome in FV-tolerant Rats by Adoptive Transfer of Spleen and Lymph Node Cells

To inhibit development of primary lymphomas in FV-tolerant rats, attempts were made to break the tolerant state by adoptive transfer of syngeneic spleen and lymph node cells. The adoptive transfer of spleen and lymph node cells from syngeneic rats immunized with WFT brought about the runting syndrome in over 80% of the tolerant rats (Table II). The tolerant state was not abrogated in any survivors, though the titer of FV in the blood decreased markedly in all tolerants rats receiving immune spleen and lymph node cells. Repeated transfer of immune spleen and lymph node cells (5 times at 3-day intervals with 5×10^7 cells/rat) into FV-tolerant rats induced a severe runting syndrome and death in almost all cases. The cytotoxic antibody to FV-specific cell-surface antigen reached its highest level from 7 to 10 days after adoptive transfer of immune lymphoid cells, just before death by the runting syndrome.

TABLE II.   Transplantation of WFT-13 in FV-tolerant Rats Inoculated with Spleen and Lymph Node Cells from Rats Preimmunized with Various Antigens

Group No.	Spleen and lymph node cells[a] from rats immunized with	No. of rats with runting syndrome/No. of rats used	Transplantation of WFT-13 cells[b] (No. died/No. used)
1	WFT-13 cells	10/12 (83)[c]	0/2 (2/2)[d]
2	AH-66 cells	4/14 (29)	7/10 (3/3)
3	SRBC	6/11 (55)	0/5 (1/5)
4	None	3/11 (27)	7/8 (1/1)
5	Nontreated	1/15 (7)	14/14

[a] Five$\times 10^7$ spleen and lymph node cells were inoculated i.p. twice at 7-day intervals.

[b] Five$\times 10^7$ WFT-13 cells were transplanted s.c. 2 weeks after the 2nd inoculation of lymphoid cells.

[c] Number in parentheses shows percentage of rats with runting syndrome.

[d] Number in parentheses shows number of rats that died of runting syndrome per number of rats rejecting the WFT-13 transplants.

Pathological Changes of Runting Rats

By macroscopic observations, the most common findings of the runted rats were atrophy of the thymus and enlargement of the spleen. However, the spleen appeared atrophic in severely runted rats or in rats that survived for a relatively long period after first exhibiting clinical symptoms. In some of the severely runted rats repeatedly transferred with immune lymphoid cells, it was not possible to identify any surviving thymic tissue at necropsy. The lymph node size varied from normal in most rats to atrophic in some extremely runted rats. Histological changes in the atrophic thymus were accompanied by a depletion of lymphocytes and a relative proliferation of reticulum cells. Histological changes of the spleen consisted of atrophy of the white pulp with a marked depletion of lymphocytes and lymphoblasts in follicular areas.

Pathogenesis of Runting Syndrome in Rats

The runting syndrome in FV-tolerant rats was induced by transfer of syngeneic immune lymphoid cells. It was postulated that an immune reaction between new cellular antigens in the virus-infected cells and transferred immune lymphoid cells occured. Development of the GVHR was measured by a local GVH technique (2) (Table III). All tolerant rats injected with immune lymphoid cells developed white nodules under the subcapsular space of the kidney, and the mean weight of the kidney increased compared with those in the tolerant rats injected with lymphoid cells from normal or tolerant donors. By microscopic examination, a marked infiltration of mononuclear cells was observed in all cases from the subcapsular space to the parenchyma on the injected kidney. These facts indicate that an immune reaction similar to the GVHR in homologous disease occured between the virus-infected cells and transferred immune lymphoid cells. For further investigation of the pathogenesis of death caused by runting, distribution of FV-infected cells in lymphoid organs of tolerant rats before and after adoptive transfer of immune lymphoid cells was tested by a complement-dependent cytotoxicity assay (Fig. 1). In the control tolerant rats, 30 to 40% of the cells in the thymus, spleen, and bone marrow were susceptible to cytotoxicity of anti-Friend tumor serum. On the other hand, these infected cells disappeared completely from the lymphoid organs on the sixth day after adoptive transfer of immune lymphoid cells and thereafter most rats died of the runting syndrome. This result

TABLE III. Local GVHR in FV-tolerant and Normal Rats by the Transfer of Syngeneic Lymphoid Cells

Transferred material	Recipient	Local GVHR	
		Mean K_i/K_c[a]	Grade[b]
Immune lymphoid cells[c]	Tolerant	1.23	I, II, II, III
	Normal	0.98	0, 0, 0, 0
Normal lymphoid cells	Tolerant	1.04	I, I, II, II
	Normal	0.84	0, 0, 0, 0
Runted lymphoid cells	Tolerant	1.11	I, I, II, II
	Normal	0.97	0, 0, 0, 0
Tolerant lymphoid cells	Tolerant	0.98	0, 0, 0, 0
	Normal	0.97	0, 0, 0, 0

[a] Weight of kidney injected with lymphoid cells/weight of collateral kidney.
[b] Grade I, noninvasive lymphoid graft; Grade II, lymphoid graft with invasive tongue; Grade III, invasive destructive reactions.
[c] Spleen and lymph node cells (5×10^7) were injected.

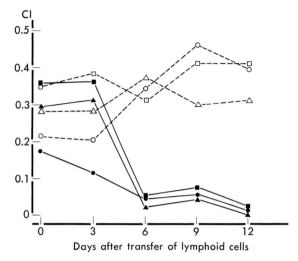

FIG. 1. Changes of FV-specific cell surface antigens in lymphoid organs of tolerant rats after an inoculation of immune spleen and lymph node cells

● Thymus cells from treated rats; ▲ spleen cells from treated rats; ■ bone marrow cells from treated rats; ○ thymus cells from nontreated rats; △ spleen cells from nontreated rats; □ bone marrow cells from nontreated rats.

indicates that the immune reaction between FV-infected lymphoid cells and newly-injected immune lymphoid cells may cause massive destruction of the lymphoid organs including the bone marrow, resulting in death by runting.

Inhibition of the Runting Syndrome and Prevention of Primary Lymphomas in FV-tolerant Rats

The adoptive transfer of immune lymphoid cells into FV-tolerant rats destroyed the virus-infected cells in the lymphoid organs and the bone marrow, and the lesions could not be repaired because of the destruction of stem cells from the bone marrow.

TABLE IV. Treatment of Runting Syndrome in FV-tolerant Rats by Inoculation of Immune Spleen and Lymph node Cells Mixed with Normal Bone Marrow Cells or Thymus Cells

Group No.	Inoculation	No. of incidence of runting syndrome/No. of rats	Transplantation of WFT-13 cells[a] (No. died/No. used)
1	ILyC[b]+NBMC	3/15 (20)[c]	0/12 (3/12)[d]
2	ILyC+NLyC	10/10 (100)	
3	ILyC+NThyC	9/9 (100)	
4	Nontreated	0/6 (0)	6/6

[a] Five×10⁷ WFT-13 cells were transplanted s.c. 2 weeks after the 4th inoculation.

[b] ILyC, immune spleen and lymph node cells; NBMC, normal bone marrow cells; NLyC, normal spleen and lymph node cells; NThyC, normal thymus cells.

[c] Number in parentheses shows percentage of rats with runting syndrome.

[d] Number in parentheses shows number of rats that died of the runting syndrome per number of rats rejecting the WFT-13 transplants.

A good supply of hematopoietic stem cells appears to be necessary to prevent or to cure the runting syndrome. In tolerant rats, adoptively transferred with immune spleen and lymph node cells and normal bone marrow cells, 3 of 15 rats died of the runting syndrome and the remaining 12 rats showed clinical symptoms of the runting syndrome such as loss of body weight, diarrhea, *etc.* (Table IV). However, all 12 survivors that were challenged with WFT 2 weeks after adoptive transfer of immune lymphoid cells rejected the tumor, but thereafter 3 of the rats died of the runting syndrome. The remaining 9 survivors did not develop primary lymphomas during more than 300 days of observation. In the rats given immune spleen and lymph node cells, and normal spleen and lymph node cells, all 10 tolerant rats died of the runting syndrome. In the rats given immune spleen and lymph node cells mixed with normal thymus cells, all 9 rats died of runting.

Induction of Tolerance to GV-induced Transplantation Antigens

Other experiments were carried out to compare GV with the FV system. We found that, like the FV system, injection of GV into newborn rats also induced immunological tolerance to GV-induced lymphomas. During a certain period after injection of the virus, the host did not show any cellular or humoral immune response to the virus-induced tumors. However, they reacted normally against nonspecific antigens such as sheep red blood cells, skin antigens for delayed type hypersensitivity, allogeneic tumors, or allogeneic skin grafts (*19*).

These results show that immunological tolerance to GV-VSTA in rats can be produced by the neonatal injection of GV. Recently, Mitchison and his colleagues (*11*) confirmed our results and demonstrated the presence of a suppression mechanism in the GV-induced tolerant rat system, which is sensitive to irradiation and abolished by trypsinization. These tolerant rats developed primary Gross lymphomas about 3

TABLE V. Lethal Growth of GV-induced Tumors Inoculated i.p. in
GV-tolerant and Normal WKA/Mk Rats

Tumor line	GV-tolerant rats[a]		No. of lethal growths in normal rats/No. tested
	No. of lethal growths/No. tested	Mean survival days	
WGT-1	8/9	15.0	0/2
WGT-2	24/25	14.0	0/15
WGT-3	15/15	18.5	0/14
WGT-4	31/31	11.1	0/13
WGT-5	4/4	19.0	
WGT-6	4/5	15.0	
WGT-7	2/2	28.0[b]	
WGT-8	2/2	16.0	
WGT-9	4/4	17.0	0/2
WGT-10	4/4	14.0	0/4
Total	98/101 (97%)		0/50 (0%)

[a] Given injections of GV at birth.

[b] Inoculated s.c.

months after the neonatal injection of GV. Histologically, GV-induced lymphomas are of the lymphocytic type. More than 10 different Gross lymphoma lines (WGT lines) were established and were maintained in the tolerant rats. These WGT lines are highly antigenic and are rejected within 2 weeks after subcutaneous (s.c.) transplantation into syngeneic adult rats (Table V).

Breakdown of GV-induced Tolerance in Rats by Adoptive Transfer of Immune Spleen and Lymph Node Cells

GV-tolerant rats were divided into 4 groups and were adoptively transferred intravenously (i.p.) 4 times at 7-day intervals, with spleen and lymph node cells, thymus cells, or bone marrow cells from rats immunized or not immunized with WGT cells. To determine whether immunological tolerance to GV-VSTA was eliminated, all rats from each group received s.c. transplants of WGT cells 2 weeks after the last inoculation of lymphoid cells (Table VI). Tolerant rats transferred with immune spleen and lymph node cells or immune thymus cells rejected the WGT transplants and none developed primary thymomas within 200 days. All tolerant rats receiving normal spleen and lymph node cells or normal thymus cells also resisted the WGT challenge but almost all rats developed primary thymomas. All tolerant rats receiving immune or normal bone marrow cells died from growth of the WGT transplants. This result shows that the adoptive transfer of immune spleen and lymph node cells or of immune thymus cells, but not of immune bone marrow cells, abrogated GV tolerance and completely inhibited the development of primary lymphomas. This differs considerably from the FV-tolerant systems described above.

TABLE VI. Breakdown of GV-tolerance in Rats by Inoculations of Syngeneic Lymphoid Cells

GV-tolerant rats inoculated with	Transplantation of WGT-4 cells[a]	Incidence of primary thymomas (survival days)
	No. died/No. used	
1) Immune spleen and lymph node cells[b]	0/9	0/9
Normal spleen and lymph node cells	0/7	6/7 (62, 65, 67, 100, 123, 138)
2) Immune thymus cells	0/8	0/8
Normal thymus cells	4/7	2/3 (104, 127)
3) Immune bone marrow cells	8/9	1/1 (111)
Normal bone marrow cells	7/7	—
4) None	6/6	—
	—	6/6 (66, 86, 97, 102, 107, 126)

[a] Five×10⁷ cells of WGT-4 were transplanted s.c. into rats 14 days after the last inoculation of cells.
[b] Immune cells obtained from rats immunized repeatedly with WGT-4 cells.

Elimination of Cells Bearing GV-induced Antigens in Lymphoid Organs of Tolerant Rats after Receiving Immune Lymphoid Cells

To elucidate the difference between the FV-tolerant and GV-tolerant state, the

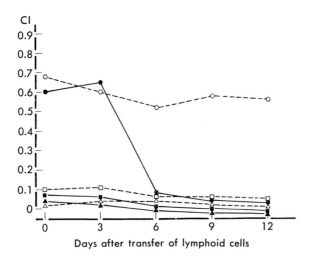

FIG. 2. Changes of GV-specific cell surface antigen in thymus, spleen, and bone marrow cells of tolerant rats after inoculation of syngeneic immune spleen and lymph node cells

● Thymus cells from treated rats; ○ thymus cells from nontreated rats; ▲ spleen cells from treated rats; △ spleen cells from nontreated rats; ■ bone marrow cells from treated rats; □ bone marrow cells from nontreated rats.

distribution of GV-infected cells in lymphoid organs of the tolerant rats was also determined before and after the transfer of immune lymphoid cells (Fig. 2). In the tolerant rats, cytotoxic sensitivity of anti-WGT serum was high only for thymus cells and low or negative for spleen and bone marrow cells on all days tested. The GV-infected cells completely disappeared from the thymus 6 days after the transfer of immune lymphoid cells. Thus, the thymus of GV-tolerant rats was destroyed first by immune cell transfer and then reconstituted by stem cells from the bone marrow. In the case of Friend-tolerant rats, the bone marrow contained more virus-infected cells than did that of the GV-tolerant rats, and was therefore attacked and destroyed by adoptively transferred immune lymphoid cells. In the Friend-tolerant system, it was not possible to save the runting rats without an additional supply of bone marrow cells from outside.

Adoptive Immunotherapy of GV-induced Lymphoma and a GV-infected Methylcholanthrene-induced Fibrosarcoma in Tolerant Rats

The next series of experiments attempted to set up an animal model for the immunotherapy of tumors in immunologically tolerant hosts by using the adoptive transfer of immune lymphoid cells. Tolerant rats were transplanted s.c. with 2×10^7 WGT cells and then were treated as follows: a) At 3 days after transplantation of the tumor, 10 tolerant rats with tumors (average tumor size, 5 mm) were adoptively transferred i.p. 3 times at 3-day intervals, with immune spleen and lymph node cells; b) at 6 days after the transplantation, 11 rats with tumors (average tumor size, 12 mm) were inoculated with immune spleen and lymph node cells; c) 8 tolerant rats were not treated. In addition to the above 3 groups, 8 tolerant rats received neither transplantation of the tumor nor injection of immune cells for the observation of primary thymomas,

TABLE VII. Treatment of WGT-4 Tumor in GV-tolerant WKA Rats by Adoptive
Transfer of Spleen and Lymph Node Cells from Syngeneic
Rats Immunized with WGT-4 cells

Group No.	Neonatal injection with GV	Lymphoid cell transfer	Challenge-transfer intervals (days)	Result of challenge with WGT-4 cells[a] (No. died/No. used)
I	+	+	3	0/10 (0/10)[b]
II	+	+	6	8/11 (0/3)
III	+	−		8/8
IV	+	−		(6/6)
V	−	−		0/10 (0/10)

[a] Two×10^7 WGT-4 cells were transplanted s.c. into the recipients.
[b] Number in parentheses shows number of rats that developed primary thymomas/number of rats used.

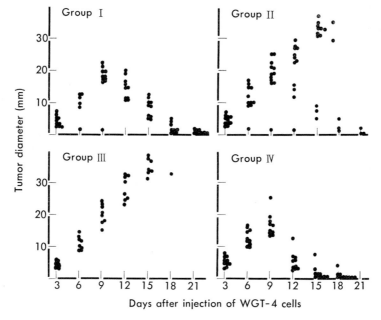

FIG. 3. Growth curves of WGT-4 tumor in tolerant rats after adoptive transfer
of immune spleen and lymph node cells

and 10 normal rats received s.c. transplants of WGT cells. The results are presented
in Table VII. In the first group, all tolerant rats completely rejected the growing
tumor by the 21st day, even though the average maximum size of the tumor reached
20 mm in diameter before beginning to regress (Fig. 3). None of the rats developed
primary thymomas within 200 days after infection. In the second group, 3 of 11 tolerant
rats rejected the growing tumors, and none developed primary thymoams. In the third
group, all tolerant rats that did not receive immune cells died from growth of the
tumor. In the 4th group, primary thymomas developed between 81 and 118 days after
infection.

Another experiment dealt with the immunotherapy of GV-infected fibrosarcoma

TABLE VIII. Treatment of GV-KMT-17 Cells in GV-tolerant WKA Rats
by Adoptive Transfer of Spleen and Lymph Node Cells from
Syngeneic Rats Immunized with WGT-4 Cells

Group No.	Status of recipient	Lymphoid cell transfer	Challenge-transfer intervals (days)	Result of challenge with GV-KMT-17 cells[a] (No. died/No. used)
I	Tolerant	+	1	0/8 (0/8)[b]
II	Tolerant	+	3	8/10 (2/2)
III	Tolerant	−		8/8
IV	Normal	−		0/6 (0/6)

[a] Five×10⁶ GV-KMT-17 cells were transplanted s.c.

[b] Number in parentheses shows number of rats that developed primary thymomas/number of rats used.

(GV-KMT-17) growing in tolerant rats. Spontaneously-developed or chemically-induced rat tumors failed to grow in syngeneic normal adult rats after they had been infected with murine leukemia viruses (7, 14). This phenomenon results from the appearance of new cell-surface antigens induced by the virus infection, a process called xenogenization. Treatment of GV-KMT-17 cells in the tolerant rats with adoptive transfer of immune spleen and lymph node cells was undertaken (Table VIII). Tolerant rats were transplanted s.c. with 5×10^6 GV-KMT-17 cells and divided into 3 groups, that were handled as follows: All rats that received immune cells i.p. 4 times at 3-day intervals, starting 1 day after transplantation, rejected the growing GV-KMT-17 tumor and none developed primary thymomas. Eight of 10 tolerant rats died from the growth of GV-KMT-17 cells when treated with immune spleen and lymph node cells starting 3 days after challenge, and the 2 survivors died later from the development of primary thymomas. In the control group, 8 tolerant rats that received no treatment died of tumor growth.

DISCUSSION

We have presented the results of our studies on two kinds of immunological tolerance to tumor-associated antigens in rats. One is FV-induced tolerance and the other is GV-induced tolerance. In order to breakdown FV-tolerance, it was necessary to provide bone marrow cells in addition to immune spleen and lymph node cells. Otherwise, the tolerant rats developed the runting syndrome, the so-called xenogenization disease. The most likely explanation for the mechanism in the prevention of runting deaths and in the abrogation of the tolerant state is that new bone marrow cells replaced the FV-infected cells and repopulated lymphoid organs that had been destroyed by the administered immune lymphoid cells. On the other hand, breakdown of GV-tolerance by the adoptive transfer of immune lymphoid cells was successful without the supply of bone marrow cells. This difference might be explained by the fact that FV and GV have different target cells in rats.

The tolerance to GV-VSTA produced by the neonatal injection of GV resembles, in certain respects, the "eclipse" of specific antitumor immune responsiveness in animals bearing tumors larger than a certain threshold size. The eclipse of tumor immunity produced by growing tumors, documented in many animal tumor systems by both *in vivo* (*12, 21*) and *in vitro* (*1, 8, 13, 20*) methods, appears to be due largely to the presence of tumor-derived substances which block the antitumor immune response at sites distant from the tumor. In a similar fashion, tolerance to GV-VSTA in rats may be maintained, at least in part, by the continuous production of circulating GV, which is analogous to circulating tumor antigens shed in soluble form from the cell surface of a growing tumor. The adoptive immunotherapy experiments show that immune lymphoid cells, administered intraperitoneally 3 days after the inoculation of GV-induced lymphoma cells in 1 case, and 1 day later in another case, brought about rejection of the growing tumor by breaking tolerance to GV-VSTA in the host. The tumor continued to enlarge to a maximum diameter of over 20 mm in 1 case and 18 mm in another case 14 days after challenge, before beginning to regress. This successful result provides evidence that adoptive immunotherapy may be effective even in the presence of immunological eclipse produced by the tumor load.

It is generally accepted that the state of immunological tolerance to tumor-specific antigens exists in the preneoplastic stage of high leukemic species of mice, hamsters, chickens, and cats. The system presented here is an experimental model for immunotherapy using antigenic tumors growing in immunologically tolerant animals.

REFERENCES

1. Barski, G. and Youn, J. K. Evolution of cell-mediated immunity in mice bearing an antigenic tumor. Influence of tumor growth and surgical removal. *J. Natl. Cancer Inst.*, **43**, 111–121 (1969).

2. Elkins, W. L. Invasion and destruction of homologous kidney by locally inoculated lymphoid cells. *J. Exp. Med.*, **120**, 329–359 (1964).

3. Gross, L. and Dreyfuss, Y. Studies on vertical transmission of leukemia virus through the male. *Proc. Am. Assoc. Cancer Res.*, **11**, 126 (1970).

4. Gross, L., Dreyfuss, Y., and Moore, L. A. Induction of leukemia in rats with mouse leukemia (passage A) virus. *Proc. Soc. Exp. Biol. Med.*, **106**, 890–893 (1961).

5. Kobayashi, H., Hosokawa, M., Takeichi, N., Sendo, F., and Kodama, T. Transplantable Friend virus-induced tumors in rats. *Cancer Res.*, **29**, 1385–1392 (1969).

6. Kobayashi, H., Kuzumaki, N., Gotohda, E., Takeichi, N., Sendo, F., Hosokawa, M., and Kodama, T. Specific antigenicity of tumors and immunological tolerance in the rat induced by Friend, Gross, and Rauscher viruses. *Cancer Res.*, **33**, 1598–1603 (1973).

7. Kobayashi, H., Sendo, F., Shirai, T., Kaji, H., Kodama, T., and Saito, H. Modification in growth of transplantable rat tumors exposed to Friend virus. *J. Natl. Cancer Inst.*, **42**, 413–419 (1969).

8. Mikulska, Z. B., Smith, C., and Alexander, P. Evidence for an immunological reaction of the host directed against its own actively growing primary tumor. *J. Natl. Cancer Inst.*, **36**, 29–35 (1966).

9. Mirand, E. A. and Grace, J. T. Induction of leukemia in rats with Friend virus. *Virology*, **17**, 364–366 (1962).

10. Moloney, J. B. Properties of a leukemia virus. *Natl. Cancer Inst. Monogr.*, **4**, 7–37 (1960).

11. Myburgh, J. A. and Mitchison, N. A. Suppressor mechanisms in neonatally acquired tolerance to a Gross virus-induced lymphoma in rats. *Transplantation*, **22**, 236–244 (1976).

12. Oren, M. E., Herberman, R. B., and Canty, J. G. Immune response to Gross virus-induced lymphoma. II. Kinetics of the cellular immune response. *J. Natl. Cancer Inst.*, **46**, 621–628 (1971).

13. Paranjpe, M. S. and Boone, C. W. Kinetics of the antitumor delayed hypersensitivity response in mice with progressively growing tumors: Stimulation followed by specific suppression. *Int. J. Cancer*, **13**, 179–186 (1974).

14. Sendo, F., Kaji, H., Saito, H., and Kobayashi, H. Antigenic modification of rat tumor cells artificially infected with Friend virus in the primary autochthonous host. *Gann*, **61**, 223–226 (1970).

15. Shirai, T., Kaji, H., Takeichi, N., Sendo, F., Saito, H., Hosokawa, M., and Kobayashi, H. Cell surface antigens detectable by cytotoxic test on Friend virus-induced tumors in the rats. *J. Natl. Cancer Inst.*, **46**, 449–460 (1971).

16. Takeichi, N., Kaji, H., Kodama, T., and Kobayashi, H. Breakdown of Friend virus-induced tolerance and development of runting syndrome in rats. *Cancer Res.*, **34**, 543–550 (1974).

17. Takeichi, N., Kuzumaki, N., Kodama, T., and Kobayashi, H. Breakdown of Gross virus-induced tolerance in rats by inoculation of lymphoid cells. *J. Natl. Cancer Inst.*, **52**, 1817–1822 (1974).

18. Takeichi, N., Kuzumaki, N., and Kobayashi, H. Immunological studies of runting syndrome in rats inoculated with Friend virus. *Cancer Res.*, **33**, 3096–3102 (1973).

19. Takeichi, N., Kuzumaki, N., and Kobayashi, H. Immunosuppression of rats infected with Friend or Gross virus. *Gann Monogr. Cancer Res.*, **16**, 27–35 (1974).

20. Youn, J. K., Le Francois, D., and Barski, G. *In vitro* studies on mechanism of the "eclipse" of cell-mediated immunity in mice bearing advanced tumors. *J. Natl. Cancer Inst.*, **50**, 921–926 (1973).

21. Vaage, J. Concomitant immunity and specific depression of immunity by residual or rejected syngeneic tumor tissue. *Cancer Res.*, **31**, 1615–1622 (1971).

XENOGENIZATION
WITH CHEMICALS AND ENZYMES

ENHANCED IMMUNOGENICITY OF CONCANAVALIN A-COATED TUMOR CELLS

W. John MARTIN and Elaine ESBER

*Division of Virology, Bureau of Biologics, Food and Drug Administration**

The immune response of C57BL/6 mice to concanavalin A (Con A)-coated EL-4 and RBL-5 leukemia cells was investigated using *in vitro* assays of cell-mediated immunity. Mice primed with X-irradiated Con A-coated EL-4 cells, and subsequently boosted with X-irradiated EL-4 cells developed high levels of anti-EL-4 lymphocyte-mediated cytotoxicity (LMC). Mice similarily inoculated with EL-4 cells alone did not develop tumor-reactive LMC. EL-4 inoculated mice did, however, possess lymphoid cells reactive with EL-4 cells in a colony inhibition assay. Furthermore LMC readily developed when spleen cells from EL-4 inoculated mice were co-cultivated for 5 days with additional X-irradiated EL-4 cells. Thus while both Con A reacted and unreacted X-irradiated EL-4 cells prime for the *in vitro* generation of LMC, only Con A-reacted EL-4 cells effectively prime for the *in vivo* generation of LMC. Both the *in vivo* and *in vitro* anti-EL-4 responses were specific for EL-4 with no evidence of cross reactivity against the Rauscher virus-induced leukemia, RBL-5. Con A coated RBL-5 cells did not prime mice for the *in vivo* development of anti RBL-5 LMC. Lymphoid cells from RBL-5 inoculated mice were active in the colony inhibition assay and LMC readily developed in spleen cells cultures from these mice. Specificity studies indicated that these responses were highly cross reactive with EL-4 cells. RBL-5 and EL-4 therefore share a common tumor-associated surface antigen. It can be concluded that the observed effect of Con A on EL-4 cells is restricted to an EL-4 unique antigen and that, in this system, Con A has no beneficial effect on the immunogenicity of the cross reactive antigen expressed by both EL-4 and RBL-5 cells.

Complex cellular interactions occur during the generation of an anti-tumor immune response. Several of these cell-to-cell interactions appear to be mediated by humoral factors acting primarily on lymphoid cell surface receptors (7). Certain natural products of plant, bacterial, and viral origin stimulate lymphocyte division and the expression of specialized immune functions (15). These compounds may be considered functional homologs of physiological immunoregulatory molecules and, as such, could conceivably be useful in attempts to evoke an effective anti-tumor response.

Several investigators have reported encouraging results using the jack bean derived T cell mitogen, concanavalin A (Con A), to increase the immunogenicity of tumor

---

* Bethesda, Maryland 20014, U.S.A.

associated surface antigens (TASA). Con A has been used either directly applied to tumor cells (4, 5, 8–14), or applied in combination with neuraminidase (1), or glutaraldehyde (6) pretreatment. This paper reviews experiments which indicate that capacity of Con A to augment the immunogenicity of EL-4 but not of RBL-5 leukemia cells in C57BL/6 mice. Analysis of this phenomenon provides an interesting insight into the complexity of antitumor immune responses.

Induction of Lymphocyte Mediated Cytotoxicity with Con A-coated Tumor Cells

The EL-4 leukemia grows readily when inoculated intraperitoneally into C57BL/6 mice. Single or repeated intraperitoneal injections of X-irradiated EL-4 cells do not evoke *in vivo* resistance to subsequent live tumor challenge. Splenic, peritoneal, and lymph node lymphocytes, obtained from mice inoculated 2 weeks previously with X-irradiated EL-4 cells were tested for cytotoxic activity against ^{51}Cr-labeled EL-4 cells in the 4-hr ^{51}Cr release cytotoxicity assay (2, 3). In repeated tests no significant lymphocyte-mediated cytotoxicity (LMC) was demonstrable (8–12).

The first indication of the possible usefulness of Con A in evoking anti-EL-4 immunity was obtained in experiments in which mice were inoculated twice with EL-4 cells exposed *in vitro* to Con A (25 μg/ml/10^7 cells at 37° for 30 min). In a number of experiments a low but significant level of LMC was generated. In other experiments there was no detectable LMC against EL-4 cells. Spleen cells from mice inoculated twice with Con A coated EL-4 were, however, capable of lysing Con A-coated EL-4 target cells. This activity appeared to be directed against Con A or a Con A-modified cell surface component, since lysis was also observed against Con A coated LSTRA cells (a Moloney virus-induced leukemia of BALB/c mice), but not against uncoated LSTRA cells (8). In the next series of experiments, mice received an initial injection of 5×10^5 Con A-coated irradiated EL-4 cells followed 3 weeks later with an injection of 5×10^7 irradiated but not Con A-coated, EL-4 cells. High levels of LMC were consistently observed when spleen cells were tested 7–10 days later (8–14). The cytotoxic cells were specific for EL-4 and did not lyse either LSTRA or RBL-5 cells (Table I).

The immunity evoked in C57BL/6 mice, using an initial injection of Con A-coated EL-4 cells followed by an injection of non-coated EL-4 cells, was confirmed in an *in vivo* assay measuring the survival of ^{125}I-iododeoxyuridine labeled EL-4 cells (8). In addition, significant prolongation of mean survival from 14 to 20 days was observed in immunized mice challenged with 10^7 viable EL-4 cells (8).

TABLE I. Specificity of LMC Evoked in Mice Pre-immunized with X-irradiated, Con A-coated EL-4 Cells, and Boosted with X-irradiated EL-4 Cells

Immunization		Cytotoxic lymphoid cell activity[a] (% lysis)		
Primary	Secondary	EL-4	LSTRA	RBL-5
5×10^5 EL-4	5×10^7 EL-4	0.5	0.6	1.0
5×10^5 Con A : EL-4	5×10^7 EL-4	38.5	2.0	1.4

[a] Lymphoid to target cell ratio of 100:1 was used in the experiments reported in Tables I–III.

Dose Response Studies Using Con A-coated Tumor Cells

Several studies were performed to test the importance of cell dose, concentration of Con A, and the need for Con A to be directly associated with the EL-4 cells (*8*). Concentrations of Con A of 5–500 μg/ml and priming cell doses from 10^4 to 10^7 effectively primed mice for subsequent generation of LMC following challenge with 5×10^7 untreated EL-4 cells. Con A injected separately from the EL-4 cells in doses of 1–100 μg and mixtures of Con A coated normal lymphoid cells and uncoated X-irradiated EL-4 cells were ineffective, indicating that Con A had to be bound with EL-4cells to achieve its effect (*8*).

Specificity of LMC Induced by Con A-coated Cells

Tissue culture studies were employed to investigate the mechanism whereby Con A-coated EL-4 cells were capable of priming mice for a subsequent *in vivo* injection of EL-4 cells. In these studies spleens of normal mice or of mice previously injected with either irradiated, or iradiated, Con A-coated EL-4 cells. Interestingly high levels of specific anti-EL-4 cytotoxic activity developed in cultures containing EL-4 cells and spleen cells from mice previously inoculated with either EL-4 or Con A-coated EL-4. Detectable levels of cytotoxic activity also developed when spleen cells from EL-4 inoculated mice were cultured in the absence of additional EL-4 cells. Normal spleen cells cultured with irradiated EL-4 cells occasionally yielded low levels of anti-EL-4 LMC (Table II). In each group the LMC was specific for EL-4 with no cross reaction observed against RBL-5 target cells (Table III).

TABLE II. *In vitro* Generation of Cytotoxic Lymphoid Cells

Immunization	Cytotoxic activity generated in culture	
	without EL-4	with EL-4
None	0	1.9
EL-4	9.9	23.3
Con A : EL-4	15.9	55.2

TABLE III. Specificity of LMC Generated in Cultured Spleen Cells
from Tumor inoculated Mice

Immunization of spleen cell donors	Cytotoxic lymphoid cell activity (% lysis)	
	EL-4	RBL-5
EL-4	33.4	2.9
Con A : EL-4	53.5	0.0
RBL-5	44.1	43.7

Colony Inhibition Assay

The development of high levels of LMC in cultured spleen cells of EL-4 inoculated mice strongly suggested that, although these mice did not readily develop LMC *in vivo*,

TABLE IV. Specificity of Colony Inhibition by Lymphoid Cells from
Mice Inoculated with EL-4 and RBL-5 cells

Immunization of lymphoid cell donor	Colony inhibition (%)	
	EL-4	RBL-5
RBL-5	20*	41*
EL-4	45*	5

* $p < 0.01$.

they had in fact, responded immunologically to an EL-4 associated tumor antigen. This conclusion was confirmed in studies employing a growth inhibition assay. In this assay 10^4 EL-4 cells were incubated in medium alone, or in medium containing 5×10^6 lymphoid cells from either normal or EL-4 inoculated C571BL/6 mice. Aliquots were removed at time zero and after 24-hr incubation. The aliquots were diluted in Agarose in petri dishes and the number of EL-4 cell colonies formed was determined by examining the dishes 7 days later. Lymphoid cells from EL-4 inoculated mice achieved highly significant colony inhibition against EL-4 (9). Lymphoid cells from EL-4 inoculated mice were similarly tested against RBL-5 leukemia cells. No significant colony inhibition of RBL-5 cells was observed (Table IV).

The nature and *in vivo* function of the lymphoid cells which mediate anti-EL-4 colony inhibition has not been determined. Possibly these cells play a role in suppressing the *in vivo* development of anti-EL-4 LMC. Whatever the mechanism of *in vivo* suppression of the generation of LMC, there is no evidence that EL-4 inoculated mice can suppress the activity of fully developed cytotoxic cells. Thus, adoptive immunotherapy in these mice using cytotoxic lymphocytes derived from *in vitro* culture of spleen cells from Con A EL-4 inoculated mice resulted in significant *in vivo* elimination of ^{125}I-iododeoxyuridine labeled EL-4 cells (9).

Lack of Efficacy of Con A on RBL-5 Tumor

In a related series of experiments the immunizing protocol using Con A-coated cells, which were found to be effective in the *in vivo* generation of anti-EL-4 LMC, was found to be ineffective when applied to the RBL-5 leukemia in C57BL/6 mice or the LSTRA leukemia in BALB/c mice. C57BL/6 mice inoculated with irradiated RBL-5 cells were tested for evidence of suppressed development of LMC. Spleen cells from RBL-5 inoculated mice readily develop anti-tumor cytotoxic lymphoid cells when cultured for 5 days with, and in most experiments even without, additional RBL-5 cells. Similarly, lymphoid cells from RBL-5 inoculated mice were capable of growth inhibition of RBL-5 cells in the colony inhibition assay. An important observation made during the course of these experiments was that both the *in vitro* generated cytotoxic lymphocytes and the cells capable of growth inhibition were highly active when tested on EL-4 cells as well as RBL-5 cells (Tables III and IV). Indeed only minor quantitative differences were observed between these target cell lines in the two assays. No activity was observed in these assays using the unrelated leukemia target cells line L1210. The finding of cross reactivity between EL-4 and RBL-5 was particularly informative because it indicated that EL-4 and RBL-5 share a common

TABLE V. Summary of Immune Activity Generated in Mice Inoculated
with Con A-coated or Uncoated EL-4 or RBL-5 Cells

Immunization	TASA	Colony inhibition	Generation of cytotoxic lymphoid cells	
			In vitro culture	In vivo boosting
EL-4	Unique	+	+	−
	Common	−	−	−
Con A : EL-4	Unique	+	+	+
	Common	−	−	−
RBL-5	Common	+	+	−
Con A : RBL-5	Common	+	+	−

TASA. This antigen was clearly not detected in studies on mice immunized against EL-4 or Con A-coated EL-4 cells. It can be concluded that although Con A was effective in diminishing the apparant *in vivo* suppression of the development of cytotoxic lymphocytes reactive with the EL-4 unique antigen, it was not effective in diminishing the *in vivo* suppression of cytotoxic lymphocyte development in RBL-5 inoculated mice nor in evoking even a suppressed response in EL-4 inoculated mice against the common TASA shared by EL-4 and RBL-5 (Table V). Furthermore, both Con A coated EL-4 and RBL-5 have shown similar properties in tests performed to date aimed at elucidating the possible mode of action of Con A. These tests have revealed that Con A-coated tumor cells i) are more readily phagocytized by macrophages, ii) bind less anti *H-2* antibody, and iii) stimulate the proliferation of spleen cells as effectively as optimal doses of soluble Con A. Although one or more of these activities may be associated for the observed enhanced immune response against the unique EL-4 TASA, additional factors must be involved to explain the inability of Con A to exert a beneficial effect on the immunogenicity of the common TASA expressed by RBL-5 and EL-4 cells.

Further exploration of the phenomena presented in the study are indicated before Con A could be applied with confidence to the immunotherapy of established tumors.

REFERENCES

1. Brugarolas, A., Takita, H., and Moore, G. E. Effect of syngeneic tumour cells bound to concanavalin A on tumour growth. *J. Surg. Oncol.*, **4**, 123–130 (1972).
2. Brunner, R. T., Mauel, J., Cerottini, J. C., and Chaupuis, B. Quantitative assay of the lytic action of immune lymphoid cells on ^{51}Cr labeled allogeneic target cells *in vitro*: Inhibition by isoantibody and by drugs. *Immunology*, **14**, 181–187 (1970).
3. Canty, T. G. and Wunderlich, J. R. Quantitative *in vitro* assay of cytotoxic cellular immunity. *J. Natl. Cancer Inst.*, **45**, 761–774 (1970).
4. Enker, W. E., Craft, K., and Wisler, R. W. Augmentation of tumour-specific immunogenicity by concanavalin A in the Morris Hepatoma 5123. *J. Surg. Res.*, **16**, 66–68 (1974).
5. Enker, W. E., Craft, K., and Wissler, R. W. Active-specific immunotherapy with concanavalin A modified tumour cells. *Transplant. Proc.*, **8** (*Suppl.* 1), 489–494 (1975).
6. Kataoka, T., Oh-hashi, F., Tasukagoshi, S., and Sakurai, Y. Induction of resistance to L1210 leukemia in (BALB/c×DBA/2Cr)F$_1$ mice, with L1210 cells treated with glutaraldehyde and Concanavalin A. *Cancer Res.*, **37**, 964–968 (1977).

7. Katz, D. H. "Lymphocyte differentiation, recognition and regulation," (1977). Academic Press, New York.

8. Martin, W. J. Use of concanavalin A to enhance immunogenicity of tumor antigens. *In* "Concanavalin A as a Tool," ed. H. Bittiger and H. P. Schnebli, pp. 563–571 (1976). John Wiley & Sons, New York.

9. Martin, W. J., Esber, E., and Wunderlich, J. R. Evidence for the suppression of the development of cytotoxic lymphoid cells in tumour immunized mice. *Fed. Proc.*, **32**, 173–179 (1973).

10. Martin, W. J. and Wunderlich, J. R. Immune response of mice to concanavalin A coated EL-4 leukemia cells. *Natl. Cancer Inst. Monogr.*, **35**, 295–299 (1972).

11. Martin, W. J. and Wunderlich, J. R. Suppressed development of cytotoxic lymphoid cells in tumour-immunized mice. *Israel J. Med. Sci.*, **9**, 324–329 (1973).

12. Martin, W. J., Wunderlich, J. R., Fletcher, F., and Inman, J. K. Enhanced immunogenicity of chemically-coated syngeneic tumour cells. *Proc. Natl. Acad. Sci. U.S.*, **68**, 469–472 (1971).

13. Meyer, A. A., Enker, W. E., Jacobitz, J. L., Wissler, R. W., and Craft, K. The tumour specific immune response of experimental active-specific immunotherapy. *Cancer*, **39**, 565–569 (1977).

14. Simmons, R. L. and Rios, A. Cell surface modification in the treatment of experimental cancer, neuraminidase or concanavalin A. *Cancer*, **34**, 1541–1547 (1974).

15. Wedner, H. J. and Parker, C. W. Lymphocyte activation. *Prog. Allergy*, **20**, 195–220 (1976).

GANN Monograph on Cancer Research 23, 1979

INDUCTION OF IMMUNE RESISTANCE TO L1210 MURINE LEUKEMIA BY LECTIN-BOUND TUMOR VACCINE

Tateshi Kataoka

*Cancer Chemotherapy Center, Japanese Foundation
for Cancer Research**

The cellular as well as immunological characteristics of glutaraldehyde-treated L1210 murine leukemic cells were examined. The possibility that malignancy of glutaraldehyde-treated tumor cells was predictable by an *in vitro* test of cell agglutinability by concanavalin A (Con A) was pointed out.

Vaccine cell-bound Con A enhanced immunogenic potency of the vaccine cells. Con A-bound L1210 vaccine cells induced the strongest immunity in mice compared with other vaccine preparations of L1210 cells.

Immunogenic potency of Con A-bound L1210 vaccine cells was enhanced by chemotherapeutic agents as well as by immunostimulants. However, the mechanisms involved were different. Chemotherapeutic agents were presumed to abrogate the suppressor cell activity whereas immunostimulants were presumed to activate amplifier cells.

Many experimental procedures for preparing tumor vaccines have been developed to induce tumor-specific immunity in laboratory animals (*6*). Before their clinical use, however, it is necessary to make certain that vaccine preparations are safe and not malignant, also that they are highly immunogenic.

From such a point of view, experimental tumor vaccines that were developed in the past should be critically evaluated. For example, X-irradiated tumor cells were repeatedly used to immunize patients as well as experimental aniamls. However, were they really safe? Retrospectively, we can tell whether they were malignant or not. Still, what is important especially in clinical trials is to know the malignancy of tumor vaccines before use. Extensive and excessive radiation would lead to the loss of immunogenic potency of tumor vaccines as well as the loss of their malignancy. Thus, it is essential to develop an *in vitro* test that will predict *in vivo* malignancy of the tumor vaccines so that the loss of immunogenic potency will be minimized. We will discuss the matter in this communication.

Many types of the tumor vaccine induced tumor-specific immunity in experimental animals. Before making any clinical trials of vaccination we have either to clarify which types of tumor vaccines are the most potent or develop a novel potent vaccine of low antigenic and highly malignant tumors such as L1210 murine leukemia. In this regard, we found that L1210 cells treated with glutaraldehyde and concanavalin A (Con A)

---

* Kami-Ikebukuro 1-37-1, Toshima-ku, Tokyo 170, Japan (片岡達治).

induced tumor-specific immune resistance in mice (*9*). We will describe some of the immunological characteristics of Con A-bound L1210 leukemic vaccine.

Malignancy of Tumor Cells Associated with Their Agglutinability by Con A

Many chemicals would suppress the malignancy of tumor cells. Glutaraldehyde, one such chemical, has been successfully used earlier in preparing tumor vaccines (*5*). When we treated L1210 cells with glutaraldehyde, the malignancy of leukemic cells was suppressed (Fig. 1). L1210 cells incubated with 0.0063% of glutaraldehyde on ice for 30 min was no longer malignant. However, we needed an *in vitro* test that would give an idea of whether the glutaraldehyde-treated leukemic cells were malignant or not, otherwise the clinical use of glutaraldehyde in preparing tumor vaccines is not feasible. It has been stressed that cell surface mobility is probably associated with malignant transformation (*7*). This led us to compare the malignancy of leukemic cells and their *in vitro* agglutinability by Con A at different concentrations of glutaraldehyde, and we found a close association (Fig. 1). Leukemic cells not agglutinable by Con A *in vitro* were not malignant either. This relationship seems true with Lewis lung carcinoma cells treated with glutaraldehyde (unpublished results by Kataoka, Okabe, and Sakurai). Further study will clarify whether they are universally associated with each other.

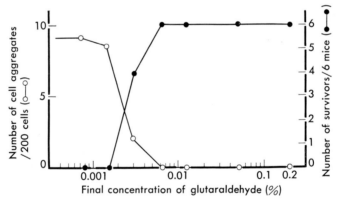

FIG. 1.   Cell agglutinability by Con A and malignancy of L1210 cells
L1210 cells incubated with glutaraldehyde on ice for 30 min were measured either for cell agglutinability by Con A (○) or for transplantability of 10^6 cells in CD2F$_1$ mice (●) (*11*).

Immunogenicity of Glutaraldehyde-treated Tumor Cells

Based on the above observation, we could safely sensitize mice with glutaraldehyde-treated L1210 cells, without the development of malignancy. The immunity induced by Con A-bound L1210 vaccine cells was examined by inoculation of the sensitized mice with live L1210 cells (Table I). The sensitized mice lived for a prolonged period compared with the control mice ($p<0.05$), although none was cured. This result contrasted with that of other investigators in which much stronger immunity was induced by glutaraldehyde-treated tumor vaccine cells prepared under

TABLE I. Induction of Immune Resistance by Glutaraldehyde-treated
L1210 Vaccine Cells[a]

Vaccination	No. of cured mice/total	Mean survival days
+	0/10	15.1[b]
−	0/10	11.9[b]

[a] A group of mice was inoculated intraperitoneally (i.p.) with 10^7 L1210 cells treated with 0.025% glutaraldehyde, three times at half-week intervals. Three weeks after the last sensitization, they were inoculated i.p. with 10^2 live L1210 cells.

[b] Significant at $p < 0.05$ by Mann-Whitney U-test.

much severer experimental conditions (5). It is assumed that low antigenicity and high malignancy of L1210 leukemic cells were liable for the apparent poor immunity induced in our experiment.

Immunogenicity of Tumor Vaccine Cells Modified by Con A

To induce stronger immunity we modified glutaraldehyde-treated L1210 cells with Con A. This stemmed from the earlier observation that inoculation of X-irradiated and Con A-bound tumor cells induced cytotoxic immunocytes in the spleen against intact tumor cells (13). We sensitized mice with Con A-bound L1210 cells pretreated with three different concentrations of glutaraldehyde (Table II). We found that the mice sensitized with Con A-bound L1210 cells prepared at 0.013 and 0.05% of glutaraldehyde not only lived for a prolonged period ($p < 0.05$) but also some were cured. This result compared with that of Table I indicates that Con A endowed the tumor cells with additional immunogenic potency.

We also noted that induction of immune resistance by ConA-bound vaccine depended on glutaraldehyde concentration, as evidenced by the fact that the vaccine cells prepared at 0.2% glutaraldehyde did not induce a detectable immune resistance. As we did not find any significant difference in the amount of bound Con A in three kinds of vaccine cells (unpublished result by Kataoka and Sakurai), it is likely that a high concentration of glutaraldehyde produced serious alteration of the tumor cell surface leading to the loss of tumor antigenicity. This is consistent with the previous finding that the cell surface of L1210 cells treated with 0.2% glutaraldehyde was dif-

TABLE II. Induction of Immune Resistance by Glutaraldehyde- and
ConA-treated L1210 Vaccine Cells[a]

Concentrations of glutaraldehyde used for vaccine preparation (%)	No. of cured mice/total	Mean survival days of dead mice
0.2	0/10	11.8
0.05	3/10	19.6[b]
0.013	3/10	18.6[b]

[a] Groups of mice were inoculated i.p. twice at 1-week intervals with 10^7 L1210 cells treated with the indicated concentration of glutaraldehyde and further with 165 μg/ml of ConA on ice for 1hr. Three weeks after the last sensitization they were inoculated i.p. with 10^2 live L1210 cells.

[b] Significant at $p < 0.05$ as compared with that of nonvaccinated animals by Mann-Whitney U test.

fered from that of the intact cells, from a physical as well as immunochemical point of view (*11*).

Immunogenic Potency of ConA-bound Vaccine Cells Enhanced by Immunostimulants or Chemotherapeutic agents

To further potentiate ConA-bound L1210 vaccine cells, we examined the effect of immunostimulants and chemotherapeutic agents on the induction of immune re- sistance by ConA-bound vaccine cells. We found that an extract of *Coriolus versicolor* (*10*), as well as other immunostimulants, such as BCG (unpublished result by Kataoka, Oh-hashi, and Sakurai) potentiated the vaccine. We also noted that chemotherapeutic agents including cyclophosphamide, mitomycin C and daunomycin potentiated the vaccine (*8*). Both types of potentiation were dependent on the vaccine-bound Con A although the mechanisms involved were supposed to be different (*9, 10*).

Immunogenicity of Tumor Vaccine Cells Prepared by Different Procedures

Under the same regimen we compared the immunogenicity of Con A-bound L1210 vaccine cells with that of other types of L1210 vaccine cells prepared by *Vibrio cholerae* neuraminidase, mitomycin C, and formaldehyde. These reagents have been repeatedly used for preparing vaccine cells of various tumor cells (*2, 3*). We found that glutar- aldehyde-treated and Con A-bound vaccine cells were the most immunogenic of all. Furthermore, we noted that Con A enhanced the immunogenic potency of mitomycin C-treated L1210 vaccine cells. This is consistent with the possibility, derived from the result of Table II, that Con A could endow the tumor vaccine cells with additional immunogenic potency.

Finally, the above study showed that vaccine-bound Con A endowed the vaccine cells with additional immunogenic potency. This could be associated with any of the various immunological activities of free, unbound Con A (*1, 4, 12*). Further study on the characterization of vaccine-bound Con A will lead us to the development of more potent tumor vaccines.

Acknowledgments

This is a part of collaborative work with F. Oh-hashi, H. Kobayashi, S. Tsukagoshi, and Y. Sakurai. Supported in part by a Grant-in-Aid for Cancer Research from the Ministry of Health and Welfare (51-8) and from the Ministry of Education, Science and Culture, Japan, and by The Princess Takamatsu Cancer Research Fund. T. K. is a recipient of Award of Society for Promotion of Cancer Research, Japan.

REFERENCE

1. Anaclerio, A., Waterfield, J. D., and Moller, G. Induction of lymphocyte-mediated cytotoxicity against allogeneic tumor cells by concanavalin A *in vivo. J. Immunol.*, **113**, 870–875 (1974).
2. Bekesi, J. G., St-Arneault, G., and Holland, J. F. Increase of leukemia L1210 immuno- genicity by *Vibrio cholerae* neuraminidase treatment. *Cancer Res.*, **31**, 2130–2132 (1971).
3. Benjamini, E., Fong, S., Erickson, C., Leung, C. Y., Rennick, D., and Scibinski, R. J.

Immunity to lymphoid tumors induced in syngeneic mice by immunization with mito-mycin C-treated cells. *J. Immunol.*, **118**, 685–693 (1977).

4. Egan, H. S., Reeder, W. J., and Ekstedt, R. D. Effect of concanavalin A *in vivo* in sup-pressing the antibody response in mice. *J. Immunol.*, **112**, 63–69 (1974).

5. Frost, P. and Sanderson, C. J. Tumor immunoprophylaxis in mice using glutaraldehyde-treated syngeneic tumor cells. *Cancer Res.*, **35**, 2646–2650 (1975).

6. Hersh, E. M., Gutterman, J. U., and Mavligit, G. "Immunotherapy of Cancer in Man," pp. 77–78 (1973). Charles C Thomas, Springfield, Ill.

7. Inbar, M., Shinitzky, M., and Sachs, L. Rotational relaxation time of concanavalin A bound to the surface membrane of normal and malignant transformed cells. *J. Mol. Biol.*, **81**, 245–253 (1973).

8. Kataoka, T., Kobayashi, H., and Sakurai, Y. Potentiation of concanavalin A-bound L1210 vaccine *in vivo* by chemotherapeutic agents. *Cancer Res.*, **38**, 1202–1207 (1978).

9. Kataoka, T., Oh-hashi, F., Tsukagoshi, S., and Sakurai, Y. Induction of resistance to L1210 leukemia in Balb/c×DBA/2CrF$_1$ mice with L1210 cells treated with glutaralde-hyde and concanavalin A. *Cancer Res.*, **37**, 964–968 (1977).

10. Kataoka, T., Oh-hashi, F., Tsukagoshi, T., and Sakurai, Y. Enhanced induction of immune resistance by L1210 vaccine and an immunopotentiator prepared from *Coriolus versicolor*. *Cancer Res.*, **37**, 4416–4419 (1977).

11. Kataoka, T., Tsukagoshi, S., and Sakurai, Y. Transplantability of L1210 cell in BALB/c×DBA/2F$_1$ mice associated with cell agglutinability by concanavalin A. *Cancer Res.*, **35**, 531–534 (1975).

12. Markowitz, H., Person, D. A., Gitnick, G. L., and Rittis, R. E., Jr. Immunosuppressive activity of concanavalin A. *Science*, **163**, 476 (1969).

13. Martin, W. J., Wunderlich, J. R., Fletcher, F., and Inman, J. K. Enhanced immuno-genicity of chemically-coated syngeneic tumor cells. *Proc. Natl. Acad. Sci. U.S.*, **68**, 469–472 (1971).

INDUCTION OF IMMUNE RESISTANCE AGAINST TUMOR BY IMMUNIZATION WITH HAPTEN-MODIFIED TUMOR CELLS IN THE PRESENCE OF HAPTEN-REACTIVE HELPER T CELLS[*1]

Toshiyuki Hamaoka, Hiromi Fujiwara, Tetsuo Tsuchida,
Toshiaki Kinouchi, and Hisakazu Aoki

Institute for Cancer Research, Osaka University Medical School[*2]

Hapten-reactive T cell activities were raised in mice by immunization with haptenated isologous mouse γ-globulin. Recent analysis of these hapten-reactive T cell activities revealed that such T lymphocytes express the biological functions of both major subtypes of regulatory T cells, namely suppressors and helpers, and that hapten-reactive suppressor and helper T lymphocytes differ in several important biological properties, including their relative susceptibility to specific inactivation by hapten conjugates of the nonimmunogenic D-amino acid copolymer, D-glutamic acid and D-lysine (D-GL).

By taking advantage of the relative susceptibility difference to hapten-D-GL, selective inactivation of hapten-reactive suppressor T cells was induced by appropriate treatment with hapten-D-GL, and the activity of hapten-reactive helper T cells was amplified. After establishing that hapten-reactive T lymphocytes can serve as amplifier cells for induction of tumor-specific killer T lymphocytes, the feasibility of utilizing this hapten-reactive T cell system for immunotherapy of the tumor was examined. The relatively weak immunogenic syngeneic plasmacytoma X5563 in C3H/He mice was used, in which the helper T cell activity against tumor-associated transplantation antigen (TATA) was never detected, in contrast to other syngeneic tumors such as the MM102 mammary adenocarcinoma. The supplement of hapten-reactive helper T cell activity to the system on immunization with X5563 with haptenation resulted in a striking augmentation of the induction of tumor-specific immunity, and a considerable number of the animals survived after challenge with viable tumor cells.

In this weak immunogenic tumor, the presence of free TATA (experimentally, this was induced by pretreatment with heavily X-irradiated tumor cells) almost completely inhibited the development of tumor immunity even after appropriate tumor-immunizing procedures. This was ascribed to the potent tolerogenic activity of an inappropriate form of TATA to the precursors of killer T cells. However, the supplement of hapten-reactive T cells to the system in conjunction with

---

[*1] This article is dedicated to the late Dr. Masayasu Kitagawa with our respect.

[*2] Fukushima 1-1-50, Fukushima-ku, Osaka 553, Japan (浜岡利之, 藤原大美, 土田哲夫, 木内利明, 青木久和).

haptenated TATA invariably inhibited this tolerance induction of killer T lymphocytes.

Thus, appropriate manipulations designed to induce potent hapten-reactive helper T lymphocytes provided a potentially very effective mode of immunotherapy against the tumor.

It has been demonstrated in our laboratory (4) that relatively weak immunogenic syngeneic plasmacytoma X5563 in C3H/He mice exclusively generated killer T cell activity without inducing any significant helper T cell activity against tumor-associated transplantation antigens (TATA). Futhermore, despite the positive killer T cell-mediated immunity, no antibody activity against the tumor was detected. The failure to induce significant helper T cell activity to the TATA of X5563 in the syngeneic system seems to be of vital importance in the following aspects. Firstly, the X5563 syngeneic tumor system failed to provide double defense mechanisms of both cell-mediated and humoral immunity related to killer and helper T cell generation, in sharp contrast to the allogeneic transplantation immunity. Furthermore, the failure to induce helper T cell activity may have some relation to the lower level of generation of killer T cell activity against syngeneic tumor cells in general. Cantor and Boyse (1, 2) reported that killer T cell development against allogeneic tumor cells was augmented by collaboration with another subset of amplifier T cells which carries a Ly-specificity different from the killer T cells, and recognizes alloantigens different from those recognized by prekiller T cells. Although this selective generation of killer T cells against TATA indicates that the generation of helper T cell activity against TATA may not be an absolute prerequisite for the effective development of killer T cell response, it is highly conceivable that if the collaborative response of helper T cells with prekiller cells can be successfully induced in the syngeneic tumor system, the T cell response against the killer determinant may be augmented. In this context, if animals are immunized with tumor cells modified by additional antigenic determinants with which the helper (amplifier) T cells may be capable of reacting, the augmentation of specific killer T cell response will be definitely expected.

In the present study, 2,4,6-trinitrophenyl (TNP) residues were introduced to the surface of tumor cells as an additional determinant because hapten-reactive helper T lymphocyte activity was easily generated in mice by immunization with TNP-modified mouse γ-globulin (MGG), and because the amplifying effect of TNP-reactive helper T cells on the TATA-reactive killer T cell generation could be analyzed by immunization with TNP-modified tumor cells. This article presents our recent results of the successful augmentation of induction of tumor-specific immunity by hapten-reactive helper T cell activity, and provides evidence that appropriate manipulations designed to induce additional determinant-reactive helper T lymphocytes afford a potentially very effective mode of immunotherapy against the tumor.

Induction of Hapten-reactive Regulatory T Cell Activities

It has been demonstrated that hapten-reactive helper T cells can be raised in mice by immunization with hapten-modified isologous mouse γ-globulin (5). These helper T cells collaborate with other hapten-specific B-lymphocytes on stimulation with isologous

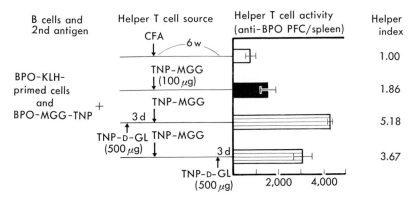

FIG. 1. Induction of TNP-reactive helper T cell activities by immunization with TNP-MGG and its amplification by TNP-D-GL treatment

Fifty $\times 10^6$ spleen cells from donor mice primed 10 weeks earlier with 100 μg of BPO-KLH in CFA were used as responding B cells, and transferred intravenously into 600 R, X-irradiated recipients together with spleen cells from either CFA-primed or TNP-MGG-primed mice. The TNP-MGG-primed mice had been immunized i.p. with 100 μg of TNP-MGG in CFA 6 weeks before the cell transfer with or without 500 μg of TNP-D-GL treatment. Secondary antigenic challenges were made by i.p. injection of 100 μg of BPO-MGG-TNP immediately after the cell transfer. Geometric means and standard error of anti-BPO-PFC responses in the spleen of the recipients 7 days after the cell transfer are illustrated.

mouse γ-globulin modified with double haptens of distinct specificities. Futhermore, under certain circumstances, the hapten-reactive helper T lymphocytes are rendered irreversibly unresponsive in a clonal fashion by treatment with nonimmunogenic hapten-D-glutamic acid-D-lysine (D-GL) copolymer (6).

We extended this hapten-reactive T lymphocyte system (8), and a system was established to enable us to detect simultaneoulsy both hapten-reactive helper and suppressor T cell activities in the above hapten-primed T cell population. The experimental system is as follows: Spleen cells from C3H/He mice immunized previously with 100 μg of TNP-MGG in complete Freund's adjuvant (CFA) or with 100 μg of benzylpenicilloyl-keyhole limpet hemocyanin (BPO-KLH) in CFA were the sources of TNP-reactive T cells and BPO-specific B cells, respectively. A mixture of spleen cells from TNP-MGG-primed and BPO-KLH-primed donors was adoptively transferred into 600 R X-irradiated syngeneic mice, and BPO-MGG-TNP or BPO-KLH-TNP was given as the stimulating antigen. As shown in Fig. 1, helper T cell activity was detected more stronger on stimulation with BPO-MGG-TNP by the greater anti-BPO antibody responses of BPO-specific B cells in the presence of TNP-MGG-primed spleen cells than in the presence of CFA-primed donor cells. On the other hands, as shown in Fig. 2, when BPO-KLH-primed cells were stimulated with 100 μg of BPO-KLH-TNP in the presence of TNP-MGG-primed cells, the anti-BPO antibody responses were significantly lower than those in the presence of CFA-primed cells. This suppressor cell effect was induced through the TNP-portion of BPO-KLH-TNP, since no suppression followed stimulation of BPO-KLH-primed cells

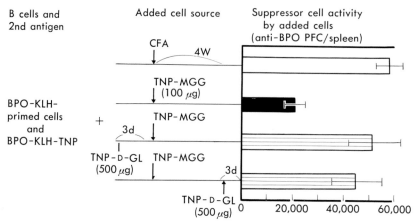

FIG. 2. Detection of TNP-reactive suppressor T cell activity in a TNP-MGG-primed cell population and its selective inactivation by TNP-D-GL treatment

The experimental protocol is essentially the same as in Fig. 1. Secondary antigenic challenge was performed with i.p. injection of 100 μg of BPO-KLH-TNP.

(in the presence of TNP-MGG-primed cells) with BPO-KLH (not conjugated with TNP, data not shown).

That the relevant cells in the TNP-MGG-primed cell population mediating the hapten-reactive helper and suppressor functions are T cells and not B cells, was indicated by the following two experimental results. First, TNP-MGG-primed spleen cells were depleted of B cells by treatment with an antiserum specific for antigens on the surface of mouse B cells, known as anti-Th-B (9). The almost complete reduction of B cell activity in the anti-Th-B-treated TNP-MGG-primed spleen cells contrasts sharply with the intact helper and suppressor cell activities. Secondly, the TNP-MGG-primed spleen cells were treated with either normal mouse serum (NMS) plus C or anti-Thy-1,2 antiserum plus component (C). Both helper and suppressor cell activities were almost completely abolished by treatment with anti-Thy-1,2 antiserum plus C (data not shown). Thus, helper and suppressor cell activities developed by immunization with TNP-MGG were both clearly mediated by Thy-1-positive T lymphocytes. Further analysis of the comparative properties of the hapten-reactive T cells revealed that the suppressor T cell activity compared with the helper activity a) develops earlier after priming, b) is more radiosensitive, and c) is distributed in separate lymphoid organs. Thus, suppressor T cells are mainly from the spleen, and helper T cells are more numerous in the mesenteric lymph nodes (8). These results indicate that the T cell population responsible for this hapten-reactive suppression is distinct from the helper T lymphocytes, and the above properties are consistent with the criteria of suppressor T cells having been reported by others in various experimental systems.

The most important observation during the course of such studies was the finding that hapten-reactive suppressor and helper T lymphocytes differ markedly in their respective susceptibilities to inactivation by exposure to the relevant hapten coupled to the non-immunogenic D-amino acid copolymer D-GL. The ability to selectively inactivate TNP-reactive suppressor T cell activity by TNP-D-GL treatment was also demonstrated by the type of experiment summarized in Figs. 1 and 2. The pretreatment of normal animals with 500 μg of TNP-D-GL 3 days prior to TNP-MGG-priming completely inhibited the development of TNP-reactive suppressor T cell activity. Likewise, the pretreatment of TNP-MGG-primed mice with TNP-D-GL, which had generated both TNP-reactive helper and suppressor T cells, also selectively abolished TNP-reactive suppressor T cell activities. In contrast to the inhibition of suppressor T cell activity, an increase in helper T cell activity was observed in both animals pretreated with TNP-D-GL. Taken collectively, these observations strongly indicate that hapten-reactive helper T cells develop or express their functions considerably more efficiently in the relative absence of hapten-reactive suppressor T cell activity.

Augmented Development of Tumor-specific Cytotoxic Killer T Lymphocytes in vivo by the Function of Hapten-reactive Amplifier T cells

Having established a reproducible system for the potent induction of hapten-reactive helper T lymphocytes in the mouse, we are now beginning to explore the feasibility of utilizing this helper T cell system to facilitate development of tumor-specific immunity. In our initial experiments, we have used TNP-modified mitomycin-attenuated X5563 cells and tested the capacity of recipient mice to develop tumor-specific cytotoxic T cells depending on whether or not such mice had been preimmunized to develop potent TNP-reactive helper T cell activities. One such experiment is summarized in Table I. C3H/He mice preimmunized with TNP-MGG 6 weeks prior to administration of TNP-conjugated tumor cells developed specific cytotoxic activity that was significantly higher than that observed in sham (CFA)-immunized control mice. Futhermore, this experiment also illustrates that the mice which had been immunized with TNP to develop more potent TNP-reactive helper T cell activities generated a striking magnitude of killer T cell activity as shown by the last two groups in Table I.

The obvious aim of this type of approach is to develop an effective method for substantially improving antitumor immunity of the host against the growth of syngeneic tumors. The following results indicate that it is possible to strikingly improve antitumor immunity by this method as reflected by the significant prolongation of host survival after inoculation of lethal viable tumor cells.

TABLE I.   Amplifing Effect of TNP-D-GL Treatment on the Generation of Killer
T Cells in the System of Hapten-TATA T-T Cell Interaction

| Exp. Group | Conditions for the generation of TNP-reactive helper T cells | | | Cytotoxic killer T cell generated[b] (%) |
	TNP-D-GL pretreatment prior to TNP-MGG-immunization (3 days)	Immunizations[a] (6 weeks duration)	TNP-D-GL treatment prior to the challenge with TNP-X5563 (3 days)	
I	None	CFA	None	0
II	None	TNP-MGG	None	8.4
III	500 μg TNP-D-GL	TNP-MGG	None	47.1
IV	None	TNP-MGG	500 μg TNP-D-GL	35.7

[a] C3H/He mice were immunized with 100 μg of TNP-MGG in CFA on day 0.

[b] Cytotoxic assay was done after 5 times i.p. challenges with 10^6 TNP-X5563 cells (MMC-treated) every 1 week, and the value represents % cytotoxity at a target effector ratio of 1 : 100.

TABLE II.   Amplifying Effect of Hapten-d-GL Pretreatment on the
Establishment of Tumor Specific Immunity[a]

| Exp. Group | C3H/He mice treated with | | | Hapten-derived tumor-immunization | Tumor growth on day[b] (μg myeloma protein/ml serum) | | Mean survival time (days) |
	TNP-d-GL pretreatment prior to TNP-MGG-immunization (3 days)	Hapten-priming	TNP-d-GL treatment prior to the challange with TNP-X5563		day 9	day 12	
1	None	CFA	None	TNP-X5563	1,228 (1.16)	3,512 (1.06)	17.8 ±0.70
2	None	TNP-MGG	None	TNP-X5563	1,424 (1.23)	5,099 (1.15)	16.3 ±1.02
3	500 μg TNP-d-GL	TNP-MGG	None	TNP-X5563	259 (1.18)	921 (1.28)	25.1 ±1.31
4	None	TNP-MGG	500 μg TNP-d-GL	TNP-X5563	1,224 (1.12)	3,187 (1.17)	17.0 ±1.34

[a] Experimental protocol is substantially the same as given in Table I, except that the mice were challenged intradermally with a lethal dose (10^6) of syngeneic tumor X5563 7 days after the last hapten modified tumor immunization.

[b] Tumor growth was quantitatively determined by the concentration of myeloma protein in serum, and this was measured by utilizing anti-idiotypic antibody to X5563 myeloma protein. The value denotes a geometric mean of 5-6 animals and the value in parentheses represents standard error.

These studies are summarized in Table II. Thus, sham (CFA)-immunized C3H/He mice failed to develop appreciable tumor-specific immune capability after immunization with TNP-coupled X5563 syngeneic tumor cells. On the other hand, the mice which had generated much potent TNP-reactive helper T cell activity before immunization with TNP-coupled X5563 displayed much higher levels of immune resistance against the challenge with viable tumor. Moreover, as shown by the mortality values of a comparable group summarized in Table II, mice subjected to this preimmunization regimen are also appreciably improved in terms of their capacity to resist tumor growth after inoculation of a lethal dose of such viable tumor cells. Other controversial observations were made in the animals pretreated with TNP-d-GL to TNP-MGG-primed mice 3 days before the commencement of TNP-tumor cell immunization to eliminate selectively the generated suppressor T cells in TNP-reactive T cell population. In this last group, the tumor-protecting activity was not appreciably augmented, compared with sham-immunized animals. The precise reason for this is not known at present, but one of the possibilities is that the affinity and specificity of TNP-reactive helper T cells generated in this condition is much lower than those generated in the absence of suppressors T cells (which was successfully accomplished by the TNP-d-GL pretreatment before TNP-MGG-immunization), and these TNP-reactive helper T cells of lower affinity may not be sufficient to augment the tumor-specific immunity efficient to protect animals from viable tumor challenge (7). At any rate, the above results clearly indicate that appropriate manipulations designed to induce potent hapten-reactive T lymphocytes provide a very effective mode of immunopotentiation against tumors.

Preventive Effect of Hapten-reactive Helper T Lymphocytes on the Tolerance Induction of Prekiller T Lymphocytes by the Presence of an Inappropriate form of TATA

The obvious goal of the application of hapten-reactive T cell activity to the tumor system is to develop an effective mode of immunotherapy to substantially improve antitumor immunity of the host against established growing tumors. For example, if one wishes to induce effective host resistance against an established tumor in this system, one approach would be to attempt to preimmunize an individual with hapten-conjugated autologous protein in conjunction with appropriate pretreatment with the relevant hapten-D-GL copolymer, followed at some later period by immunization of the individual with hapten-coupled attenuated tumor cells. Such tumor cells can either be obtained by surgical extirpation in the case of solid tumors or from peripheral blood in the case of leukemias; alternatively, hapten coupling can be accomplished by *in situ* conjugation by direct exposure of a given tumor to reactive chemicals. As demonstrated in our experiments described in earlier sections, the hapten-specific T cells induced by previous immunization in this manner facilitated the development of tumor-specific cytotoxic T lymphocytes or other forms of relevant effector mechanisms and thus resulted in tumor rejection.

However, our further preliminary experiments to demonstrate the above hapten-reactive helper T cell system to suppress the established tumor so far have been unsuccessful. One of the reasons for these frustrating results may be that the development of potent antitumor cytotoxic T lymphocytes is significantly depressed in the later

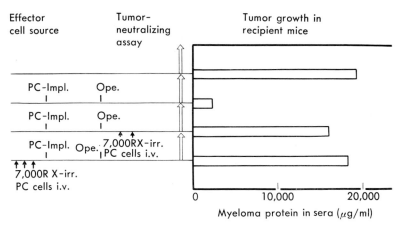

Fig. 3. Tolerance induction of prekiller T lymphocytes by administration of an inappropriate form of TATA

For immunization of the host with TATA, 10^7 of viable X5563 tumor cells were intradermally inoculated and surgically extirpated 7 days later. For the tolerance induction of the host to TATA, 10^7 of 7,000 R, X-irradiated tumor cells were given intravenously 3 times over consecutive 2-day intervals, either immediately after the surgical extirpation of tumor or before viable tumor implantation for the immunization. Two weeks after the surgical operation, the tumor-neutralizing activity of the spleen cells from respective groups was tested by mixing with 10^6 of viable tumor cells and transfered i.p. into another group of recipient mice.

stage of tumor-bearing animals, and that one of the mechanisms of this depression may be the presence of a large quantity of tumor antigen derived from the tumor mass. As a matter of fact, in the X5563 system, the immune capability of the cells from tumor-bearing mice to prevent tumor growth was strikingly suppressed, as tested by their tumor-neutralizing activity *in vivo*, and induction of this suppression of the tumor-bearing state could be successfully inhibited by the complete surgical removal of the tumor (*3*). Moreover, the specific immunosuppression observed in the tumor-bearing animals could also be induced by consecutive intravenous administrations of heavily (7,000 R) X-irradiated tumor cells, which were completely attenuated and did not induce a tumor in the host after implantation. The suppressive effect of such tumor antigen administration on the subsequent development of antitumor immunity is shown in Fig. 3. In this experiment, intradermal tumor-implantation followed by the surgical extirpation of the tumor 7 days later was utilized as the effective immunization procedure of the host with TATA. As evident from Fig. 3, consecutive intravenous treatments of the host with completely attenuated tumor cells either immediately after surgical extirpation of the tumor or before viable tumor implantation for immunization, completely suppressed the subsequent development of effective antitumor immunity, as revealed by the tumor-neutralization activity of the host lymphoid cells (Fig. 3) as well as by the direct challenge of the host with viable tumor cells (data not shown).

Another detailed analysis of the underlying mechanism for this tumor-specific immunosuppression revealed that clonal deletion of TATA-specific prekiller T lymphocytes was induced by such treatment. This conclusion was derived from the following observations.* (1) Besides the negative tumor-neutralizing activities of the cells from such a pretreated host, the cells failed to confer any effective tumor immunity on the host even when transferred into other X-irradiated recipients. (2) Such a failure to induce effective tumor immunity was not ascribed to the generation of suppressor cell activity as tested by mixed-type experiments. (3) The failure to induce tumor immunity by such lymphoid cells or the absence of suppressor cell activity did not revert to positive even after surface treatment of lymphoid cells with papain or trypsin *in vitro*. Thus, the pre- or coexistence of inappropriate forms of TATA inhibits the subsequent induction of antitumor immunity by the clonal deletion mechanisms of T cells responsible for conferring effective tumor resistance on the host, and this suppressive mechanism may be operating in the specific immunosuppression of tumor-bearing animals.

Based on the above consideration, we next explored the feasibility of the utilization of the hapten-reactive helper T lymphocyte system in the prevention of this type of tolerance induction of T cell lineage. If one can prevent T cell tolerance induced by the presence of an inappropriate form of TATA with hapten-reactive helper T cell activities, this approach may provide some premise for the circumvention of TATA-specific immunodepression frequently observed in tumor-bearing animals. In addition, the aforementioned line of approach by the hapten-reactive helper T cell system may be potentially applicable to the suppression of the established tumors. Precise details of the experimental protocol to demonstrate the potent preventive activity of hapten-

---

* Fujiwara, H., Tsuchida, T., Mizuochi, T., Kohmo, T. and Hamaoka, T. Unresponsiveness in effector T cell clones against tumor specific transplantation antigens. I. The mechanism of unresponsiveness induced by intravenous presensitization with X-irradiated tumor cells (Submitted for publication).

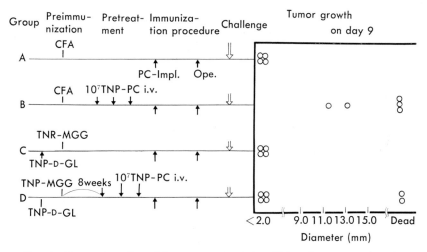

FIG. 4. Preventive effect of hapten-reactive helper T lymphocytes on the tolerance induction of the host to TATA

TNP-modified and 7,000 R X-irradiated X5563 tumor cells (10^7) were injected intravenously to induce TATA-specific tolerance. The protocols for TNP-MGG-immunization and tumor immunization were substantially the same as in Figs. 1 and 3. Ten days after the surgical operation, 10^6 viable tumor cells were challenged intradermally, and the sizes of tumor growth on day 9 were measured.

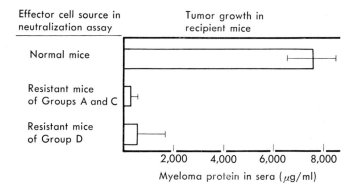

FIG. 5. Potent tumor-neutralizing activity of lymphoid cells from the animals that escaped from tolerance induction by hapten-reactive helper T cell activity

Five$\times 10^7$ spleen cells from each corresponding group of mice in Fig. 4 were individually mixed with 10^6 of viable tumor cells on day 14 after the tumor challenge, and submitted to tumor-neutralizing assay by transferring them intraperitoneally into other recipient mice. Tumor growth in recipient mice on day 10 is depicted.

reactive helper T cells for tolerance induction of T cells by TATA are given in Fig. 4.

In this experiment, as shown in Group B 10^7 of 7,000 R X-irradiated tumor cells with TNP-derivatization had been given intravenously to inhibit the subsequent development of antitumor immunity in the host. For immunization, hosts were intradermally inoculated with the tumor and subsequently the tumor was extirpated. In these experimental conditions, the generation of potent TNP-reactive helper T lymphocyte activity in group D, by preimmunization with TNP-MGG in conjunction with TNP-D-GL, resulted in the effective prevention of tolerance induction of host killer T cell lineage; a considerable number of the animals survived after the challenge with viable tumor cells. This sharply contrasted with the immune capability of group B animals, in all of whom the challenged tumors progressively grew, as in nonimmune animals. Consistent with the above immune resistance of the host against the challenged tumor, the development of tumor-neutralizing activity in the spleen of the resistant mice of group D was comparable to that of groups A and C. Further analysis of the nonresistant mice of group B and of a part of group D revealed that the predominant outgrowth of metastasized tumors in the spleen was observed in all the animals, and that this was caused by the failure to develop neutralizing activity in the spleen in these immuno-suppressed animals.

All these results clearly indicate that appropriate manipulations designed to induce hapten-reactive helper T cell activity successfully augmented the development of host antitumor immunity and provided a potentially effective mode of immunotherapy against tumor cells. We are now further extending this system to the analysis of tumor tissues in a variety of mouse strains, and of representative tissue origins, to fully establish the feasibility of this approach for eventually inducing effective *de novo* antitumor immunity in animals harboring established autochthonous tumors.

Finally, it should be pointed out that although we assume that a major mechanism of antitumor immunity developed in such systems will involve the function of cytotoxic T lymphocytes, it is also possible that hapten-reactive helper T cells may, in some instances, promote the development of antitumor antibodies that could exert either protective or deleterious effect on the host's resistance to tumor growth. Therefore, all of the forthcoming studies should include routine screening procedures for the presence of such antibodies and, if found, the role they may play in the host's tumor resistance should be ascertained.

REFERENCES

1. Canter, H. and Boyse, E. A. Functional subclasses of T lymphocytes bearing different Ly antigens. I. The generation of functionally distinct T-cell subclasses in a differentiative process independent of antigen. *J. Exp. Med.*, **141**, 1376–1389 (1975).
2. Cantor, H. and Boyse, E. A. Functional subclasses of T lymphocytes bearing different Ly antigen. II. Cooperation between subclasses of Ly^+ cells in the generation of killer activity. *J. Exp. Med.*, **141**, 1390–1399 (1975).
3. Fujiwara, H., Hamaoka, T., Nishino, Y., and Kitagawa, M. Inhibitory effects of tumor-bearing state on the generation of *in vivo* protective immune T cells in a syngeneic murine tumor system. *Gann*, **68**, 589–601 (1977).
4. Fujiwara, H., Hamaoka, T., Teshima, K., Aoki, H., and Kitagawa, M. Preferential generation of killer or helper T-lymphocyte activity directed to the tumor-associated transplantation antigens. *Immunology*, **31**, 239–248 (1976).
5. Hamaoka, T., Inada, T., Yamashita, U., and Kitagawa, M. Preventive effect of hapten-reactive thymus-derived helper lymphocytes on the tolerance induction in hapten-specific precursors of antibody forming cells. *J. Immunol.*, **114**, 676–683 (1975).
6. Hamaoka, T., Yamashita, U., Takami, T., and Kitagawa, M. The mechanism of tolerance induction in thymus-derived lymphocytes. I. Intracellular inactivation of hapten-reac-

tive helper T lymphocytes by hapten-nonimmunogenic copolymer of D-amino acids. *J. Exp. Med.*, **141**, 1308–1328 (1975).

7. Hamaoka, T., Yoshizawa, M., Yamamoto, H., Kuroki, M., and Kitagawa, M. Regulatory functions of hapten-reactive helper and suppressor T lymphocytes. II. Selective inactivation of hapten-reactive suppressor T cells by hapten-nonimmunogenic copolymers of D-amino acids and its application to the study of suppressor T-cell effect on helper T-cell development. *J. Exp. Med.*, **146**, 91–106 (1977).

8. Yamamoto, H., Hamaoka, T., Yoshizawa, M., Kuroki, M., and Kitagawa, M. Regulatory functions of hapten-reactive helper and suppressor T lymphocytes. I. Detection and characterization of hapten-reactive suppressor T-cell activity in mice immunized with hapten-isologous protein conjugate. *J. Exp. Med.*, **146**, 74–90 (1977).

9. Yutoku, M., Grossberg, A. L., Stout, R., Herzenberg, L. A., and Pressman, D. Further studies on Th-B, a cell surface antigenic determinant present on mouse B cells, plasma cell and immature thymocytes. *Cell. Immunol.*, **23**, 140–157 (1976).

GANN Monograph on Cancer Research 23, 1979

DIRECT AND LIPOSOME-MEDIATED INTRODUCTION OF A FLUORESCENT HAPTEN AND A HAPTEN-CONJUGATED PROTEIN INTO TUMOR CELL MEMBRANE, AND INDUCTION OF TUMOR-SPECIFIC TRANSPLANTATION IMMUNITY WITH THE HAPTEN-CONJUGATED TUMOR CELLS

Yoshiyuki HASHIMOTO,[*1] Banri YAMANOHA,[*2] Hiroo ENDOH,[*1]
and Taiko ISHIZUKA[*1]

Pharmaceutical Institute, Tohoku University[*1] *and*
Tokyo Biochemical Research Institute[*2]

Modification of tumor cell membranes was carried out by the direct reaction of a fluorescent chemical, 5-dimethylamino-naphthalene-1-sulfonyl (dansyl) chloride, or by fusion of liposomes conjugated with a dansyl group or dansyl-bound protein.

A dansyl group was effectively introduced into the cell membrane by the use of a water-soluble dansyl chloride-cyclohepta-amylose complex without destroying the tumor cells. Transplantation immunity against EL4 leukemia cells was induced by intraperitoneal injections of dansyl-conjugated EL4 cells in syngeneic C57BL/6 mice. Although serum and spleen cells of the mice immunized with dansyl-conjugated EL4 cells and EL4 cells were cytotoxic against both EL4 cells and dansyl-conjugated EL4 cells, neither were cytotoxic to dansyl-conjugated allogeneic leukemia cells.

A dansyl group or dansyl-bound protein was introduced into tumor cell membranes by incubation of tumor cells with liposomes conjugated with the reagent. The incorporation of the reagent into the cell membranes was shown by fluorescence microscopy and by complement-dependent lysis of the tumor cells with anti-dansyl or anti-protein antibody.

The presence of an antigen which is specific for a tumor and responsible for host-mediated immunological rejection has been widely demonstrated in variety of experimental tumors. For such tumors, immunotherapy has been found to be successful. However, the degree of immunogenicity of many animal and human tumors is not always high enough to respond to immunotherapy. Therefore, modification of tumor cells with an alien substance has been attempted in order to give the tumor such immunogenicity as to induce host immunity not only to the modified antigen but also to the tumor-associated antigen.

[*1] Aramaki, Sendai 980, Japan (橋本嘉幸, 遠藤弘郎, 石塚泰子).
[*2] Takada 3-41-8, Toshima-ku, Tokyo 171, Japan (山之端万里).

Modification of tumor cell surface antigen has been accomplished either with viruses or chemicals. Chemical modification of tumor cells, carried out usually by the direct reaction of a chemical with tumor cells, results in a covalent binding of the chemical to the tumor cells, and the chemical may act as a hapten in the immunological reactions (2, 9, 12, 13). For obtaining chemically-modified tumor cells applicable to immunological studies, it is desirable that the chemical does not reduce the immunogenicity of the tumor-associated antigen. In order to introduce a substance into the tumor cell membrane, liposomes, vesicles of an artificial lipid membrane, can be used alternatively, by taking advantage of fusion of hapten-conjugated or protein-incorporated liposomes with the plasma membrane of the viable cells (6, 11).

This paper describes 1) the introduction of a fluorescent chemical, 1-dimethylaminonaphthalene-5-sulfonyl group (dansyl group) into tumor cell membranes and the application of dansyl-conjugated tumor cells for the induction of tumor transplantation immunity against syngeneic tumor cells, and 2) preliminary studies on the introduction of a dansyl group or dansyl-conjugated protein into tumor cell membranes by using liposomes.

Tumor cells used in the present experiments were EL4 leukemia cells of C57BL/6 mouse origin, RADA1 leukemia cells of A mouse origin, Meth-A sarcoma cells of BALB/c mouse origin. These tumors were donated by the Sloan Kettering Institute for Cancer Research, New York, and have been serially passed in the corresponding syngeneic mice. A rat ascites tumor, Yoshida sarcoma, also was used.

Introduction of a Dansyl Group into Tumor Cells (7)

Dansyl chloride, which originally is hardly soluble in water, was altered to a water-soluble form by treatment with an aqueous solution of cyclohepta-amylose according to the method of Kinoshita et al. (8). A saturated aqueous solution of dansyl chloride-cyclohepta-amylose complex (CDC) containing 84 μg/ml dansyl chloride was serially diluted with water. To nine volumes quantity of tumor cell suspension containing $1-5 \times 10^6$ cells/ml of pH 7.4 isotonic phosphate buffered saline, one volume of CDC solution was added and the suspension was kept for 30 min at 22° with stirring, and the washed cells were used for experiments. By treatment with CDC solution, tumor cells and normal lymphoid cells, but not erythrocytes, reacted with dansyl chloride. As shown in Table I, fractionation of the homogenate of dansyl-conjugated EL4 leu-

TABLE I.   Distribution of Fluorescence Quantum in Subfraction
of Dansyl-conjugated EL4 Cells

Fraction	Fluorescence[b] (I_{FL} dansyl/μg protein)
Homogenate	1.07
Supernatant	0.62
Pellet[a]	2.14
Plasma membrane	2.18
Vesicles	1.25
Nucleus	1.41

[a] Pellet fraction was fractionated by centrifugation in sucrose density gradient solution.
[b] I_{FL}, Arbitrary unit of fluorescence intensity.

kemia cells revealed that dansyl chloride was highly reactive with the plasma membrane and less reactive with cytoplasm, subcellular vesicles and nuclei. A cytotoxicity test with antidansyl-KLH serum raised in a rabbit, and the activity determined by immuno-precipitation and by fluorescence enhancement of dansyl-lysine, resulted in the lysis of dansyl-conjugated RADA1 leukemia and Meth-A sarcoma cells in the presence of guinea pig complement, indicating the dansyl group bound to a tumor cell membrane was functioning as a hapten.

Induction of Transplantation Immunity by Dansyl-conjugated EL4 Leukemia Cells to Syngeneic Mouse (7)

Male C57BL/6 mice were immunized by intraperitoneal injections of dansyl-conjugated EL4 leukemia cells. When mice were injected with EL4 cells, which had been treated with CDC whose concentration in the reaction mixture was 1/20 to 1/80 of saturated CDC solution, many mice survived, rejecting the tumor. However, mice that received EL4 cells untreated or treated with 1:160 diluted CDC died of tumor growth (Table II). Nearly all the mice that survived from the injection of dansyl-conjugated EL4 cells rejected the subsequently challenged untreated EL4 cells, indicating that these mice acquired transplantation immunity against the syngeneic EL4 leukemia cells. Similar to dansyl-conjugated EL4 cells in the syngeneic mouse, dansyl-conjugated Yoshida sarcoma cells induced transplantation immunity in Donryu rats against untreated Yoshida sarcoma cells. In this case, it required a higher concentration of CDC to obtain immune rats than that to EL4 cells (7).

In order to see whether immunization with dansyl-conjugated tumor cells induced cytotoxic serum or lymphocytes specific for the dansyl group, we investigated the cytotoxicity of serum and spleen cells obtained from mice which had been repeatedly immunized with dansyl-conjugated EL4 and EL4 or with dansyl-conjugated EL4 alone. Serum from the former mice showed cytotoxicity against EL4 cells as well as to dansyl-conjugated EL4 cells in the presence of the complement, but not to untreated or dansyl-conjugated allogeneic leukemia cells (Table III). Similarly, spleen cells of EL4-immune mice were cytotoxic both to EL4 and dansyl-conjugated EL4 cells but not to untreated or dansyl-conjugated allogeneic leukemia cells. Neither the serum nor

TABLE II. Immunization Effect of Dansyl-conjugated EL4 Leukemia Cells in C57BL/6 Mice Syngeneic to the Tumor

Dilution of CDC[a]	No. of survivors/test with successive injection of[b]				
	DNS-EL4		EL4		
	10^6	5×10^6	10^5	10^6	10^7
1/20	10/10	6/10	6/6	6/6	6/6
1/40	10/10	6/10	6/6	6/6	6/6
1/80	6/10	3/6	3/3	3/3	3/3
1/160	0/10				
Control[c]	0/5	0/5	0/2	0/2	0/2

[a] Dilution of CDC in the cell suspension for treating to saturated CDC solution.
[b] Cells were injected successively at 3-week intervals. DNS, Dansyl-conjugated.
[c] Mice received the same number of untreated EL4 cells each time as the experimental animals.

TABLE III. Cytotoxicity of Serum and Spleen Cells from C57BL/6 Mice Immune
to Dansyl-conjugated and Untreated EL4 Leukemia Cells

Donors of serum and spleen cells[a]	Target cells[b]			
	EL4	DNS-EL4	RADA1	DNS-RADA1
Cytotoxicity of serum (titer)				
DNS-EL4 and EL4 immune	1/8	1/16	>1/4	>1/4
DNS-EL4 immune	>1/4	>1/4	>1/4	>1/4
Cytotoxicity of spleen cells (% lysis)				
DNS-EL4 and EL4 immune	33.6	58.0	−16.6	−5.8
DNS-EL4 immune	−5.4	4.8	−0.6	−5.8

[a] D NS-EL4 and EL4 immune: Mice were immunized with DNS-EL4 (10^6 and EL4 cells (10^5, 10^6, and 5×10^7). DNS-EL4 immune: Mice were immunized with DNS-EL4 cells (10^6, 10^7, and 5×10^7). Sera and spleen cells were obtained 7 days after the last immunization.
[b] Dansylation of target leukemia cells was carried out at 22° for 30 min with 1 : 80 diluted CDC solution.
[c] Cytotoxicity test of the serum was performed by the semi-micromethod using 1 : 3 diluted fresh guinea pig serum as complement.
[d] Cytotoxicity of spleen cells was determined by the ^{3}H-uridine method. Target cells were incubated with 5-fold spleen cells for 18 hr at 37°.

spleen cells from mice which had been immunized with dansyl-conjugated EL4 alone were cytotoxic to any test cells.

From these results, two possibilities are likely for the mechanism of induction of transplantation immunity with dansyl-conjugated tumor cells: 1) The dansyl group acts as a hapten and augments the production of hapten-specific helper T cells which help the induction of antibody or cytotoxic lymphoid cells specific for the tumor-associated antigen and thus induce an effective immunity to the untreated tumor cells and 2) dansyl modification may merely attenuate tumor cells and inhibit their growth in the recipient animal. Transplantation immunity in the mouse is induced by these attenuated tumor cells.

Introduction of a Dansyl Group into Tumor Cells through the Aid of Liposomes (3)

As an alternative method for introducing a substance into a cell membrane, liposomes can be used (6, 11). We prepared liposomes from a 1 : 1 mixture of phosphatidylcholine and dansyl-conjugated phosphatidylethanolamine by a method similar to that reported by Uemura and Kinsky (14). Presence of the dansyl group on the liposome membrane was proved by fluorescence microscopy and aggulutination of the liposomes to anti-dansyl-KLH antibody as well as by release of ^{14}C-glucose included in the liposomes with the antibody and complement. The extent of the agglutination was quantitatively determined using ^{14}C-labeled liposomes by trapping the agglutinated liposomes on a glass fiber filter paper.

In order to fused the liposomes with tumor cells, sonicated dansyl-conjugated liposomes (10^8 vesicles to a tumor cell) were incubated with tumor cells suspended in pH 7.4 phosphate-buffered saline containing 5% fetal calf serum for 45 to 60 min at 37°. The tumor cells treated with the liposomes showed fluorescence mainly at the plasma membrane and they were sensitive to agglutination and to complement-dependent cytolysis with anti-dansyl-KLH serum. This suggests the presence of a dansyl group on the cell membrane.

Introduction of Dansyl-conjugated Bovine Serum Albumin (BSA) into Tumor Cell Membrane (4)

Introduction of a protein into liposomes has been attempted in several ways (1, 5). We prepared liposomes conjugated with dansyl-conjugated bovine serum albumin (BSA) by the treatment of phosphatidylethanolamine-phosphatidylcholine liposomes with toluene-2,4-diisocyanate, followed by dansyl-conjugated BSA according to the method of Mahan and Copeland (10) for the preparation of antigen-conjugated erythrocytes. These liposomes were agglutinated by the addition of anti-BSA serum or with anti-dansyl-KLH serum (Fig. 1), and were also sensitive to complement-dependent ^{14}C-glucose release (Fig. 2), suggesting the presence of dansyl-conjugated BSA on the liposome surface. Fusion of the dansyl-BSA-conjugated liposomes with Meth-A sarcoma cells by a method similar to the above, resulted in the introduction of dansyl-BSA into tumor cell membranes. The treated tumor cells were destroyed with anti-BSA serum and complement.

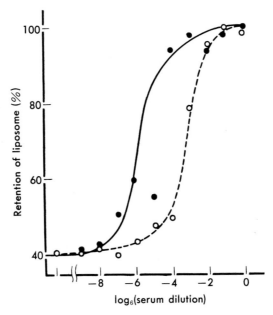

FIG. 1. Agglutination of dansyl-BSA-conjugated liposomes with anti-dansyl-KLH serum and anti-BSA serum

^{3}H-labeled liposomes conjugated with dansyl-conjugated BSA were incubated with antiserum for 60 min at 37°. The reaction mixture was filtered through a glass fiber paper, and the retained radioactivity was determined as an indication of agglutination. ● anti-BSA; ○ anti-DNS.

Y. HASHIMOTO ET AL.

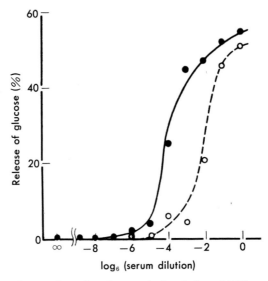

FIG. 2. Complement-dependent immunolysis of dansyl-BSA-conjugated liposomes

Dansyl-BSA-conjugated liposomes including ^{14}C-glucose in the vesicle were treated as given in Fig. 1, in the presence of a guinea pig serum. The mixture was filtered with a Millipore filter (0.22 μm pore size), and the retained radioactivity was measured as an indication of the release of glucose from the liposomes. ● anti-BSA; ○ anti-DNS.

CONCLUSION

The present paper reported that 1) viable tumor cells can be labeled with a fluorescent dansyl group by the use of a water-soluble dansyl chloride-cyclic sugar complex and that transplantation immunity against the syngeneic tumor can be induced by dansyl-conjugated tumor cells. However, neither immune serum nor immune lymphoid cells specific for the dansyl group were induced in the animals immunized with dansyl-conjugated tumor cells. 2) Chemical substances as well as proteins can be introduced into a tumor cell membrane by the aid of liposomes.

The application of these chemically-modified liposomes and tumor cells for immunotherapy and for basic immunological reactions are currently being investigated.

Acknowledgment

This work was supported in part by Grant-in-Aid for Cancer Research from the Ministry of Education, Science and Culture.

REFERENCES

1. Curman, B., Östberg, L., and Peterson, P. A. Incorporation of murine MHC antigens into liposomes and their effect in the secondary mixed lymphocyte reaction. *Nature*, **272**, 545–547 (1978).
2. Dennert, G. and Halten, L. E. Induction and properties of cytotoxic T cells specific for hapten-coupled tumor cells. *J. Immunol.*, **114**, 1705–1712 (1975).

3. Endoh, H., Kawashima, Y., Suzuki, Y., and Hashimoto, Y. Quantitative determination of immunological agglutination of hapten-coupled liposomes. *Abstr. 98th Annu. Meet., Pharm. Soc. Jpn.*, p. 87 (1978) (in Japanese).

4. Endoh, H., Suzuki, Y., and Hashimoto, Y. Unpublished data.

5. Gergoriadis, G. and Neerujun, E. D. Comparative effect and fate of non-entrapped and liposome-entrapped neuraminidase injected into rats. *Biochem. J.* **140**, 323–330 (1974).

6. Gregoriadis, G. and Neerunjun, E. D. Homing of liposomes to target cells. *Biochem. Biophys. Res. Commun.*, **61**, 537–544 (1975).

7. Hashimoto, Y. and Yamanoha, B. Induction of transplantation immunity by dansylated tumor cells. *Gann*, **67**, 315–319 (1976).

8. Kinoshita, T., Iinuma, F., and Tsuji, A. Fluorescent labeling of proteins and a plasma membrane using cyclohepta-amylose-dansyl chloride complex. *Anal. Biochem.*, **61**, 632–637 (1974).

9. Koren, H. S., Wunderlich, J. R., and Inmer, J. K. T cell menory for the cytotoxic response to hapten-modified target cells. *J. Immunol.*, **116**, 403–408 (1976).

10. Mahan, D. E. and Copeland, R. L. Method using toluene-2,4-diisocyanate and glutaraldehyde to stabilize and conjugate antigens to erythrocytes for use in passive hemagglutination test. *J. Immunol. Methods*, **19**, 217–226 (1978).

11. Martin, F. J. and Macdonald, R. C. Lipid vesicle-cell interactions III. Introduction of a new antigenic determinant into erythrocyte membrane. *J. Cell Biol.*, **70**, 515–526 (1976).

12. Parker, C. W., Yoo, T. J., Johnson, M. C., and Codt, S. M. Fluorescent probes for the study of the antibody-hapten reaction. I. Binding of the 5-dimethylaminonaphthalene-1-sulfonamide group by homologous rabbit antibody. *Biochemistry*, **6**, 3408–3416 (1976).

13. Shearer, G. M., Rhen, T. G., and Garearino, C. A. Cell-mediated lymphocytolysis of trinitrophenyl-modified autologous lymphocytes. Effector cell specificity to modified cell surface components controlled by H-2K and H-2D serological regions of the major histocompatibility complex. *J. Exp. Med.*, **141**, 1348–13 (1975).

14. Uemura, K. and Kinsky, S. Active *vs.* passive sensitization of liposomes towards antibody and complement by dinitrophenylated derivatives of phosphatidylethanolamine. *Biochemistry*, **22**, 4085–4095 (1972).

GANN Monograph on Cancer Research 23, 1979

IMMUNOPROPHYLAXIS AND THERAPY WITH LIPID CONJUGATED LYMPHOMA CELLS

Morton D. Prager and William C. Gordon

Departments of Surgery and Biochemistry, University of Texas Health Science Center*

Dimethyldioctadecylammonium bromide (DDA) was selected as an agent for antigen modification because of the possibility of complexing the lipophilic cation with negatively charged lymphoma cells. Increasing the lipid content of certain antigens led to cellular responses to native antigen without a concomitant humoral response, a result of potential value in cancer immunotherapy. Lymphoma cells were first modified by reaction with iodoacetamide (IAd). Immunoprophylaxis with four different syngeneic mouse lymphoma systems was examined using suboptimal immunization to facilitate evaluation of DDA. In groups challenged after vaccination with IAd-lymphoma cells with DDA there were 71% survivors compared to 29% for mice similarly vaccinated without DDA. The enhanced protection was dependent on DDA dosage and was most striking when DDA was complexed to the modified tumor cells. DDA also enhanced response to antigen prepared by sonication of P1798 cells, especially at low antigen dose. With sheep erythrocytes (SRBC) as a non-proliferating particulate antigen, DDA increased both cellular and humoral responses, again particularly at low SRBC dose. Giving DDA prior to SRBC especially stimulated a humoral response. Macrophages are activated by DDA and presumably contribute to the heightened immune responses. In therapy experiments BALB/c mice bearing P1798 were treated with methotrexate (MTX) followed by immunotherapy with IAd-P1798 alone or complexed to DDA. With 1, 2, and 3 cycles of treatment, MTX alone yielded 0, 5, and 13% survivors, respectively, while adding immunotherapy with the DDA complex produced survival rates of 38 (with 2 immunotherapeutic injections), 63, and 71%. Chemoimmunotherapy in the absence of DDA produced intermediate results. In the absence of antigen, DDA was ineffective in either immunoprophylaxis or therapy.

A rational basis for cancer immunotherapy derives from several critical observations. 1) Antigens not demonstrable in normal adult tissue are often found in tumors. 2) The host frequently responds immunologically against its tumor-associated antigens (TAA). 3) Host immune competence relates, albeit imperfectly, to prognosis. 4) Immunologically mediated resistance to tumor growth can be induced. In contrast to chemotherapy and radiotherapy, the number of malignant cells which can be handled by the immune system seems rather small. Nevertheless the two former therapeutic modalities in exhibiting first-order kinetics with respect to cell kill theoretically will

* Dallas, Texas 75235, U.S.A.

leave a residuum of malignant cells, a limitation that does not apply to immunological destruction. These considerations have led to exploration of chemoimmunotherapy in experimental models using specific TAA for immunological stimulation.

The question of how to present TAA to a syngeneic host is a major one. Many studies have utilized X-irradiated tumor cells which retain immunogenicity while exhibiting reduced growth capacity. Chemical modification of malignant cells has also been extensively explored (14) and adds a dimension of increased foreignness which can lead to immunological response in an otherwise minimally responsive tumor-host system (15). Despite the widespread use of irradiated cells for immunization, chemically modified malignant cells were more immunogenic for several syngeneic tumor-host systems (1, 10, 13, 18). However, it should be noted that by overtreatment cells may lose capacity to protect against subsequent tumor implants. Solubilized TAA may also be used for immunization without the accompanying concern of producing tumors (8). Aggregated or otherwise high molecular weight TAA may induce stronger anti-tumor responses with decreased risk of producing immunologic enhancement of tumor growth, but more information on this point would be welcome.

In prior studies in this laboratory, mouse lymphoma cells treated with iodoacet-amide (IAd) have been favored for immunization because of their effectiveness and ease of preparation and use (13, 17). Although the ease of achieving resistance varies with the tumor-host system, IAd-modified lymphoma cells were successfully used to immunize C3H mice to 6C3HED lymphoma, BALB/c to P1798, DBA/2 to L1210, and A/Sn to YAC. Recent studies have been directed toward increasing the lipoidal character of the IAd-lymphoma cells (16) because of observations that immunization with protein antigens acylated with long-chain fatty acids gave delayed hypersensitivity (DH) responses to the native antigen but little or no antibody (4–6). A reason for at-tempting to achieve this response pattern to TAA comes from observations of im-munosuppression by antigen-antibody complexes. Obviously such complexes cannot form in the absence of antibody. There are also reports of selective induction of delayed hypersensitivity responses to acetoacetylated antigens prepared by diketene treatment; these include soluble and cellular antigens including TAA (3, 11, 12). It may be argued that acetoacetylation also increases the lipoidal nature of the antigens. However, since carboxymethylation of lysozyme, which cannot be considered a lipophilic modification, also leads primarily to cell-mediated immunity (20), lipid cannot be the only factor influencing this selectivity. An alternate view is that good inducers of cellular immunity may be small antigens or larger molecules that are sparse in determinants (2), and modification may act to decrease the number of determinants perceived by the host.

Effects of DDA on the Immune System

To investigate the effect on immunogenicity of increasing the lipoidal character of a particulate, but non-proliferating, antigen, sheep erythrocytes (SRBC) were treated with dimethyldioctadecylammonium bromide (DDA). It was anticipated that the posi-tively charged lipid cation would interact with sufficient strength with the negatively charged cell surface to lend stability to a complex. When 10^8 SRBC were exposed to 0.2 μmol DDA for 5 min at 37°C and then washed to remove excess, they bound to an adherent layer of macrophages more avidly than untreated cells. Many remained

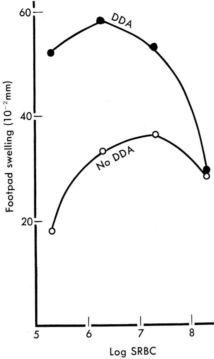

FIG. 1.   Effect of DDA on delayed hypersensitivity response to SRBC
    BALB/c mice were injected i.p. with SRBC (○) or SRBC mixed with 0.2 μmol
DDA (●) on day 0. SRBC (10^8) were injected into the left rear footpad on day 5
and 24 hr footpad swelling was determined. Data points represent the average of
two mice.

tightly bound even after jetting the preparations in a stream of saline. The effect of
DDA on a DH response was determined by the footpad swelling assay and on antibody
response by measuring splenic plaque-forming cells (PFC) by the Jerne technique.
To evaluate the effect on delayed hypersensitivity, varying numbers of SRBC were
injected i.p. either without or with 0.2 μmol DDA on day 0; on day 5 a challenge dose
of 10^8 SRBC was injected into the footpad, and 24 hr later foot thickness was measured
with calipers. With a marginal amount of antigen for DH (2×10^5 SRBC), DDA increased swelling over 2 fold, but as antigen dose increased to 2×10^8 SRBC, the DDA
effect diminished as did the DH response (Fig. 1). The PFC response was evaluated
on day 4 after i.p. injection of varying numbers of SRBC. With large sensitizing doses
of 2×10^8 and 2×10^9 SRBC, simultaneous administration of 0.2–0.4 μmol DDA had
only a modest effect, increasing PFC 1.2–1.5 times. A more pronounced effect was
again observed with numbers of SRBC ($2–5 \times 10^7$) marginal for a PFC response, the
increase being 5–11 fold. Several experiments were performed in which DDA was
injected i.p. 4 hr prior to SRBC (also i.p.) instead of being mixed with antigen. While
the DH response to 2×10^7 SRBC remained about the same, *i.e.*, about a 2-fold increase,
the humoral response was markedly increased from 23-fold to as much as 95 times in
one experiment. Approximately equivalent results were obtained when DDA was
incubated with SRBC for 30 min at 25° or for 5 min at 37°. However, prolonged in-

cubation for 60 min at 37° led to reduction of both cellular and humoral responses. Under the latter conditions there was substantial lysis of the SRBC suggesting that in addition to its stimulatory activity part of the DDA effect on the immune response may involve altering the effective antigen concentration (perhaps even under conditions not giving obvious lysis). The latter effect could contribute to the difference in PFC response when SRBC and DDA were given separately (4 hr apart) compared to that when they were mixed prior to administration. Although these studies clearly indicate that DDA enhances immune responses to SRBC, especially at low antigen dose, they do not demonstrate selective induction of delayed hypersensitivity.

Other studies were concerned with effects of DDA on the host. Between days 2 and 4 after i.p. injection of 0.2–0.4 μmol DDA, the number of cells recoverable from the peritoneum increased 3 fold. On day 1, when cell number had increased 2.5 times, the adherent cells increased 8 fold and were 66% of the population; on day 4 the adherent cells were still increased 3 fold (44% of population) and were mostly mononuclear. Cytochemical staining for peroxidase was distinctly positive for the early monocyte-macrophage population compared to non-induced PC but by day 4 had markedly diminished. The day 4 adherent cells exhibited increased rate of spreading on a glass surface and heightened capacity to phagocytose SRBC sensitized with a sub-

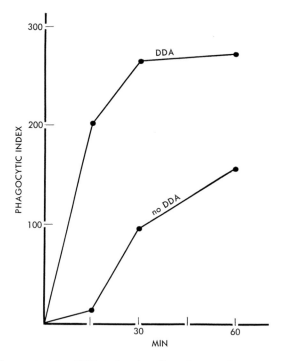

FIG. 2.   Phagocytosis by DDA-induced peritoneal macrophages
    Glass-adherent peritoneal cells from normal mice or mice injected i.p. 4 days prior with 0.2 μmol DDA were cultured with SRBC sensitized with mouse anti-SRBC serum. At each time point, adherent cells were scored according to the number of internalized SRBC, as follows: no SRBC ingested=0, one SRBC=1, two or three SRBC=2, three or more SRBC=3. Phagocytic index is the cumulative score per 100 adherent cells.

agglutinating amount of mouse antibody (Fig. 2). Thus DDA induced an influx of activated macrophages which appear to be heterogeneous in agreement with the findings of Lee and Berry (9) following *Corynebacterium parvum* injection.

Effect of DDA on Anti-tumor Immunoprophylaxis

IAd-modified mouse lymphoma cells employed for immunoprophylaxis included 6C3HED, P1798, L1210, and YAC. These were used for vaccination of the respective syngeneic host with or without complexing to DDA (10^7 cells and 0.2–0.4 μmol DDA/ injection) (16). To permit evaluation of the effect of DDA, immunization was deliberately suboptimal prior to challenge with a dose of tumor cells, which was lethal for nonimmunized animals. Among mice immunized with IAd lymphoma cells plus DDA, there were 71% (69/97) survivors while survival among those immunized with IAd treated cells alone was 29% (26/91). This difference is significant at the 1% probability level (Wilcoxon paired-ranks test). Vaccination with DDA alone has not afforded protection.

The relationship between dose of DDA/injection and degree of protection afforded by vaccination of BALB/c mice with IAd-P1798 was examined. Cells were suspended in DDA solution so that 0.2 ml given i.p. delivered 10^7 cells and the desired amount of DDA. Three vaccinations with IAd-P1798 alone followed by challenge with 10^3 P1798 cells gave 38% survivors. When 0.04, 0.2, or 1.0 μmol DDA was added to each vaccination, survival was, respectively, 50, 100, and 44%. Washing treated cells to remove excess DDA had no adverse effect on those treated with an optimal amount and improved the protective capacity of those treated with a larger quantity. In an experiment in which vaccination with IAd-P1798 and DDA given together produced 6/8 survivors, giving DDA 4 hr or 4 days before antigen decreased survival to 3/8 and 0/8, respectively. Therefore intimate association of DDA and TAA appear important for the antitumor effect.

An experiment was performed to determine the relationship between protection and development of cytotoxic anti-YAC antibody in A/Sn mice immunized with IAd-YAC cells alone or complexed to DDA. Six weekly vaccinations were given with blood drawn 3 days following each vaccination after the third; challenge with 10^3 YAC cells was one week after the sixth injection. In the DDA group, antibody was detected after the fourth vaccination and continued to increase whereas antibody was detected only after the sixth immunizing injection in the group not receiving DDA. Only 2 of 10 mice in the DDA group failed to reject the YAC implant, and they had the smallest amount of antibody. However this correlation did not hold in the non-DDA group; 7 of 12 survived challenge, but the 5 succumbing to tumor growth had both large and small amounts of antibody relative to those which rejected tumor.

Membrane fragments prepared by sonication of P1798 cells have also been used for immunization with and without added DDA. Antigen dose was expressed in blocking units (BU) where one BU is the amount of antigen which reduces the complement-dependent cytotoxicity of a BALB/c anti-P1798 antiserum for 10^7 P1798 cells by 50%; *i.e.*, one BU is equivalent to the amount of antigen on 5×10^6 intact P1798 cells. Mice received 3 weekly vaccinations followed by challenge one week later with 10^3 P1798 cells. Mice vaccinated with 0.4, 2.0, or 10.0 BU/injection exhibited survival of 0, 13, and 75%, respectively; when the same antigen doses were given with DDA (0.2 μmol), survival increased to 25, 63, and 88%. Like results with SRBC, the greatest effect of DDA was at low antigen dose.

Chemoimmunotherapy

Methotrexate (MTX), which prolongs survival of BALB/c mice bearing P1798, was selected for therapeutic trials. Cytoreductive therapy was begun on day 3 or 4 after tumor implantation with 30 mg MTX/kg. Immunotherapy, given 3 days after MTX, was with 10^7 IAd-P1798 alone or mixed with 0.2 μmol DDA. A single dose of MTX alone or followed by a single injection of IAd-P1798 with or without DDA was not curative. However, when drug treatment begun on day 3 was followed twice by immunotherapy in the presence of DDA (Table I, Group 3A), 6 of 16 (38%) survived. When treatment was delayed to day 4, there were again survivors (2 of 6, 33%, Group 3B), but the number of mice are not large enough to have statistical significance. When IAd-P1798 was given without DDA, immunotherapy by this protocol was without benefit (Groups 2A and 2B). For mice succumbing to tumor growth, mean survival time was increased less than 25% for chemoimmunotherapy groups relative to that for Groups 1A and 1B receiving MTX only. An alternate protocol in which immunotherapy was initiated on day 1 followed by MTX on day 4 and immunotherapy again on days 6 and 9 failed to produce survivors, but the group receiving DDA with IAd-P1798 had a significantly increased mean survival time of 31.2 days compared to 25.0 days for MTX alone. This latter study was performed because of a report that immunological stimulation prior to chemotherapy was of benefit (7).

With an inoculum of 10^4 P1798 cells and two therapeutic cycles, survival was further improved. MTX alone yielded 1 survivor of 19 (Table II, Group 1A); survival increased to 4 of 16 (Group 2A) by including immunotherapy with IAd-P1798 and increased further to the highly significant 18 of 32 (Group 3A) when DDA was included in the protocol ($p<0.001$). Following implantation of 10^6 cells, therapy did not produce survivors, and Group 3B exhibited a mean survival time only 15% greater than Group 1B.

TABLE I. Immunotherapy of BALB/c Mice Bearing P1798 Lymphoma[a]
Following a Single Administration of Methotrexate

Group	Day of treatment with			No. of survivors/ Total No.
	MTX (25-30 mg/kg)	IAd-P1798 (10^7)	IAd-P1798 (10^7) +DDA (0.2 μmol)	
0	—	—	—	0/12
1 A	3	—	—	0/12
1 B	4	—	—	0/6
2 A	3	6,9	—	0/16
2 B	4	6,9	—	0/6
3 A	3	—	6,9	6/16[b]
3 B	4	—	6,9	2/6

[a] 10^4 P1798 cells injected on day 0.

[b] $p=0.02$ compared to mice treated with MTX alone; Fisher exact probability test (19).

TABLE II.   Results of Two Cycles of Chemoimmunotherapy
of BALB/c Mice Bearing P1798 Lymphoma

| Group | Inoculum | Day of treatment with | | | No. of survivors/ Total No. |
		MTX[a] (30 mg/kg)	IAd-P1798 (10^7)	IAd-P1798 (10^7) +DDA (0.2 μmol)	
0 A	10^4	—	—	—	0/12
0 B	10^6	—	—	—	0/4
1 A	10^4	3,12	—	—	1/19
1 B	10^6	3,12	—	—	0/8
2 A	10^4	3,12	6,15	—	4/16
3 A	10^4	3,12	—	6,15	18/32[b]
3 B	10^6	3,12	—	6,15	0/8

[a] Mice in B groups received 50 mg/kg of MTX on day 12.
[b] $p<0.001$ compared to mice treated with MTX alone; Fisher exact probability test (19).

When 3 cycles of therapy were used, MTX was given on days 3, 12, and 19 with immunotherapy again given 3 days after MTX injection. Immunotherapy with IAd-P1798 either without or with DDA improved survival in a statistically significant way to 63% and 71%, respectively, compared to 13% for mice treated by chemotherapy only.   Mean survival time for the few mice dying in the two immunotherapy groups was increased by 29% and 75%.

Mice surviving 90 days were always tumor free and were considered cured. Upon subsequent challenge with 10^3 P1798 cells, a dose lethal for nonimmune BALB/c mice, all rejected the implant. Unlike studies with BCG and other experimental tumors, DDA without antigen conferred no therapeutic benefit.

Acknowledgment
This report is aided by grant IM-167 from the American Cancer Society, and by a grant from the Blanche Mary Taxis Foundation.

REFERENCES

1. Bekesi, J. G., St-Arneault, G., and Holland, J. F. Increase of leukemia L1210 immunogenicity by *Vibrio cholerae* neuraminidase treatment. *Cancer Res.*, **31**, 2130–2132 (1971).
2. Brunda, M. J. and Raffel, S. Macrophage processing of antigen for induction of tumor immunity. *Cancer Res.*, **37**, 1838–1844 (1977).
3. Chao, H., Peiper, S. C., Aach, R. D., and Parker, C. W. Introduction of cellular immunity to a chemically altered tumor antigen. *J. Immunol.*, **111**, 1800–1803 (1973).
4. Coon, J. and Hunter, R. Selective induction of delayed hypersensitivity by a lipid conjugated protein antigen which is localized in thymus dependent lymphoid tissue. *J. Immunol.*, **110**, 183–190 (1973).
5. Dailey, M. O. and Hunter, R. L. The role of lipid in the induction of hapten-specific delayed hypersensitivity and contact sensitivity. *J. Immunol.*, **112**, 1526–1534 (1974).
6. Dailey, M. O., Post, W., and Hunter, R. L. Induction of cell-mediated immunity to chemically modified antigens in guinea pigs. II. The interaction between lipid-conjugated antigens, macrophages, and T lymphocytes. *J. Immunol.*, **118**, 963–970 (1977).
7. Houchens, D. P., Bonmassar, E., Gaston, M. R., Kende, M., and Goldin, A. Drug-

mediated immunogenic changes of virus-induced leukemia *in vivo. Cancer Res.,* **36**, 1347–1352 (1976).

8. Kahan, B. D. Solubilization of allospecific and tumor-specific cell surface antigens. *Methods Cancer Res.,* **9**, 283–338 (1973).

9. Lee, K-C. and Berry, D. Functional heterogeneity in macrophages activated by *Corynebacterium parvum*: Characterization of subpopulations with different activities in promoting immune responses and suppressing tumor cell growth. *J. Immunol.,* **118**, 1530–1540 (1977).

10. Martin, W. J., Wunderlich, J. R., Fletcher, F., and Inman, J. K. Enhanced immunogenicity of chemically-coated syngeneic tumor cells. *Proc. Natl. Acad. Sci. U.S.,* **68**, 469–472 (1971).

11. Parish, C. R. Immune response to chemically modified flagellin. II. Evidence for a fundamental relationship between humoral and cell-mediated immunity. *J. Exp. Med.,* **134**, 21–47 (1971).

12. Parish, C. R. Preferential induction of cell-mediated immunity by chemically modified sheep erythrocytes. *Eur. J. Immunol.,* **2**, 143–151 (1972).

13. Prager, M. D. Immune response to modified tumors cells. *In* "Cellular Membranes and Tumor Cell Behavior," pp. 523–540 (1975). The Williams and Wilkins Co., Baltimore, Md.

14. Prager, M. D. and Baechtel, F. S. Methods for modification of cancer cells to enhance their antigenicity. *Methods Cancer Res.,* **9**, 339–400 (1973).

15. Prager, M. D., Baechtel, F. S., Ribble, R. J., Ludden, C. M., and Mehta, J. M. Immunological stimulation with modified lymphoma cells in a minimally responsive tumor-host system. *Cancer Res.,* **34**, 3203–3209 (1974).

16. Prager, M. D. and Gordon, W. C. Enhanced response to chemoimmunotherapy and immunoprophylaxis using tumor associated antigens with a lipophilic agent. *Cancer Res.,* **38**, 2052–2057 (1978).

17. Prager, M. D., Gordon, W. C., and Baechtel, F. S. Immunogenicity of modified tumor cells in syngeneic hosts. *Ann. N. Y. Acad. Sci.,* **276**, 61–74 (1976).

18. Ray, P. K., Thakur, V. S., and Sundaram, K. Antitumor immunity. I. Differential response of neuraminidase-treated and X-irradiated tumor vaccine. *Eur. J. Cancer,* **11**, 1–8 (1975).

19. Siegel, S. "Nonparametric Statistics," pp. 96–104 (1956). McGraw-Hill, New York.

20. Thompson, K., Harris, M., Benjamini, E., Mitchell, G., and Noble, M. Cellular and humoral immunity: A distinction in antigenic recognition. *Nature New Biol.,* **238**, 20–21 (1972).

GANN Monograph on Cancer Research 23, 1979

ALTERATION OF IMMUNOSENSITIVITY IN NITROGEN MUSTARD-RESISTANT YOSHIDA SARCOMA CELLS

Shigeru Tsukagoshi[*1] and Yoshiyuki Hashimoto[*2]

*Cancer Chemotherapy Center, Japanese Foundation for Cancer Research[*1] and Pharmaceutical Institute, Tohoku University[*2]*

Yoshida sarcoma cells acquired resistance to nitrogen mustard (HN_2) on repeated contact *in vitro*. When Donryu rats were inoculated subcutaneously in the hind footpad with highly HN_2-resistant Yoshida sarcoma cells (resistance index, 2,500) without any treatment, the initial tumor growth was followed by regression and all the rats survived. Inoculation of tumor cells in the footpad usually induces lymph node and organ metastases. Among these animals inoculated with HN_2-resistant cells, size of the right footpad enlarged, accompanying lymph node metastasis, but the tumors began to regress from about 2 weeks after inoculation and disappeared completely after 1 month.

With antiserum or peritoneal lymphoid cells obtained from animals immunized with either HN_2-sensitive or -resistant Yoshida sarcoma cells, it was found that the immunosensitivity of drug-resistant Yoshida sarcoma cells increased compared with the cells of the original sensitive line. It was suggested that the increased immunosensitivity could account for the greater chemotherapeutic response to 6-mercaptopurine for rats inoculated intraperitoneally with HN_2-resistant cells as compared with those inoculated with the original sensitive line.

Experimentally, it has been reported that the antigenicity of animal tumor cells may increase with the acquisition of drug resistance (*2, 6, 14, 18, 20, 25*) and that such drug-resistant tumors may be more susceptible to treatment with different types of drugs other than those used for the induction of resistance. Attention has not been focused, however, on the possibility of increased immunosensitivity of tumor cells, accompanying the origin of drug resistance. Recently, we observed that Yoshida sarcoma cells (YSc) that had acquired a high resistance to nitrogen mustard did not grow progressively or cause the death of rats inoculated with tumor cells in the footpad, which is a good site for the experimental induction of lymph node and organ metastases. For the purpose of clarifying this phenomenon, immunological assays of the drug-resistant cells were carried out. In the current study an increase in immunosensitivity was observed for tumor cells that had become highly resistant to nitrogen mustard as compared with the original sensitive Yoshida sarcoma cells.

In a nitrogen mustard-resistant subline of Yoshida sarcoma, Tsukagoshi (*23*) observed that ATPase activity of the plasma membrane was markedly elevated during

---

*[*1] Kami-Ikebukuro 1-37-1, Toshima-ku, Tokyo 170, Japan (塚越　茂).
*[*2] Aramaki, Sendai 980, Japan (橋本嘉幸).

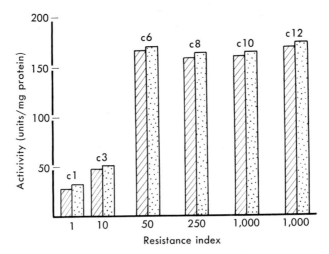

FIG. 1. Increase in membrane ATPase activity of Yoshida sarcoma cells in the process of acquiring resistance to nitrogen mustard

     Total ATPase activity;   Mg-ATPase activity c1-c12, resistant sublines of Yoshida sarcoma.

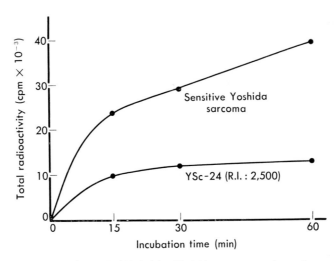

FIG. 2. Uptake of ^{3}H-HN$_2$ (10^{-4}M) by Yoshida sarcoma and a resistant subline YSc-24

     The cells of each subline were incubated at 37° with ^{3}H-HN$_2$ in Hanks' saline solution for various lengths of time. The ordinate expresses total radioactivity found in 2×10^7 cells washed once (by Inaba *et al.* (*10*)).

the process of acquiring resistance against nitrogen mustard (Fig. 1). Inaba (*10–12*) also found that transport of nitrogen mustard into the resistant cells was suppressed considerably during induction of drug resistance, as shown in Fig. 2. From these results together with a previous study (*4*) on the incorporation of labeled antitumor compounds into the resistant cells, we thought that certain biological or chemical changes would be produced in the cell membrane of the resistant cells during acquisition of drug resistance.

Induction of Nitrogen Mustard-resistance

Sensitive and drug-resistant Yoshida sarcoma cells were maintained in female Donryu rats weighing 120 to 140 g by intraperitoneal (i.p.) passage weekly. Drug-resistant sublines of Yoshida sarcoma were obtained by repeated contact of the tumor cells with dilute nitrogen mustard solution according to the method reported by Sakurai and Moriwaki (*21*). The degree of drug resistance was expressed as YSc*n*, in which *n* expresses the number of *in vitro* contacts for Yoshida sarcoma cells with nitrogen mustard (*17*). The relationship of the contact number and the drug and resistance indices is indicated in Table I, in which resistance indices were calculated by dividing minimum effective concentration (MEC) for resistant Yoshida sarcoma cells by MEC for sensitive Yoshida sarcoma. MEC is defined as the minimum concentration causing 50% abnormal mitosis 48 hr after *in vitro* culture of Yoshida sarcoma with an antitumor agent, as reported by Ishidate *et al.* (*13*). Usually, these resistance indices were stable, without further exposure to the drug, for at least 2 months after their establishment.

TABLE I.   Change of Resistance Index of Nitrogen Mustard-resistant
Sublines of Yoshida Sarcoma

Cell line	Resistance index[a]	Cell line	Resistance index
Original Yoshida sarcoma	1		
YSc1	5	YSc11	1,000
YSc2	5	YSc12	1,000
YSc3	10	YSc13	2,500
YSc5	10	YSc15	2,500
YSc6	25	YSc18	2,500
YSc7	50	YSc22	2,500
YSc8	250	YSc24	2,500
YSc9	500	YSc25	2,500
YSc10	1,000		

[a] Obtained by dividing the MEC of nitrogen mustard determined *in vitro* for the resistant Yoshida sarcoma cells by the MEC for the original Yoshida sarcoma cells.

Fate of Rats Inoculated s.c. with Original or Drug-resistant Yoshida Sarcoma in the Footpad (24)

One million original sensitive or nitrogen mustard-resistant Yoshida sarcoma cells, suspended in 0.5 ml of Hanks' solution, were inoculated subcutaneously (s.c.) in the footpad of the right hind leg of Donryu rats. With this inoculation system, tumor cells metastasized to various lymph nodes as well as to organs. In the original sensitive Yoshida sarcoma, this inoculation system caused death of the rats within about 15 days. Rats inoculated with Yoshida sarcoma cells died with progressive growth of a tumor in the lymph nodes. However, almost all of the rats inoculated with drug-resistant Yoshida sarcoma with a drug contact number of 18 or more (YSc18), for which resistance indices were 2,500, showed only transient tumor growth and did not succumb (Fig. 3).

Change in size of the right footpad of rats inoculated with 10^6 cells of YSc24

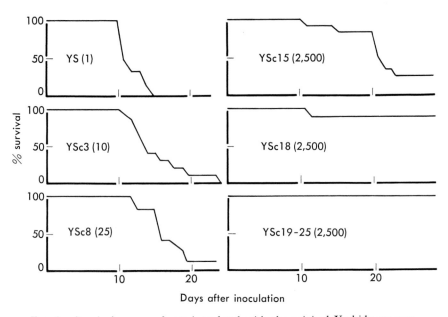

Fig. 3. Survival curves of rats inoculated with the original Yoshida sarcoma (YS) or nitrogen mustard-resistant Yoshida sarcoma into the right footpad

Number in parentheses shows resistance index (see legend to Table I).

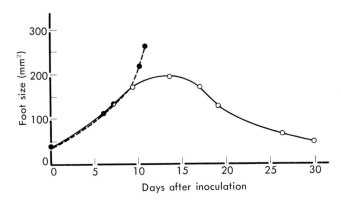

Fig. 4. Change in foot size of rats inoculated with the original (YS) or nitrogen mustard-resistant Yoshida sarcoma (YSc24) (resistance index, 2,500), into the right footpad

Foot size (mm²) was calculated by multiplying the width (mm) at the root of toe by maximum thickness (mm) of the right hind leg in which tumor cells were inoculated s.c. The width and thickness were measured by calipers. Each point represents an average value of foot size of 5 rats except the last point of that of Yoshida sarcoma-bearing rats, which is an average of 3 rats. All control rats inoculated with Yoshida sarcoma expired before day 12. ● YS; ○ YSc24.

after s.c. inoculation is shown in Fig. 4. For YSc24, the footpad enlarged until 2 weeks after inoculation, shrinking gradually thereafter to the normal size. Table II indicates that drug-resistant Yoshida sarcoma cells were growing and had infiltrated the lumbar lymph node before regression.

TABLE II. Bioassay of Lymph Nodes of Rats Inoculated with Original or
Nitrogen Mustard-resistant Yoshida Sarcomas, YSc19 or YSc24

Sarcoma	Rat 1			Rat 2			Rat 3		
	Foot size (mm)	Re (mm)	Life-span (days)	Foot size (mm)	Re (mm)	Life-span (days)	Foot size (mm)	Re (mm)	Life-span (days)
Yoshida	16×12	$12 \times 6 \times 5$	14	15×12	$12 \times 6 \times 6$	15	15×13	$12 \times 6 \times 6$	15
YSc19	15×11	$11 \times 4 \times 3$	30	15×12	$11 \times 4 \times 4$	28	15×12	$12 \times 4 \times 3$	20
YSc24	15×12	$10 \times 4 \times 3$	26	16×12	$12 \times 4 \times 3$	30	14×12	$11 \times 4 \times 3$	30

The lumbar lymph node (Re) was removed 7 days after s.c. injection into the footpad of the right
hind leg, and then minced in 1 ml of Hanks' solution. Whole lymph node suspension was inoculated
i.p. into normal rats for measurement of lifespan. Three rats each were used as the donors and recipients. Measurements were made of the width at the root of the toe and of the maximum thickness
in mm with calipers. Lymph node size was also determined by measuring length, width, and thickness.

TABLE III. Number of Survivors and Average Lifespan of Rats Inoculated
i.p. with Yoshida Sarcoma or Nitrogen Mustard-resistant Yoshida
Sarcoma, YSc19 (Resistance index, 2,500)

No. of tumor cells inoculated/ rat	Yoshida sarcoma		YSc19			
			Exp. 1		Exp. 2	
	No. of 60-day survivors/ total No. of test animals[a]	Av. lifespan of animals that died before day 60 (days)	No. of 60-day survivors/ total No. of test animals[a]	Av. lifespan of animals that died before day 60 (days)	No. of 60-day survivors/ total No. of test animals[a]	Av. lifespan of animals that died before day 60 (days)
10^3	0/5	14.8	2/5	15.3	3/5	16.3
10^4	0/5	12.0	0/5	12.0	1/5	15.0
10^5	0/5	8.8	1/5	11.5	2/5	13.0
10^6	0/5	8.6	0/5	10.0	1/5	13.0

[a] Five rats/group.

In the next experiment, varying number of drug-resistant cells ranging from 10^3
to 10^6 (YSc19) were inoculated intraperitoneally (i.p.) into normal Donryu rats to determine the extent of regression of cell growth in the peritoneal cavity. A comparison was
made with the results obtained using original Yoshida sarcoma cells (Table III). On

TABLE IV. Effect of X-irradiation on the Lifespan of Rats Inoculated
with Yoshida Sarcoma or Nitrogen Mustard-resistant Yoshida
Sarcoma into the Right Hind Leg

Sarcoma	Av. lifespan of animals that died before day 60 (days)	60-Day survivors/total test animals[b]
Yoshida sarcoma	10.5	0/10
YSc19	15.0	1/10
YSc24	16.0	0/10

[a] Resistance index, 2,500.

[b] Ten rats/group.

i.p. inoculation, growth of the resistant tumor was evidently more progressive than
that after s.c. inoculation. Nevertheless, in this experiment, an increase of average
lifespan and decrease of tumor deaths were found in the drug-resistant subline, YSc19.

Although all rats inoculated in the footpad with YSc19 or YSc24 cells showed
complete regression of the tumor, as indicated above, X-irradiation (300 rads) 2 days
before footpad inoculation permitted progressive tumor growth and resulted in death
in all but one of the irradiated rats (Table IV).

Increase of Immunosensitivity of Nitrogen Mustard-resistant Yoshida Sarcoma Cells (24)

In the nitrogen mustard-resistant subline of Yoshida sarcoma possessing a resistance index of more than 2,500, tumors started to grow and then regressed completely following the footpad inoculation system described above. Immune serum or
peritoneal fluid cells were obtained from rats after immunization with the drug-resistant subline, YSc22 (Table I). The first challenge was s.c. inoculum of 10^6 cells
into the footpad, and the tumors regressed completely following an initial period of
growth. The second challenge of 10^6 cells (i.p.) was carried out 2 months after the
initial s.c. inoculation of YSc22 when the rats were completely devoid of tumors, and
subsequent challenge with 10^7 and 10^8 cells was made i.p., each after an interval of 2
weeks. Serum and peritoneal fluid cells were obtained 4 and 7 days, respectively, after
the last challenge with 10^8 cells. Sera were inactivated at 56° for 30 min. Peritoneal
fluid cells were fractionated by the method described previously (7), and the purified
lymphocytes were used for the experiments.

The antigenicity of the drug-resistant cells, cytocidal activity of immune serum,
and destruction of tumor cells by peritoneal lymphoid cells (PLC) obtained from immunized rats were examined, comparing the sensitive and drug-resistant subline YSc24

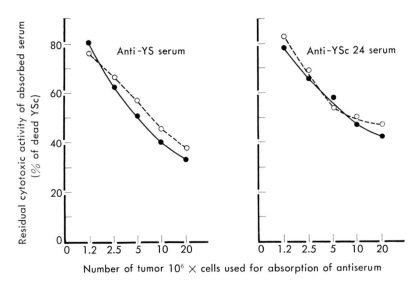

FIG. 5. Quantitative absorption test of immune serum with Yoshida sarcoma
cells (YS) (●) or with nitrogen mustard-resistant Yoshida sarcoma cells (YSc24)
(O)

(Tables V and VI). In these experiments YSc22 cells were used for the initial immunization of rats, and YSc24 cells were used for rechallenge in order to obtain immune serum and lymphocyte target cells.

Then, a cytotoxicity test for immune serum was carried out by the method described by Geering et al. (5), and the amount of cell surface antigen absorbed by the humoral antibody was measured by the quantitative absorption technique described by Boyse et al. (3).

Yoshida sarcoma-immune or YSc24-immune serum produced an equivalent decrease of cytotoxic activity following absorption with an equal volume of packed Yoshida sarcoma cells or YSc24 cells at 4° for 2 hr, indicating that cell surface antigens in these 2 cell lines have the same specificity, at least in accordance with the criterion of cytotoxicity. As shown in Fig. 5, the result of quantitative absorption tests suggests that the amount of cell surface antigens of a Yoshida sarcoma cell and of a YSc24 cell is essentially equal.

However, immune sera obtained for both sensitive and resistant cells yielded greater

TABLE V. Cytotoxicity Test of the Immune Serum[a] Obtained from Rats Immunized with the Original or Nitrogen Mustard-resistant Yoshida Sarcoma

Immune serum donors	Test cells	Titer
Yoshida sarcoma immune	Yoshida sarcoma	1/128
Yoshida sarcoma immune	YSc24	1/256
YSc24 immune	Yoshida sarcoma	1/16
YSc24 immune	YSc24	1/64

[a] Obtained 4 days after the last challenge with 10^8 cells.

TABLE VI. Cytotoxic Activity of Immune PLC

7-Day-immune PLC donors	PLC (No./ml $\times 10^6$)	Labeled target cells	Retained radioactivity (cpm)		
			0 hr	5 hr	24 hr
		Yoshida sarcoma	1881 ± 23[a]	3445 ± 115	3654 ± 257 (100)[b]
		YSc24	2456 ± 64	3857 ± 33	4361 ± 18 (100)
Yoshida sarcoma	2.5	Yoshida sarcoma		2730 ± 118	1342 ± 70 (36.7)
Yoshida sarcoma	2.5	YSc22		2651 ± 35	531 ± 3 (12.2)
YSc24	5.0	Yoshida sarcoma		2208 ± 294	947 ± 7 (25.9)
YSc24	5.0	YSc22		2250 ± 140	566 ± 48 (13.0)
YSc24	2.5	Yoshida sarcoma		2970 ± 119	2044 ± 101 (55.9)
YSc24	2.5	YSc24		2832 ± 26	657 ± 50 (15.1)
YSc24	1.25	Yoshida sarcoma		3180 ± 277	2793 ± 121 (76.3)
YSc24	1.25	YSc24		3338 ± 70	2095 ± 232 (48.0)

A mixture of 0.25 ml of a suspension containing immune PLC (1.25 to 5×10^6/ml) and 0.25 ml of a suspension containing ^{3}H-uridine-labeled target cells (1×10^6/ml) was placed in a test tube and incubated at 37° in a CO_2 incubator. As a control, target cells alone were cultured. Radioactivity retained in the cell mixture was measured after washing with cold 5% trichloroacetic acid solution. Percentage [%=(cpm of tumor cells+PLC−background)/(cpm of tumor cells alone−background)×100] reveals the extent of viable tumor cells. (The detailed in vitro experiments on the cytotoxicity of immune lymphocytes against Yoshida sarcoma cells have been reported in Ref. 7.)

[a] Mean±S.D.

[b] Number in parentheses shows percentage.

cytotoxicity against drug-resistant cells, YSc24, as indicated by the titration values (Table V). This result indicates that the drug-resistant YSc24 cells were more immunosensitive than the drug-sensitive Yoshida sarcoma.

For the purpose of further ascertaining the increase in immunosensitivity of the drug-resistant cells, the cell-mediated cytotoxic reaction of tumor cells was examined by measuring retained radioactivity of ³H-uridine in the target cells (8).

When PLC obtained from donors immunized with sensitive or resistant cell lines were placed in contact with sensitive or resistant cells, damage of target cells was greater in the resistant line, irrespective of the source of PLC. The percentage of retained radioactivity for resistant cells was about one-half to one-third of that of sensitive cells (Table VI). Thus, the drug-resistant tumor cells were apparently more immunosensitive than the original tumor cells, not only to humoral antibodies but also to immune lymphocytes.

Application of Chemotherapy to Rats Inoculated with the Drug-resistant Subline

In order to determine whether the nitrogen mustard-resistant cells were subject to collateral sensitivity, 6-mercaptopurine (6-MP) was injected i.p. into rats inoculated with either the sensitive or drug-resistant YSc24 cells, starting 3 days after inoculation. As shown in Fig. 6, 6-MP was more effective in the treatment of rats bearing drug-resistant YSc24 cells.

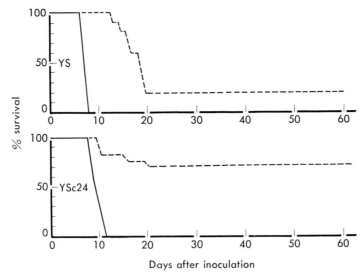

Fig. 6. Effect of 6-MP on rats inoculated i.p. with the original (YS) or nitrogen mustard-resistant Yoshida sarcoma cells (YSc24)

Resistance index of YSc24 was 2,500. 6-MP was given i.p. starting 3 days after inoculation at 20 mg/kg/day. —— control; - - - 6-MP.

DISCUSSION

Increase of antigenicity has been found in certain instances for drug-resistant mouse leukemia L1210 cells (2, 14, 18–20, 25) and an increase of antigenicity by artificial means has been observed (*1, 5, 15, 16, 26*). Hashimoto and Sudo (*7*) demonstrated that Donryu rats acquired transplantation resistance to Yoshida sarcoma cells when the rats were immunized with attenuated tumor cells by nitrogen mustard or X-irradiation. The present studies suggest that, alternatively to an increase in antigenicity of Yoshida sarcoma cells, an increase in immunosensitivity may also occur as a result of drug therapy, accompanying the origin of drug resistance.

Recently, Ishidate (personal communication) found that there was a partial change of karyotype in YSc19–25 but that the chromosomal mode was the same as that of the original Yoshida sarcoma. However, as illustrated in the present study, there were no qualitative antigenic differences evidenced in the absorption test for the original and drug-resistant Yoshida sarcomas, indicating no significant difference in the cell-surface antigens.

Increased immunosensitivity of resistant tumor cells as well as increased antigenicity may account for the phenomenon of collateral sensitivity observed for drug-resistant tumor cells (*22*). For drug-resistant Yoshida sarcoma, existence of collateral sensitivity has been reported by Hoshino (*9*) and was also observed in the present study. It is not clear, however, whether the increase in immunosensitivity of nitrogen mustard-resistant sublines of Yoshida sarcoma demonstrated *in vitro* would manifest itself *in vivo* or whether it is a common phenomenon accompanied by the acquisition of drug resistance by various tumor cells. Nevertheless, the studies indicate the possibility that an increase in sensitivity of the resistant tumor to another type of drug (collateral sensitivity), such as that for the drug-resistant Yoshida sarcoma, may have as an additional basis for the increased immunosensitivity of resistant cells.

Acknowledgment

We extend our appreciation to Dr. Ayako Moriwaki for the supply of nitrogen mustard-resistant sublines of Yoshida sarcoma.

REFERENCES

1. Bekesi, J. G., St.-Arneault, G., and Holland, J. F. Increase of leukemia L1210 immunogenicity by *Vibrio cholerae* neuraminidase treatment. *Cancer Res.*, **31**, 2130–2132 (1971).

2. Bonmassar, E., Bonmassar, A., Vadlamudi, S., and Goldin, A. Immunological alteration of leukemic cells *in vivo* after treatment with an antitumor drug. *Proc. Natl. Acad. Sci. U.S.*, **66**, 1089–1095 (1970).

3. Boyse, E. A., Miyazawa, M., Aoki, T., and Old, L. J. Ly-A and Ly-B. Two systems of lymphocyte isoantigens in the mouse. *Proc. Roy. Soc. London, Ser. B*, **170**, 175–193 (1968).

4. El-Merzabani, M. M. and Sakurai, Y. Distribution of N-methyl[^{14}C]-bis(3-mesyloxy-propyl)amine hydrochloride and its metabolites in normal and tumor-bearing rats. *Gann*, **59**, 481–488 (1968).

5. Geering, G., Old, L. J., and Boyse, E. A. Antigens of leukemias induced by naturally occurring murine leukemia virus: Their relation to the antigens of Gross virus and the leukemia viruses. *J. Exp. Med.*, **124**, 753–772 (1966).

6. Goldberg, A. I. and Glynn, J. P. Adoptive immunotherapy following chemotherapy against AKR lymphoma. *Proc. Am. Assoc. Cancer Res.*, **13**, 56 (1972).

7. Hashimoto, Y. and Sudo, H. Studies of acquired transplantation resistance. III. Cyto-

cidal effect of sensitized peritoneal lymphocytic cells of Donryu rats against the target Yoshida sarcoma cells *in vitro*. *Gann*, **59**, 7–18 (1968).

8. Hashimoto, Y. and Sudo, H. Evaluation of cell damage in immune reactions by release of radioactivity from ^{3}H-uridine labeled cells. *Gann*, **62**, 139–143 (1971).

9. Hoshino, A. Combination chemotherapy from the standpoint of drug resistance. *Nippon Gan Chiryo Gakkaishi* (*J. Jpn. Soc. Cancer Ther.*), **4** (*Suppl.*), 28–34 (1969) (in Japanese).

10. Inaba, M. and Sakurai, Y. Mechanism of resistance of Yoshida sarcoma to nitrogen mustard. *Int. J. Cancer*, **7**, 430–435 (1971).

11. Inaba, M., Moriwaki, A., and Sakurai, Y. Mechanism of resistance of Yoshida sarcoma to nitrogen mustard. II. Further evidence for suppressed transport of nitrogen mustard. *Int. J. Cancer*, **10**, 411–417 (1972).

12. Inaba, M. Mechanism of resistance of Yoshida sarcoma to nitrogen mustard. *Int. J. Cancer*, **11**, 231–236 (1973).

13. Ishidate, M., Sakurai, Y., Imamura, H., and Moriwaki, A. Studies on carcinostatic substances. XXII. Screening method for antimitotic substances using the *in vitro*-cultured Yoshida sarcoma cells. *Chem. Pharm. Bull. Tokyo*, **7**, 873–877 (1959).

14. Kitano, M., Mihich, E., and Pressman, D. Antigenic differences between leukemia L1210 and a subline resistant to methylglyoxal-bis(guanylhydrazone). *Cancer Res.*, **32**, 181–186 (1972).

15. Martin, J. W., Wunderlich, J. R., Fletcher, F., and Inman, J. K. Enhanced immunogenicity of chemically-coated syngeneic tumor. *Proc. Natl. Acad. Sci. U.S.*, **68**, 469–472 (1971).

16. Mihich, E. Modification of tumor regression by immunologic means. *Cancer Res.*, **29**, 2345–2350 (1969).

17. Moriwaki, A. Determination of resistance index of tumor cells to antitumor agents. *Gann*, **54**, 323–329 (1963).

18. Nicolin, A., Vadlamudi, S., Bonmassar, E., and Goldin, A. Antigenic properties induced in L1210 leukemic cells by antitumor agents. *Proc. Am. Assoc. Cancer Res.*, **12**, 13 (1971).

19. Nicolin, A., Vadlamudi, S., and Goldin, A. Increased immunogenicity of drug-resistant L1210 leukemias in CDF$_1$ mice. *Arch. Ital. Pathol. Clin. Tumori*, **13**, 125–133 (1970).

20. Nicolin, A., Vadlamudi, S., and Goldin, A. Antigenicity of L1210 leukemic sublines induced by drugs. *Cancer Res.*, **32**, 653–657 (1972).

21. Sakurai, Y. and Moriwaki, A. The *in vitro* induction of drug resistance of Yoshida sarcoma to alkylating agents. *Gann*, **54**, 473–479 (1963).

22. Schmid, F. A. and Hutchison, D. J. Collateral sensitivity of resistant lines of mouse leukemia L1210 and L5178Y. *Cancer Res.*, **32**, 808–812 (1972).

23. Tsukagoshi, S., Moriwaki, A., and Sakurai, Y. Increase of adenosine triphosphatase activity of Yoshida sarcoma cells in the process of acquiring resistance to alkylating agents. *Gann*, **62**, 65–66 (1971).

24. Tsukagoshi, S. and Hashimoto, Y. Increased immunosensitivity in nitrogen mustard-resistant Yoshida sarcoma. *Cancer Res.*, **33**, 1038–1042 (1973).

25. Venditti, J. M., Goldin, A., Kline, I., and Sheldon, D. R. Evaluation of antileukemic agents in the treatment of drug resistant variants of leukemia L1210. *Cancer Res.*, **23**, 1011–1084 (1963).

26. Wu, C. Y. and Cinader, B. Increase in hapten-specific plaque-forming cells after preinjection with structurally unrelated macromolecules. *J. Exp. Med.*, **134**, 693–712 (1971).

RECOGNITION OF CELL SURFACE ANTIGENS UNDERGOING XENOGENIZATION

NON-ENVELOPED VIRUS-INDUCED SPECIFIC CELL-SURFACE ANTIGEN AND ITS ROLE IN CELL-MEDIATED IMMUNITY

Hisao Uetake, Toshiki Inada, and Shoichi Hasegawa

*Department of Serology and Immunology Institute for Virus Research, Kyoto University**

Mouse adenovirus-induced specific antigen(s) appeared on the surface of infected cells at an early stage of infection in the absence of viral DNA and capsid antigen synthesis. Cell-mediated immunity (CMI) was induced against the infected cells. The infected cells were killed by immune spleen cells (ISC), in which the effector cells were T cells. The S antigen proved to serve as a target site for CMI. Cell-mediated cytolysis occurred when the effector (more exactly sensitizing) and target cells were H-2 compatible. The cell-mediated cytolysis was blocked by anti-S, anti-H-2 or anti-β_2m serum but not by anti-θ or by anti-Ig serum. The S antigens were co-capped with H-2 antigens either by anti-S or by anti-H-2 serum, but not with θ antigens or immunoglobulins either by anti-S or by anti-θ or by anti-Ig serum. The S antigens were co-precipitated with H-2K or H-2D antigens either by anti-S or by anti-H-2 serum. It was indicated that one infected cell carries at least two forms of S antigen, one associated with H-2K antigens and the other associated with H-2D antigens. It remains to be determined, however, whether the S antigen is bound to the heavy or light chain or to both of the H-2 antigen molecule. The co-precipitation of S and H-2 antigens favors the "altered self" hypothesis to explain the H-2 compatibility requirement for T cell-mediated cytolysis.

The above findings are consistent with our previous findings in other *in vitro* experiments, inhibition of capsid antigen synthesis by ISC and macrophage migration inhibition, and also give support to our hyphothesis concerning the mechanism of induction of CMI to virus infections.

It is now well known that cell-mediated immunity (CMI) is also very important in the host defense against virus infections, although its exact role in recovery from or protection against virus infections remains to be elucidated. The importance of CMI was realized at first from clinical observations of virus infection in immunodeficient patients (*6, 11, 34, 35, 37*), then from experimental findings in virus infections of thymectomized or anti-lymphocyte serum-treated animals (*6, 11, 34, 37*) and in the frequent occurrence of delayed hypersensitivity in clinical and experimental virus infections (*1, 34, 35*). However, as to the mechanisms of its induction and its mode of action, it is only 12 years since an hypothesis was proposed for the first time by

---

* Kawara-cho, Shogoin, Sakyo-ku, Kyoto 606, Japan (植竹久雄, 稲田敏樹, 長谷川捷一).

Uetake (*34, 35*). It was stated that a virus may induce virus-specific structural changes on the surface of infected cells, which may be recognized as a new antigen that may serve as a target site for CMI similar to transplantation immunity.

Since then, in order to gain support for this hypothesis, we have been experimenting with human (*7, 24, 29, 30, 31*) and mouse adenoviruses (M-Ad) (*8, 9, 12–23, 25, 26, 36*). The reason for employing non-enveloped viruses as the experimental material was to avoid viral envelope antigens appearing on the surface of infected cells, which might cause difficulties in isolating, purifying, and characterizing the antigen concerned. We present here with some of the results with mouse adenovirus, especially confined to *in vitro* T cell-mediated cytolysis of infected cells.

Appearance of S Antigen(s) on M-Ad-infected Cells at an Early Stage of Infection

Antisera against a virus-induced specific antigen that was expected to appear on the surface of M-Ad-infected cells, were prepared in mice by intraperitoneal immunization with infected mouse embryonic (ME) cells or with infected 5-fluoro deoxyuridine riboside (FUdR)-treated ME cells (*12, 20*). Both sera stained the cell surface in more than 80% of the 24-hr infected cells at a dilution of 1:2 (Fig. 1). Since the antiserum prepared with infected, FUdR-treated ME cells contained no detectable neutralizing antibodies, it can be said to be a specific anti-S serum (*20*).

As shown in Fig. 2, the S antigen became detectable at 6 hr after infection and was demonstrated in about 90% or more of infected cells at 24 to 36 hr later. When infected cells were incubated in the presence of FUdR at a concentration of 10^{-5} M/ml to prevent viral DNA and subsequent virion protein synthesis (*9, 10*), the S antigen became detectable in a time course similar to that observed in infected ME cells in the absence of FUdR, but capsid antigens were not demonstrable at any time. These findings indicate that the S antigen is synthesized at an early stage of infection in the absence of viral DNA synthesis (*20*).

The anti-S serum did not stain the surface of ME or HeLa cells that were infected

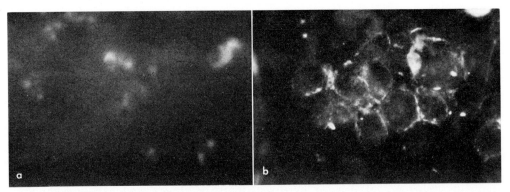

FIG. 1.   S antigens on M-Ad-infected cells

ME cell monolayers were infected with M-Ad at an moi of about 20 plaque-forming unit (PFU)/cell, washed with minimum essential medium (MEM), and incubated at 37°. Samples shown were stained before (a) and 24 hr, after infection.

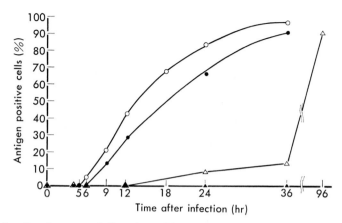

FIG. 2.   Development of S and capsid antigens in M-Ad-infected ME cells in the presence or absence of FUdR (10^{-5} M/ml)

S antigen(s) in the presence (●) or absence (○) of FUdR; capsid antigens in the presence (▲) or absence (△) of FUdR.

with human adenovirus type 2, 3, or 12, indicating that the S antigen(s) is specific for M-Ad (20).

CMI Induced against M-Ad-infected Cells

In vitro CMI was investigated by inhibition of intracellular capsid synthesis in infected cells (9, 24), by macrophage migration inhibition test (13, 22, 36), and by ^{51}Cr-release from labeled infected cells (14, 21, 23, 36). The results are summarized in Table I. Here, only the results of ^{51}Cr-release experiments are explained in some detail.

M-Ad-infected cells were killed by exposure to immune spleen cells (ISC). The killing was demonstrated by the Trypan Blue dye exclusion test (9) and by the ^{51}Cr-release test (14, 21, 36). In the former case, ISC were added to infected cells incubated

TABLE I.   Summarized data of CMI to M-Ad Infection

	Virion antigen synthesis ($\downarrow$)	MMI	^{51}Cr-release	S antigen
Without virion antigen · synthesis	+	+	+	+
Antigen appearance at stage	Early	Early	Early	Early
in cells	Surface	Surface	Surface	Surface
Effect of ISC	Killing		Killing	
Effector cell	T cell	T cell	T cell	
CMI development	Rapid rise	Rapid rise	Rapid rise	
	Rapid fall	Rapid fall	Rapid fall	
M-Ad specificity	Yes	Yes	Yes	Yes
Blocking by anti-S serum		+	+	
by anti-allo serum		+	+	
by anti-β_2m serum			+	+
by anti-Ig serum			−	−
by anti-θ serum			−	−

in the presence of 10^{-5} M FUdR, under which conditions infected cells were kept alive more than 4 days in the absence of ISC while more than 70% of infected cells were killed by ISC in 4 days.

When ISC were pretreated with anti-θ serum and complement, their cytolytic activity was abrogated, whereas it was not inhibited when ISC were pretreated with anti-mouse Ig serum and complement or when they were deprived of adhesive cells. These results indicated that effector cells in ISC are T cells (*23, 24, 36*).

CMI Induced against S Antigen(s) as a Target Site

The following findings indicated that CMI was induced against S antigen(s) as a target site.

1) When anti-S serum was added to a reaction mixture of ISC and infected target cells, cytolysis was significantly inhibited, whereas it was not inhibited when anti-θ or anti-mouse Ig serum was added (Table II).

2) Infected cells became sensitive to ISC even when they were incubated in the presence of FUdR. As mentioned above, under these conditions, S antigens were synthesized but not capsid antigens.

3) Infected cells became sensitive to ISC at an early stage of infection, and their sensitivity increased with increasing time of incubation in parallel with the development of S antigens (Fig. 3).

TABLE II.   Inhibitory Effect of Anti-S or Anti-H-2 Serum on Cytolysis by ISC

ISC derived from		M-Ad-infected target cells		
		C3H spleen cells	C3H/He thymus cells	C57BL/6 spleen cells
C3H/He	—	12.8 ± 2.9	17.0 ± 3.3	
	10% normal C57BL/6 serum	13.7 ± 1.7		
	10% C57BL/6 anti-C3H/He serum	$6.2\pm1.8\ (51.5)$**		
	10% anti-S serum	$2.6\pm0.8\ (79.7)$*	$2.3\pm2.0\ (86.5)$*	
	10% anti-M-Ig serum	$11.3\pm2.6\ (11.7)$[a]		
	10% anti-Thy, 1.2 serum		$16.7\pm3.0\ (\ 1.8)$[a]	
C57BL/6	—			26.7 ± 2.6
	10% normal C3H/He serum			28.1 ± 2.2
	10% C3H/He anti-C57BL/6 serum			$14.8\pm1.0\ (44.6)$*
	10% anti-S serum			$2.9\pm2.2\ (89.1)$*
	10% anti-human β_2m serum (rabbit)			$2.4\pm2.4\ (91.0)$*
	10% normal rabbit serum			$23.8\pm2.8\ (10.9)$[a]
(C3H/He× C57BL/6)F_1	—	10.6 ± 2.0		11.1 ± 1.7
	C3H/He anti-C57BL/6	$9.3\pm1.9\ (12.3)$[a]		$6.8\pm2.5\ (38.7)$***
	C57BL/6 anti-C3H/He	$4.3\pm2.4\ (59.4)$*		12.8 ± 5.1

* $p<0.001$,   ** $p<0.005$,   *** $p<0.025$,   [a] Not significant.

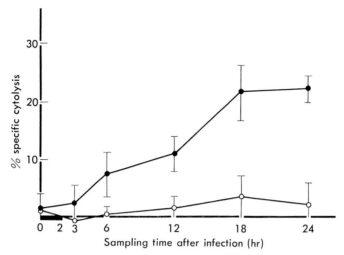

FIG. 3. Development of susceptibility to T cell-mediated cytolysis in M-Ad-infected cells

^{51}Cr-labeled spleen cells were infected with M-Ad at an moi of about 50 PFU/cell and incubated at 37°. At the indicated period, samples were removed, and exposed to ISC at the ratio of 1 : 60 at 37° for 6 hr. The supernatants were removed and their radioactivity was determined. ——, adsorption period.

Major Histocompatibility Complex (MHC) Restriction in T Cell-mediated Cytolysis

The cytolytic activity of ISC was assayed in various combinations of effector and target cells with respect to H-2 compatibility. Table III shows the summarized data (*16, 23, 36*).

ISC from immune H-2^k mice were shown to be cytotoxic against infected H-2^k and F$_1$ target cells but not against infected H-2^b or H-2^d target cells, or uninfected

TABLE III. Effector and Target Cell H-2 Compatibility Requirement
for Cytolysis of Infected Cells

M-Ad-infected target spleen cells	Effector cells from M-Ad-infected mice		
	C3H/He (H-2^k)	C57BL/6 (H-2^b)	(C3H/He× C57BL/6)F$_1$
C3H/He (H-2^k)	⧣	−	⧺
C57BL/6 (H-2^b)	−	⧣	+
BALB/c (H-2^d)	−	−	−
A/J (H-2^a)	⧺	−	NT
AKR (H-2^k)	NT	NT	⧺
(C3H/He×C57BL/6)F$_1$	⧣	⧺	
L (H-2^k)	NT	NT	⧣
Uninfected cells[a]	−	−	−

[a] Uninfected cells of each haplotype tested were used as controls.

⧣ $p < 0.001$; ⧺ $p < 0.005$; + $p < 0.01$; − not significant; NT, not tested. Statistical calculations were made between infected and uninfected cells. Twenty-four-hr infected spleen cells were labeled with ^{51}Cr, washed with MEM, resuspended, mixed with effector cells at the ratio of 1 : 50, and incubated at 37° for 6 hr. The supernatants were removed and their radioactivity was determined.

target cells regardless of H-2 haplotype. Conversely, ISC from immune H-2^b mice were cytolytic against infected H-2^b and F$_1$ target cells but not against infected H-2^k or H-2^d cells, or uninfected cells of any H-2 haplotype. ISC from immune F$_1$ mice were cytolytic against infected cells carrying H-2^k or H-2^b antigens, and not against infected H-2^d cells or uninfected cells of any haplotype.

These findings indicate that T cell-mediated cytolysis occurs only when the effector (more exactly sensitizing) and target cells share all or some of the same H-2 antigens.

Association of S and H-2 Antigens

Based on the above results additional experiments were carried out in order further to clarify the relationships between S and H-2 antigens. The results indicated that S and H-2 antigens are closely associated as shown in the following experiments.

1) Blocking of T cell-mediated cytolysis by antisera against S antigen(s), H-2 antigens, or β₂-microglobulin

As shown in Table II, the cytolysis of infected cells by ISC was found to be blocked when anti-S, anti-H-2, or anti-β_2m serum was added to the reaction mixture of effector and infected target cells. It was not inhibited when anti-θ, anti-mouse Ig, or normal (mouse or rabbit) serum was added (17)

When ISC from immune F$_1$ mice were employed as effectors, blocking of the cytolysis was observed when antiserum against H-2 antigens of target cells was added to the reaction mixture and not observed when antiserum against H-2 antigens, that were carried by F$_1$ effector cells and not by target cells, was added. This result indicates that antibodies inhibit cytolysis by binding to antigens on the target cell surface and not to antigens on the effector cell surface. Most important is the fact that the T cell-mediated cytolysis can be inhibited not only by anti-S serum but also by anti-H-2 or by anti-β_2m serum.

TABLE IV. Co-capping of S Antigen(s) and H-2 Antigens on M-Ad-Infected Cells

Serum against the antigens to be capped	Capped cells (%)	Rhodamine-labeled antiserum to test co-capping	Presence or absence of the rhodamine florescence after cap formation
—	—	Anti-S	⧾⧾⧾
Anti-H-2, 23, 32	>90	Anti-S	—
Anti-H-2, 8, 9, 37	>90	Anti-S	+
Anti-H-2, 32	>90	Anti-S	+
—	—	Anti-H-2, 23, 32	⧾⧾⧾
Anti-S	>95	Anti-H-2, 23, 32	—
—	—	Anti-S	⧾⧾⧾
Anti-β_2m	>95	Anti-S	—
Anti-Thy, 1, 2	>80	Anti-S	⧾⧾
Anti-Ig^a	≒40	Anti-S	⧾⧾

^{a} M-Ad-infected C3H spleen cells.

2) Co-capping of S and H-2 antigens

The topological relationship between S and H-2 antigens on the surface of infected cells was examined by the effect of capping of one antigen upon subsequent immunofluorescent antibody staining of the other. Twenty-four to 36-hr infected ME or mouse spleen cells were employed. The results are summarized in Table IV.

When private H-2 antigens were capped on the infected cells by anti-H-2 plus anti-mouse Ig sera, S antigens became undetectable by immunofluorescent antibody staining. Similar results were also obtained when the infected cells were pretreated with anti-β_2m plus anti-mouse Ig sera. Conversely, when S antigens were capped by anti-S plus anti-mouse Ig sera, H-2 antigens became undetectable by immunofluorescent antibody staining. In contrast, when θ antigens or immunoglobulins were capped by anti-θ or by anti-mouse Ig serum, subsequent immunofluorescent antibody staining of S antigens was little affected.

3) Co-precipitation of S and H-2 antigens

If S and H-2 antigens were associated, it would be expected that the antigens

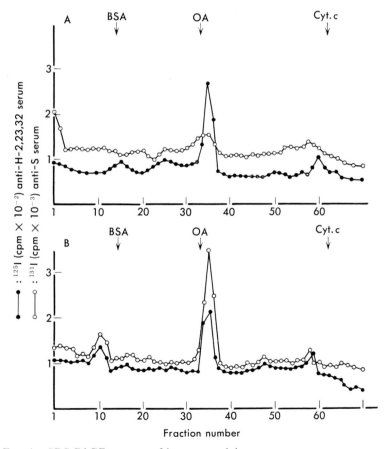

FIG. 4. SDS-PAGE patterns of immunoprecipitates

From extracts of uninfected (A) and M-Ad-infected (B) C3H/He thymus cells, precipitates were formed by anti-S (○) plus anti-mouse Ig sera or by anti-H-2, 23, 32 (●) plus anti-mouse Ig sera, and subjected to SDS-PAGE.

could be co-precipitated either by anti-S serum alone or by anti-H-2 serum alone. This was tested by the following experiments and the results proved to be as expected.

C3H/He mouse thymus cells were infected with M-Ad at 37° for 24 hr, then enzymically labeled with ^{125}I or ^{131}I at 37° for 10 min, and lysed with 0.5% NP40. The supernatant was obtained by centrifugation at 105,000 g for 30 min, reacted with either anti-H-2 or anti-S serum for 20 min at 4°, followed by incubation with anti-Ig serum at 37° for 20 min. The immune precipitate was collected by centrifugation, solubilized with 2% sodium dodecyl sulfate (SDS), and 8M urea containing 2ME in boiling water for 2 min, and electrophoresed in polyacrylamide gel. One of the results of these experiments is shown in Fig. 4 (25).

The precipitate from M-Ad-infected cells by anti-H-2, 23, 32 serum gave three major peaks corresponding to about 80,000, 40,000, and 12,000 daltons. The precipitate from anti-S serum gave similar patterns as above.

As controls, the immune precipitate made from uninfected cells by anti-H-2, 23,

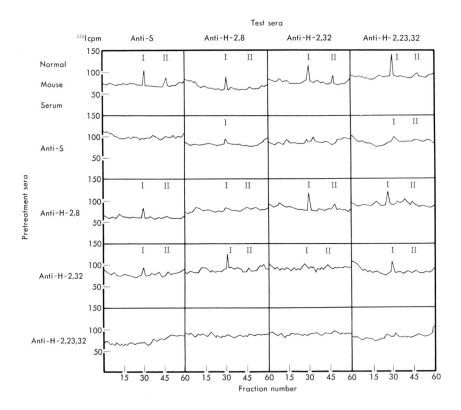

FIG. 5.   Sequential immunoprecipitation
Antigenic extract was prepared from 24-hr infected and radioiodine-labeled C3H/He thymus cells. It was divided into five portions, one was pretreated with one of the sera listed on the left-hand side of the graph and anti-Ig serum, respectively, and the resulting precipitates were removed by centrifugation. The supernatants received one of the sera listed on the top of the graph and anti-Ig. The resulting precipitates were subjected to SDS-PAGE. I, Peak I (MW *ca.* 40,000 daltons); II, Peak II (MW *ca.* 12,000 daltons)

32 serum gave similar patterns as above but no corresponding peaks were observed in the immune precipitate made from uninfected cells by anti-S serum.

These results suggest that the S antigenicity is associated with 80,000 daltons molecules or with either one or both polypeptides of 40,000 and 12,000 daltons, both of which correspond to component molecules that are precipitable by anti-H-2 serum, and are possibly identical to those of two constituent polypeptides of the H-2 antigens reported by Peterson *et al.* (*32*).

To further confirm the above experimental results, sequential immunoprecipitation tests were carried out by using anti-S serum and antisera specific for H-2K.8, H-2K.23, H-2D.32, or H-2, 23, 32. The antigenic extract was prepared from 24-hr infected and radioiodine-labeled C3H/He thymus cells as described above, and sequential immunoprecipitations were carried out according to the method of Cullen *et al.* (*3*). Figure 5 shows the results (*26*).

After pretreatment with normal mouse serum, the extract reacted with anti-S, anti-H-2,8, anti-H-2,32 or anti-H-2, 23, 32, and all the precipitates showed in SDS-PAGE (sodium dodecyl sulfatepolyacrylamide gel electrophoresis) almost the same patterns of two peaks, I and II, at positions of polypeptides of apparent molecular weight (MW) *ca.* 40,000 and 12,000 daltons, respectively. From the extract which was pretreated with anti-S serum no more precipitates were formed by additional anti-S serum or by anti-H-2, 32 but some precipitates were formed by anti-H-2, 8 or by anti-H-2, 23, 32, which showed similar but lower one (I) or two (I, II) peaks by SDS-PAGE. This indicated that some of H-2 antigens were co-precipitated with an S antigen. The extract that was pretreated with anti-H-2, 8 (or anti-H-2, 32) serum reacted only slightly with the same serum whereas it still reacted well not only with anti-H-2, 32 (or anti-H-2, 8) serum but also with anti-S serum. The extract pretreated with anti-H-2, 23, 32 serum did not react with any of the anti-H-2 sera or with anti-S serum. The above findings indicate that S antigens are co-precipitated with H-2K or H-2D antigens. This implies that one infected cell carries at least two forms of S antigen, one associated with H-2K antigens and the other with H-2D antigens.

DISCUSSION

The above results are summarized as follows:

1) M-Ad-induced specific antigen appeared on the surface of infected cells at an early stage of infection in the absence of viral DNA and capsid protein synthesis. 2) CMI was induced against the infected cells. 3) The infected cells were killed by ISC. 4) Effector cells in ISC were T cells. 5) The S antigen proved to serve as a target site for CMI. 6) The cell-mediated cytolysis occurred when the effector (more exactly sensitizing) and target cells were H-2 compatible. 7) The cell-mediated cytolysis was blocked by anti-S, anti-H-2, or anti-β_2m serum but not by anti-θ or by anti-Ig serum. 8) S antigens were co-capped with H-2 antigens either by anti-S serum or by anti-H-2 serum, but not with θ antigens or immunoglobulins, either by anti-S or by anti-θ or by anti-Ig serum. 9) The S antigens were co-precipitated with H-2K or H-2D antigens either by anti-S or by anti-H-2 serum. 10) It was indicated that one infected cell carries at least two forms of S antigen, one associated with H-2K antigens and the other associated with H-2D antigens. It remains to be determined, however, whether the S anti-

gen is bound to the heavy or light chain or both of the H-2 antigen molecules, and/or whether it is bound covalently or noncovalently.

The above-mentioned findings indicate that at an early stage of M-Ad infection, virus-specific S antigen is induced on the surface of infected cells, CMI may be induced against this antigen, and immune T cells destroy infected cells, resulting in the interruption of intracellular virus multiplication. It is consistent with our findings in other *in vitro* experiments, inhibition of capsid antigen synthesis by ISC (*9, 10*), and macrophage migration inhibition (*13, 22*). It also gives support to our hypothesis on the mechanism of induction of CMI to virus infections (*9, 34, 35*). The appearance of virus-induced surface antigens on virus-infected cells is not restricted to M-Ad-infected cells and has been observed in cells infected with a variety of viruses except parvoviruses (*2, 34, 35*).

The H-2 compatibility requirement for T cell-mediated cytolysis is consistent with recent reports on lymphocytic choriomeningitis (*38, 39*), ectromelia (*5*), vaccinia (*27, 28*), and Sendai viruses (*4, 39*), also with chemically modified cells (*cf. 33*). In order to explain this phenomenon, two hypotheses have been proposed, "dual recognition" and "altered self" (or "interaction antigen"). Our finding that S and H-2 antigens were co-precipitated either by anti-S serum or by anti-H-2 serum seems more favorable for the latter than for the former, though the exact nature of the association between S and H-2 antigens remains to be determined

Acknowledgment

The authors are grateful to Prof. T. Tachibana, Tohoku University, for his kind supply of private antigen-specific alloantisera. This work was partly supported by a Grant-in-Aid for Cancer Research from the Ministry of Education, Science and Culture, Japan.

REFERENCES

1. Allison, A. C. Cell-mediated immune responses to virus infections and virus-induced tumours. *Br. Med. Bull.*, **23**, 60–65 (1967).
2. Burns, W. H. and Allison, A. C. Surface antigens of virus-infected cells. *In* "Virus Infection and the Cell Surface," ed. G. Poste and G. L. Nicolson, pp. 213–247 (1977). Elsevier/North-Holland Biomed. Press, Amsterdam.
3. Cullen, S. E., Schwartz, B. D., Nathenson, S. G., and Cherry, M. The molecular basis of codominant expression of the histocompatibility-2 genetic region. *Proc. Natl. Acad. Sci. U.S.*, **69**, 1394–1397 (1972).
4. Doherty, P. C. and Zinkernagel, R. M. Specific immune lysis of paramyxovirus-infected cells by H-2-compatible thymus-derived lymphocytes. *Immunology*, **31**, 27–32 (1976).
5. Gardner, I. D., Bowern, N. A., and Blanden, R. V. Cell-mediated cytotoxicity against ectromelia virus-infected target cells. III. Role of the H-2 gene complex. *Eur. J. Immunol.*, **5**, 122–127 (1975).
6. Glasgow, L. A. Cellular immunity in host resistance to viral infections. *Arch. Intern. Med.*, **126**, 125–134 (1970).
7. Hamada, C., Nakajima, S., and Uetake, H. Detection of a specific surface antigen(s) in adenovirus type 12-transformed cells by fluorescent antibody technique. *Jpn. J. Microbiol.*, **17**, 297–302 (1973).
8. Hamada, C. and Uetake, H. Studies of the effects of immune cells on mouse cells infected with mouse adenovirus. *Annu. Rep. Inst. Virus Res. (Kyoto Univ.)*, **11**, 25–27 (1968).

9. Hamada, C. and Uetake, H. Mechanism of induction of cell-mediated immunity to virus infections: *In vitro* inhibition of intracellular multiplication of mouse adenovirus by immune spleen cells. *Infect. Immun.*, **11**, 937–943 (1975).

10. Hamada, C., Uetake, H., and Inada, T. Interruption of intracellular virus multiplication by immune spleen cells. *Proc. 1st Intersect. Congr. IAMS, 1974*, **4**, 42–49 (1975).

11. Hoyer, J. R., Cooper, M. D., Gabrielsen, E. E., and Good, R. A. Lymphopenic forms of congenital immunologic deficiency diseases. *Medicine*, **47**, 201–226 (1968).

12. Inada, T. and Uetake, H. Cell-mediated immunity to mouse adenovirus infection: Fluorescent antibody staining of S antigen(s) on mouse adenovirus-infected cells. *Annu. Rep. Inst. Virus Res. (Kyoto Univ.)*, **18**, 111–113 (1975).

13. Inada, T. and Uetake, H. Cell-mediated immunity to mouse adenovirus infection: Macrophage migration inhibition from peritoneal exsudate cells by exposure to virus-infected cells. *Annu. Rep. Inst. Virus Res. (Kyoto Univ.)*, **18**, 114–118 (1975).

14. Inada, T. and Uetake, H. Cell-mediated immunity to mouse adenovirus infection: Release of ^{51}Cr from infected cells by exposure to immune spleen cells. *Annu. Rep. Inst. Virus Res. (Kyoto Univ.)*, **18**, 119–124 (1975).

15. Inada, T. and Uetake, H. Cell-mediated immunity to mouse adenovirus infection: Cocapping of S antigen(s) and alloantigen(s) on mouse adenovirus-infected mouse embryonic cells. *Annu. Rep. Inst. Virus Res. (Kyoto Univ.)*, **18**, 124–127 (1975).

16. Inada, T. and Uetake, H. H-2 compatibility requirement for mouse adenovirus-specific T-cell-mediated cytolysis. *Annu. Rep. Inst. Virus Res. (Kyoto Univ.)*, **19**, 46–49 (1976).

17. Inada, T. and Uetake, H. Cell-mediated cytotoxicity to mouse adenovirus-infected cells: Blocking experiments. *Annu. Rep. Inst. Virus Res. (Kyoto Univ.)*, **20**, 48–50 (1977).

18. Inada, T. and Uetake, H. Reciprocal inhibition of immunofluorescence staining of S and H-2 antigens by noncorresponding antibodies. *Annu. Rep. Inst. Virus Res. (Kyoto Univ.)*, **20**, 50–52 (1977).

19. Inada, T. and Uetake, H. Reduction of the amount of H-2 antigens on the mouse adeno-virus-infected cell surface. *Annu. Rep. Inst. Virus Res. (Kyoto Univ.)*, **20**, 52–54 (1977).

20. Inada, T. and Uetake, H. Virus-induced specific cell surface antigen(s) on mouse adeno-virus-infected cells. *Infect. Immun.*, **18**, 41–45 (1977).

21. Inada, T. and Uetake, H. Cell-mediated immunity assayed by ^{51}Cr release test in mice infected with mouse adenovirus. *Infect. Immun.*, **20**, 1–5 (1978).

22. Inada, T. and Uetake, H. Cell-mediated immunity to mouse adenovirus infection: Macrophage migration inhibition test. *Microbiol. Immunol.*, **22**, 391–401 (1978).

23. Inada, T. and Uetake, H. Nature and specificity of effector cells in cell-mediated cytolysis of mouse adenovirus-infected cells. *Microbiol. Immunol.*, **22**, 119–124 (1978).

24. Inada, T., Hamada, C., and Uetake, H. Inhibition of intracellular virus multiplication by immune lymphocytes: Effects of anti-thymocyte and anti-immunoglobulin sera. *Annu. Rep. Inst. Virus Res. (Kyoto Univ.)*, **17**, 33–35 (1974).

25. Inada, T., Hasegawa, S., and Uetake, H. Polypeptides of mouse adenovirus-induced cell surface antigen(s). *Annu. Rep. Inst. Virus Res. (Kyoto Univ.)*, **19**, 49–52 (1976).

26. Inada, T., Hasegawa, S., and Uetake, H. Association of mouse adenovirus-induced surface antigen(s) with H-2K or H-2D antigen molecule on infected mouse cells. *Annu. Rep. Inst. Virus Res. (Kyoto Univ.)*, **20**, 45–48 (1977).

27. Koszinowski, U. and Ertl, H. Lysis mediated by T cell and restricted by H-2 antigen of target cells infected with vaccinia virus. *Nature*, **255**, 552–554 (1975).

28. Koszinowski, U. and Thomssen, R. Target cell-dependent T cell-mediated lysis of vaccinia virus-infected cells. *Eur. J. Immunol.*, **5**, 245–251 (1975).

29. Nakajima, S., Hamada, C., and Uetake, H. Prevention of tumor induction in hamsters

by immunization with adenovirus-infected cells. *Annu. Rep. Inst. Virus Res. (Kyoto Univ.)*, **12**, 117–120 (1969).

30. Nakajima, S., Hamada, C., and Uetake, H. Alternate changes of surface antigen(s) in adenovirus type 12-transformed and tumor cells. *Jpn. J. Microbiol.*, **17**, 303–311 (1973).
31. Nakajima, S., Hamada, C., and Uetake, H. Tumor-specific transplantation antigen activity of freshly adenovirus-infected cells. Intercurrent immunization against viral tumorigenesis with virus-infected cells. *Jpn. J. Microbiol.*, **18**, 243–252 (1974).
32. Peterson, P. A., Rask, L., Sege, K., Klareskog, L., Anundi, H., and Östberg, L. Evolutionary relationship between immunoglobulin and transplantation antigens. *Proc. Natl. Acad. Sci. U.S.*, **72**, 1612–1616 (1975).
33. Shearer, G. M., Schmitt-Verhulst, A.-M., and Rehn, T. G. Significance of the major histocompatibility complex as assessed by T-cell-mediated lympholysis involving syngeneic stimulating cells. *Contemp. Top. Immunobiol.*, **7**, 221–243 (1977).
34. Uetake, H. Biological defense mechanisms and lymphocytes. *Kagaku (Science)*, **39**, 206–214 (1969) (in Japanese).
35. Uetake, H., Hamada, C., and Nakajima, S. Mechanisms of induction of immunity to virus infections: Interruption of intracellular virus multiplication. *Tanpakushitsu Kakusan Koso (Protein, Nucleic Acid, and Enzyme)*, **17**, 835–847 (1972) (in Japanese).
36. Uetake, H. and Inada, T. Mechanism of induction of cellular immunity to virus infections: Experiments with adenoviruses. *Ann. Microbiol. (Inst. Pasteur)*, **128B**, 517–530 (1977).
37. Wheelock, E. F. and Toy, S. T. Participation of lymphocytes in viral infections. *Adv. Immunol.*, **16**, 123–184 (1973).
38. Zinkernagel, R. M. and Doherty, P. C. Restriction of *in vitro* T cell-mediated cytotoxicity in lymphocytic choriomeningitis within a syngeneic or semi-allogeneic system. *Nature*, **248**, 701–702 (1974).
39. Zinkernagel, R. M. and Doherty, P. C. Major transplantation antigens, viruses, and specificity of surveillance T cells. *Contemp. Top. Immunobiol.*, **7**, 179–220 (1977).

GANN Monograph on Cancer Research 23, 1979

DEVELOPMENT AND ALTERNATE CHANGES OF SURFACE ANTIGEN IN ADENOVIRUS TYPE 12-TRANSFORMED CELLS

Chuya Hamada and Yasunobu Maeta

*School of Medicine, Niigata University**

A virus-specific surface (S) antigen in adenovirus type 12 (Ad12)-transformed cells underwent alternate changes *in vitro* and *in vivo*. In a fluorescent antibody test, while all of the hamster and mouse cells transformed *in vitro* with Ad12 were positive for the S antigen, tumor cells *in vivo*, produced by grafting the transformed cells, were negative (S(+) and S(−), respectively). Conversely, the S(−) cells could be converted to S(+) by repeated subcultures *in vitro* or by Ad12 infection. In addition, H-2 antigens in Ad12-transformed mouse cells became undetectable by allografting. These various phenotypes of Ad12-transformed cells, thus obtained, were examined for their immunological properties. S(+) cells were more immunosensitive and less tumorigenic than S(−) cells. Co-existence of the S and H-2 antigens was required for cells to be injured by immune spleen cells. These findings were discussed from the viewpoint of tumor immunity.

A virus-specific surface (S) antigen in adenovirus type 12 (Ad12)-transformed cells is characteristic in its mode of behavior in that the antigen undergoes alternate changes *in vitro* and *in vivo*. In a fluorescent antibody (FA) test, while all of the cells transformed *in vitro* with Ad12 were positive for the S antigen, the tumor cells *in vivo*, produced by grafting the transformed cells, were negative (4). Conversely, the tumor cells *in vivo*, negative for the S antigen, could be converted to positive, stably by repeated subcultures (10), and transiently by Ad12 infection. In addition, Ad12-transformed mouse cells displayed a specific shift in their activity of H-2 (murine major histocompatibility) antigens by allografting (8). When a transformed cell line exhibiting H-2 antigens was grafted into allogeneic mice, cells in the grown tumors did not bear any detectable level of H-2 activity.

Thus, by employing an appropriate method for passage, we were able to prepare a number of Ad12-transformed cell lines in various combinations of the activities of the S and H-2 antigens, and had an opportunity to examine the role of these antigens in defining the immunological properties of the cell lines by comparing their immunosensitivity and oncogenicity. This paper deals with the results of these experiments.

---

* Asahimachi 1-757, Niigata 951, Japan (浜田忠弥, 前田裕伸).

Detection of S Antigen in Ad12-transformed Cells by the FA Technique

Antisera to the S antigen were those of C3H/He mice immunized with their syngeneic spleen cells infected abortively with Ad12. The resulting antisera were reactive exclusively to the S antigen without preabsorption. All the experiments described in this paper were carried out by the direct FA technique using mouse antisera tagged with fluoresceinisothiocyanate (FITC).

Recent results of FA staining of the S antigen in Ad12-transformed and tumor cells are given in Table I. While all of the hamster (HT-4, HT-101–105) and mouse (C3AT-1, -2; C57AT-1--4) cell lines transformed *in vitro* with Ad12 were positive for the S antigen (S(+)), no activity for the antigen was detectable in *in vivo* tumor cells (S(−)). These findings were a reconfirmation of our previous observations (*4, 10*), and seem ubiquitous for the range of Ad12-transformed and tumor cells regardless of their original species or strains.

TABLE I. Fluorescent Antibody Staining of S Antigen in Ad12-transformed Hamster and Mouse Cell Lines

Cells and cell lines examined	S antigen
Ad12-transformed cell lines *in vitro*	
Hamster cell lines	
HT-4	+
HT-101	+
HT-102	+
HT-103	+
HT-104	+
HT-105	+
C3H/He mouse cell lines	
C3AT1	+
C3AT2	+
C57BL/6 mouse cell lines	
C57AT1	+
C57AT2	+
C57AT3	+
C57AT4	+
Ad12-primary tumors *in vivo*	
Hamster tumors (10 cases)	−
C3H/He mouse tumors (10 cases)	−

All the cells and cell lines were examined by direct FA technique using mouse antisera tagged with FITC. + and −: 1:1-1:16 serum dilutions stained more than 90% and less than 0.5% of cells in a given specimen, respectively.

Alternate Changes of S Antigen in vitro and in vivo

After these findings, our next inquiry was whether the S(+) property was confined to the *in vitro* transformed cells genetically, and conversely whether the S(−) property was confined to the *in vivo* tumor cells. The question in this line was examined once with S(+) hamster cells (*10*); the cells converted to S(−) when grown as tumor cells *in vivo*, and the resultant S(−) cells converted again to S(+) after repeated sub-

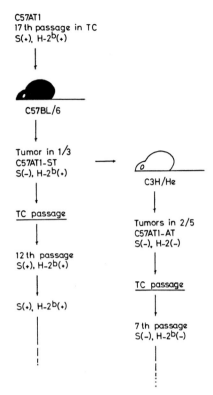

FIG. 1.   Alternate changes of S and H-2^b antigens in C57AT1 cells *in vitro* and *in vivo*

C57AT1: An Ad12-transformed cell line derived *in vitro* from C57BL/6 mouse cells. C57AT1-ST: Tumor cells grown by grafting C57AT1 cells into C57BL/6 mice; when 10^7 C57AT1 cells were grafted subcutaneously on their backs, 1 out of 3 animals developed tumors. C57AT1-AT: Tumor cells grown by grafting C57AT1-ST cells into C3H/He mice; when 10^7 C57AT1-ST cells were grafted subcutaneously on their backs, 2 out of 5 animals developed tumors.

cultures *in vitro*. These observations were also the case for a mouse cell line, C57AT1, an Ad12-transformant of C57BL/6 mouse cells (Fig. 1). Its S(+) property converted to S(−) when grown in syngeneic mice, and then turned to S(+) after 12 subcultures *in vitro*. Thus, the S(+) and S(−) properties were interconvertible in the same cell line, and not destined genetically by their origin.

Disappearance of H-2 Antigens by Allografting

Besides the S antigen, C57AT1 cells bear H-2^b antigens specific to the original mouse strain (S(+), H-2^b(+) in Fig. 1). In contrast to the conspicuous changes of the S antigen between the *in vitro* and the *in vivo* cells, activity of the H-2^b antigens was fairly constant, as long as the cells were propagated in syngeneic mice (Fig. 1). When, however, tumor cells in syngeneic mice (S(−), H-2^b(+)) were grafted into allogeneic mice (C3H/He), cells in the growing tumors, as well as those in their tissue culture descendants, within 7 times of subculture at least, were negative for both the S and

H-2^b antigens (S(−), H-2^b(−) in Fig. 1). Thus, in addition to the S antigen, the H-2 antigens in Ad12-transformed mouse cells were also convertible in the same cell line in the allogeneic host.

Development of S Antigen in S(−) Cells by Ad12 Infection

As mentioned above, S(−) tumor cells *in vivo* could be converted to S(+) cells by repeated subcultures *in vitro*. The S(+) property, thus acquired, was inherited stably in its *in vitro* descendants. Another method of converting S(−) cells to S(+) cells is by virus infection. When C57AT1-ST cells (S(−), H-2^b(+)) in Fig. 1 were infected with Ad12, more than 90% developed the S antigen 24–36 hr after infection. Likewise, C57AT1-AT cells (S(−), H-2^b(−)) came to produce the S antigen after Ad12 infection, though at low efficiency compared to that in the infected C57AT1-ST cells. Activity of the S antigen induced by Ad12 in S(−) cells, however, was transient in its duration, and became undetectable after several subcultures. The H-2^b antigens in the S(−) cells, on the other hand, were not affected by virus infection and the antigenic activity remained in them unaltered throughout, whether positive or negative.

Immunological Properties of Various Phenotypes of Ad12-transformed Cells

As exemplified in the foregoing paragraphs and with respect to the activities of the S and H-2 antigens, various phenotypes of Ad12-transformed mouse cell lines could arbitrarily be made available by employing the appropriate method of propagation. These cell lines can be used as antigenic variants for examining the role of these antigens

TABLE II. Cell-mediated Cytotoxicity by ISC Exerted on C57AT1 Cell Line and Its Derivatives

ISC derived from	Target cells				
	C57AT1 *in vitro* Ad12-transformed C57BL/6 mouse cells	C57AT1 grafted into a syngeneic mouse (C57AT1-ST$_1$)	C57AT1-ST$_1$ infected with Ad12	C57AT1 grafted into an allogeneic mouse (C57AT1-AT$_1$)	C57AT1-AT$_1$ infected with Ad12
	S (+) H-2 (+)	S (−) H-2 (+)	S (+) H-2 (+)	S (−) H-2 (−)	S (+) H-2 (−)
Ad12 immunized C57BL/6	41.4±3.3*	0.7±1.5	10.7±2.3*	1.8±3.7	1.9±1.7
Ad12 immunized C3H/He	5.1±2.6	0.8±1.5	2.5±2.0	2.8±1.2	1.2±1.8
Nonimmunized C57BL/6	2.9±1.9	−1.7±2.0	0.6±1.1	0.5±1.0	1.5±1.1
Nonimmunized C3H/He	2.8±2.4	0.4±2.2	−0.3±0.8	−0.2±2.8	1.5±1.2

^{51}Cr-labeled cells were exposed to ISC in a target: Effector ratio of 1:40 for 18 hr. Values for the specific ^{51}Cr-release were calculated by the formula: Specific ^{51}Cr-release (%)=(counts in supernatant) −(counts of spontaneous release)/(counts in supernatant after water lysis)−(counts of spontaneous release)×100.

* $p<0.001$; means and standard deviations were determined from 4 samples per specimen and compared by Student's t-test to those that were obtained with nonimmune spleen cells. For the designations of cell lines, see the legend to Fig. 1 and text.

in tumor immunity. An attempt was made in this respect to examine the susceptibility of various cell lines to immune spleen cells (ISC) *in vitro*. The cell lines tested were the derivatives of C57AT1 cells. ISC were those of C57BL/6 and C3H/He mice immunized with Ad12. Results are presented in Table II as values of the specific ^{51}Cr-release from labeled target cells. When the cell lines were exposed to the ISC, the S(+), H-2^b(+) cells were injured, whereas the S(+), H-2^b(−), the S(−), H-2^b(+), and the S(−), H-2^b(−) cells were refractory. The activity of both the S and H-2^b antigens were required for cells to be injured. Cell injury was virus-specific (data not shown), and caused restrictedly by the syngeneic ISC, whose activity was abolished by treatment of the ISC with antiserum to mouse θ-antigen with a complement (data not shown). A test was also made for the tumorigenic activity of various cell lines. When tested in syngeneic mice (C57BL/6), while cell number for the 50% tumor-producing dose (TPD$_{50}$) of the S(+), H-2^b(+) and the S(+), H-2^b(−) cells were $10^{7.2-7.5}$, those for the S(−), H-2^b(+) and the S(−), H-2^b(−) cells were $10^{5.0-5.5}$. S(−) cells were more tumorigenic than S(+) cells *in vivo*.

DISCUSSION

All the Ad12-transformed cells *in vitro* were S(+). These S(+) cells converted to S(−) when grown as tumor cells *in vivo*. S(+) cells were less tumorigenic, probably due to their greater immunosensitivity. Some other virus-transformed cells *in vitro* are rarely tumorigenic (*3, 5–7, 9, 11, 13, 15*). The above may be one of explanations for this. Similarly, activity of H-2^b antigens in Ad12-transformed mouse cells became undetectable through allografting. When, however, the S(+), H-2^b(+)cells were grafted into nude mice, cells in the growing tumors retained both the original antigenic activities (*14*). Some immunological factor(s), relevant to T cell function, may be involved in H-2^b (+)→(−) as well as S(+)→(−) conversion. Antigenic modulation by Old *et al.* was induced by humoral antibody (*12*). If the same is true for our observations has yet to be proved.

Of note is the observation that the S(+), H-2^b(+) cells were injured by syngeneic ISC, but the S(+), H-2^b(−) cells were not. This finding is explained by dual recognition or the altered-self hypotheses (*2*). Recently, however, major histocompatibility antigens have been postulated to have a receptor function for the male-specific Y-chromosome-associated histocompatibility (H-Y) antigen and for viral antigens as well (*1*). That H-2^b(−) cells might not fix the S antigen stably enough to be recognized and injured by the ISC is another explanation. This question is now being studied in our laboratory.

Acknowledgment

A part of this study was supported by a Grant-in-Aid for Cancer Research (No. 301537) from the Ministry of Education, Science and Culture of Japan.

REFERENCES

1. Beutler, B., Nagai, Y., Ohno, S., Klein, G., and Shapiro, I. M. The HLA-dependent expression of testis-organizing H-Y antigen by human male cells. *Cell*, **13**, 509–513 (1978).

2. Doherty, P. C., Blanden, R. V., and Zinkernagel, R. M. Specificity of virus-immune effector T cells for H-2K or H-2D compatible interactions: Implications for H antigen diversity. *Transplant. Rev.*, **29**, 89–124 (1976).

3. Freeman, A. E., Black, P. H., Vanderpool, E. A., Henry, P. H., Austin, J. B., and Huebner, R. J. Transformation of primary rat embryo cells by adenovirus type 2. *Proc. Natl. Acad. Sci. U.S.*, **58**, 1205–1212 (1967).

4. Hamada, C., Nakajima, S., and Uetake, H. Detection of a specific surface antigen(s) in adenovirus type 12-transformed cells by fluorescent antibody technique. *Jpn. J. Microbiol.*, **17**, 297–302 (1973).

5. Kit, S., Dubbs, D. R., and Somers, K. Strategy of simian virus 40. *In* "Strategy of the viral genome," ed. by G.E.W. Wolstenholm and M. O'Connor, pp. 229–265 (1971). A Ciba Foundation Symposium, Churchill Livingstone, Edinburgh and London.

6. Kryukova, I. N., Babkova, O. V., and Obukh, I. B. Malignant and transforming activity of Rous sarcoma virus (RSV). III. Detection of tumor-specific transplantation and membrane antigens in mouse cell lines transformed *in vitro* by RSV. *J. Natl. Cancer Inst.*, **47**, 819–827 (1971).

7. Kryukova, I. N., Obukh, I. B., and Biryulina, T. I. Tumour production in adult mice by syngeneic embryonic cultured cells containing the incomplete Rous virus. *Nature*, **219**, 174–176 (1968).

8. Maeta, Y. and Hamada, C. A specific surface antigen in Ad12-infected and -transformed cells. *Abstr. 25th Gen. Meet. Jpn. Virologist*, p. 228 (1977).

9. McAllister, R. M., Nicolson, M. O., Lewis, A. M., Jr., Macpherson, I., and Huebner, R. J. Transformation of rat embryo cells by adenovirus type 1. *J. Gen. Virol.*, **4**, 29–36 (1969).

10. Nakajima, S., Hamada, C., and Uetake, H. Alternate changes of surface antigen(s) in adenovirus type 12-transformed and tumor cells. *Jpn. J. Microbiol.*, **17**, 303–311 (1973).

11. Negroni, G. and Hunter, E. Antigenic heterogeneity in cell populations of cloned polyoma, virus-induced tumour lines. *Nature New Biol.*, **230**, 18–20 (1971).

12. Old, L. J., Stockert, E., Boyse, E. A., and Kim, J. H. Antigenic modulation. Loss of TL antigen from cells exposed to TL antibody. Study of the phenomenon *in vitro*. *J. Exp. Med.*, **127**, 523–539 (1968).

13. Rabson, A. S., Kirschstein, R. L., and Legallais, F. Y. Autologous implantation of Rhesus monkey cells "transformed" *in vitro* by Simian virus 40. *J. Natl. Cancer Inst.*, **35**, 981–991 (1965).

14. Torii, Y. and Hamada, C. Unpublished observation.

15. Walls, E. J. and Negroni, G. The properties of cell clones derived from a polyoma induced mouse tumour. *Europ. J. Cancer*, **2**, 221–225 (1966).

HETEROGENIZATION AND MAJOR HISTOCOMPATIBILITY COMPLEX-RESTRICTED T CELLS

Rolf M. Zinkernagel

*Department of Immunopathology, Scripps Clinic and Research Foundation**

Heterogenization may heighten the immunogenicity of tumor-associated antigens by providing better T cell help as follows: 1) by promoting oncolysis and, thus, subsequent processing of tumor-associated antigens by antigen-presenting cells; this mechanism may be most effective for non-lymphohemopoietic tumors; and 2) by introducing antigenic determinants that enhance induction of T cell help, a mechanism which may be particularly effective for lymphohemopoietic tumors.

Over the last few years, research has shown that T cells express dual specificity; that is, specificity for a cell-surface "self" determinant coded by the major histocompatibility gene complex (MHC, *H-2* in mice, *HLA* in humans) and for a foreign antigenic determinant (reviewed in *3, 7–10*). It is unclear whether this duality reflects the presence of one or two recognition sites on T cells. If two sites exist, the first could recognize "foreign" and the second self MHC antigens; whereas one recognition site could recognize a complex formed between self and foreign antigens (also called altered-self). In general, *cytotoxic* T cells are restricted so that they recognize only self-determinants coded by the MHC regions, which also code the serologically defined major transplantation antigens (H-2K, D; HLA-A-B). Yet, *nonlytic* T helper cells or T cells involved in delayed type hypersensitivity or macrophage activation are restricted so as to recognize only determinants of the *H-2I* or *HLA-D* regions (*10*). Accordingly, K, D determinants function as receptors for lytic signals and, *I* region determinants seem to function as receptors of cell-specific differentiation signals. When I determinants are triggered on B cells they initiate the synthesis of immunoglobulin or the switch from IgM to IgG production; on macrophages they induce an increase and modification of enzymic, digestive activities, *etc.*

Interestingly, the same MHC regions seem to contain genes that regulate the immune responsiveness of various types of effector T cells (*1, 2, 10*). Thus *K* or *D* region genes regulate the immune responsiveness of cytotoxic T cells, but *I* region genes control that of nonlytic T helper cells, *etc.* The capacity of both types of T cells to recognize MHC determinants as restriction specificities and the regulatory rule of *Ir* genes are dictated by the thymus (*2, 10*). During T cell maturation precursor T cells are selected to express a restriction specificity for the MHC products expressed by the thymic epithelial cells. Similarly the *Ir* genes as expressed by the thymus determine the phenotype of T cells in terms of their subsequent immune responsiveness.

Mature T cells are primed and triggered by antigen when that antigen is present

* La Jolla, California 92037, U.S.A.

on "immunogenic" cells (probably Ia-positive cells in mice), apparently all belonging to the lymphoreticular system and derived from lymphohemopoietic stem cells (10). For example, viral antigen expressed on infected liver or skin cells does not seem to sensitize cytotoxic T cell responses; to initiate a T cell response, the viral antigen must be expressed on cells of the lymphoreticular system. Whether this recognition of I-associated antigen is mandatory in activating T cells because T cell help is needed to trigger effector T cells or B cells is unclear.

Thus, to summarize: 1) Cell-mediated immunity and the MHC are intimately interrelated; 2) the thymus plays a major role in selecting the receptor repertoire for self-MHC recognition; 3) lymphoreticular cells seem to be specialized in presenting antigens in an immunogenic fashion; other somatic cells not belonging to the lympho-hemopoietic lineage cannot readily sensitize T cells but can only serve as target cells for T cell effector functions; and 4) T cell help is necessary to induce effector T or B cells. From an immunologic point of view, therefore, one can divide a higher vertebrate into three major cellular compartments: 1) Lymphohemopoietic cells, 2) thymus epi-thelial cells, and 3) other somatic cells. Consequently, tumor cells can escape immune surveillance not only by mimicking, tolerance, suppression, *etc.*, but also by the follow-ing two mechanisms: 1) Tumor cells of nonlymphohemopoietic origin can avoid pro-cessing by macrophages and therefore remain nonimmunogenic or, 2) tumor cells of lymphohemopoietic origin may simply not express antigenic determinants that induce T cell help. Heterogenization (5, 9), the process of introducing foreign antigenic deter-minants (viral antigens or haptens) onto tumor cells, therefore, may promote the im-munogenicity of otherwise nonimmunogenic tumor-associated antigens; presumably, T cells play a major role in this process. In this light, understanding how the MHC and lymphoreticular cells may be involved in triggering T cell immunity during hetero-genization may well improve one's evaluation of heterogenization and its application to immunotherapy against cancer. From the facts summarized here, many immunologic factors may be manipulated by heterogenization. Only two obvious examples will be discussed briefly; antigen presentation and T cell help.

Heterogenization and Antigen Presentation

If antigen presentation *via* macrophages or other Ia-positive cells is crucial for the induction of T cell immunity, then tumor cells that are not lymphohemopoietic cells must be processed to become immunogenic. For example, murine allogeneic fibroblasts cannot stimulate an alloresponse *in vitro* or *in vivo* to generate alloreactive cytotoxic T cells. In contrast, allogeneic lymphoid cells are extremely potent in inducing allo-reactive T cell responses (4). Therefore, if fibrosarcomas or carcinomas proliferate during early development and few decay, these cells would not be immunogenic despite the fact that they may express tumor-associated antigens.

Heterogenization would be a way to improve macrophage processing of tumor cells so that tumor-associated antigens are presented immunogenically. Introduction of dispersed tumor cells alone is apparently not sufficient, nor is the use of irradiated and or Formalin-fixed cells. The introduction of new antigenic determinants certainly renders tumor cells more immunogenic. Whether this is mediated by more avid phago-cytosis and/or by more efficient induction of T cell help is unclear as yet. Heterogenization with cytolytic viruses could well be very effective in boosting immunogenicity of a tumor because virus may 1) lyse tumor cells (oncolysis), creating a vast amount of membrane fragments that are phagocytized and thus become immunogenic, and 2) infect tumor cells *in vivo*, and therefore have an avalanche effect, at least temporarily.

Once a T cell immune response is triggered, its maintenance or boosting may depend much less on the combined presentation of tumor-associated antigens and *I* region products. If this were the case (and experimental precedence exists), heterogenization would be needed only to push the immune response over the initial trigger threshold; thereafter, reactivity could be propagated by tumor-associated antigen alone.

Heterogenization and T Cell Help

Tumor cells of lymphohemopoietic origin often express the structures required for presenting tumor-associated antigens in an immunogenic form. For example, many such tumor cells can induce alloreactivity. Heterogenization may therefore not necessarily improve immunogenic antigen display, but may reveal these tumor-associated antigens better or may introduce new antigenic determinants that serve as helper determinants. Why tumor-associated antigens should not provide good helper determinants is unknown; *Ir* gene defects (at the T cell or the antigen presenting level), tolerance, or mimicking may be responsible. In any case, introduction of an immunogenic helper determinant could induce and provide the initial T cell help that appears to be necessary to trigger T or B effector cell function. The work of A. N. Mitchison has been outstanding in defining the mechanisms involved in inducing T cell help to antigens on cell membranes (see A. N. Mitchison this volume and Ref. 6).

CONCLUSION

Heterogenization may introduce foreign antigenic determinants so as to circumvent the failure of tumor-associated antigens to induce a specific immune response. T cell help seems to be the crucial limiting factor. Such helper activity could be introduced or augmented for instigating the response to tumor-associated antigens on nonlymphohemopoietic tumor cells (*e.g.*, fibrosarcomas, carcinomas) by forcing macrophages to process, (*e.g.*, by viral oncolysis) these antigens. Alternatively, on lymphohemopoietic tumor cells, strongly immunogenic helper determinants may be introduced directly and could trigger T cells or B cells specific for the tumor-associated antigen.

This is obviously a very simplified and restricted view of the problem of immune surveillance and of heterogenization. The question of the T cell helper response is studied extensively (see N. A. Mitchison and T. Hamaoka, this volume) in models that involve lymphohemopoietic cells. The results of this work support the general idea that augmentation of T cell help may be crucial in improving immune protection against tumors. Whether macrophage processing is equally important because it enhances induction of T help remains to be seen.

Acknowledgment

I thank Ms. Elizabeth Sinclair and Phyllis Minick for their excellent help in preparing this manuscript. Some of the experimental work summarized here was supported by USPHSG

A1-07007, A1-13779, and A1-00-278. This is publication number 1571 of the Immunology Departments, Scripps Clinic and Research Foundation, La Jolla, California 92037, U.S.A.

REFERENCES

1.   Benacerraf, B. and Germain, R. N. The immune response genes of the major histocompatibility complex. *Immunol. Rev.*, **38**, 71–119 (1978).

2.   von Boehmer, H., Haas, W., and Jerne, N. K. Major histocompatibility complex-linked immune-responsiveness is acquired by lymphocytes of low-responder mice differentiating in thymus of high responder mice. *Proc. Natl. Acad. Sci. U.S.*, **75**, 2439–2442 (1978).

3.   Katz, D. H. "Lymphocyte Differentiation, Recognition and Regulation," (1977). Academic Press, New York.

4.   Lafferty, K. J. and Cunningham, A. J. A new analysis of allogeneic interactions. *Aust. J. Exp. Biol. Med.*, **53**, 27–42 (1976).

5.   Lindenmann, J. and Klein, P. Viral oncolysis. *Rec. Result. Cancer Res.*, **8**, 1–85 (1967).

6.   Mitchison, N. A. and Lake, P. Latent help. *In* "Immune System: Genetics and Regulation," ed. E. Sercarz, L. A. Herzenber, and C. F. Fox, pp. 555–558 (1977). Academic Press, New York.

7.   Munro, A. J. and Bright, S. Products of the major histocompatibility complex and their relationship to the immune response. *Nature*, **264**, 145–152 (1976).

8.   Paul, W. E. and Benacerraf, B. Functional specificity of thymus-dependent lymphocytes *Science*, **195**, 1293–1300 (1977).

9.   Svet-Moldavsky, G. A. and Hamburg, V. P. Quantitative relationships in viral oncolysis and the possibility of artificial heterogenization of tumors. *Nature* **202**, 303–304 (1964).

10. Zinkernagel, R. M. Thymus and lymphohemopoietic cells: Their role in T cell maturation, in selection of T cells' *H-2*-restriction-specificity and in *H-2* linked *Ir* gene control. *Immunol. Rev.*, **42**, 224–270 (1978).

ASSOCIATIVE RECOGNITION IN THE RESPONSE TO ALLOANTIGENS (AND XENOGENISATION OF ALLOANTIGENS)

J. Bromberg, M. Brenan, E. A. Clark, P. Lake, N. A. Mitchison, I. Nakashima, and K. B. Sainis

ICRF Tumour Immunology Unit, Department of Zoology, University College*

Primary immunization against allo-antigen may fail in congenic hosts due to lack of helper activity. The requirement for help is relatively stringent for certain antigens (H-$2D^d$, Thy-1, and Ly) immunoglobulin classes (IgG), and Ir genes (I^b). To be effective, helper determinants must be carried on the same cell, but not necessarily on the same molecule (intra-structural, inter-molecular help). Genetic analysis identifies a small number of effective helper allo-antigens. Viruses (herpes, vaccines, and Sendai) generate effective help.

Secondary immunization of successfully primed animals requires similar help. A wider range of allo-antigens are effective as judged by genetic analysis. Following hyperimmunization the antigens Thy-1.2, H-$2K^q$, and H-$2K^s$ generate help, although they do not do so initially, a phenomenon termed "latent help." Latency is interpretable in terms of processing of antigen by host macrophages. Major histocompatibility system (MHC) restriction data indicate that host processing occurs. It is proposed that limitations on host processing constitutes an important mechanism of self-tolerance.

We are engaged in a study of the role of helper T cells (T_h cells) in regulating the immune response to cell surface antigens. This type of antigen is important in immunopathology and in protective immunity to viruses, and may also matter in cancer. Through manipulation of T_h cell activity it should be possible to control these responses. A greater understanding of naturally occurring helper determinants should tell something about the principles of their structure, and thus enable us to design effective molecules for the purpose of immunological intervention.

Why analyse antigens of the cell surface when so much can be done with soluble ones? Quite apart from questions of relevance to the ultimate aims of our study, it is now clear that antigens of the cell surface are handled by the immune system in certain unique ways. Thus i) macromolecules carried on cell surfaces encounter the immune system in the form of assemblies, in which one type of molecule can regulate the response to another if they are present on the same assembly. An example of this type of phenomenon is intermolecular, intrastructural help (*11*), in which T cell activity directed at one molecule regulates the response of B cells to another molecule on the

---

* London, WC1E 6BT, U.K.

same cell surface. Thus also ii) macromolecules carried on cell surfaces may enter the immune system through alternative routes (2). Through the direct route, they are recognised by lymphocytes in association with their own major histocompatibility system (MHC) molecules. Through the indirect or reprocessing route, they are re-processed by macrophages so that they are then recognised in association with host MHC molecules.

T_h cells can act in two distinct ways, and our discussion of their activity will become confused unless this distinction is clear. In one, help is specific in its generation but not in its effect. A T_h cell reacts with its specific antigen, but then generates activity, presumably in the form of a non-specific factor of the allogeneic effect factor (AEF) type, which can affect other lymphocytes, irrespective of their specificity. In the other, help is specific both in its generation and in its effect. A T_h cell reacts with its specific antigen, and can then affect other lymphocytes only if they are specific for determinants carried on the same antigenic structure—"associative help." In that case, it is believed that either the helper and effector cells have to be linked by a physical bridge, or the helper cells' receptors are released and forms a bridge between the effector cell and a third party cell. In practice the crucial experiment is to compare the activity of an antigen carrying two determinants, one specific for helper and the other for effector cells, with a mixture carrying the two specificities separately.

The question of recognition of Ia molecules on effector cells is also important in this discussion. It is now generally accepted that T cells can recognise antigens only in association with MHC products, and that for T_h cells the recognition is in association with Ia molecules. Accordingly, if antigens form a bridge between T_h cells and effectors, the T_h cells would be expected to need to recognise Ia molecules on the effector cells in order for help to be effective. Just such a result has been obtained in cell transfer experiments (18). This finding is not in accord with the demonstration in vitro of an antigen-specific helper factor which lacks the ability to recognise Ia molecules (4). One way to reconcile this difference would be if helper action started with the formation of a T_h-effector cell-cell bridge, and then proceeded to expand locally through factor release. The information at present available does not permit any firm conclusion about mechanism to be reached. Clearly the findings which have been made in vitro will need to be carefully evaluated in vivo.

Most of the evidence for associative help has been made with B cells as effectors. From the point of view of cancer research it is important to know whether the same rules apply to other types of effector, particularly cytotoxic T cells (T_c cells). At present we have only hints. Thus i) non-associative help appears to dominate the generation of T_c cells in vitro (15). This may be misleading, because ii) non-associative help also dominates B cell responses in vitro (19) although this does not apply in vivo. If we examine other T cell subsets, we find that iii) associative help operates in the generation of T_h cells themselves in vitro (5) and that iv) suppressor T cells (T_s cells) operate through an associative mechanism in vitro (1). Recent work v) on thymus grafts indicates that T_h cells control the generation of T_c cells in vivo (24). vi) The provisional evidence from this kind of system is that the T_h cells involved do not recognise Ia molecules on the precursors of T_c cells, or at least that a search for evidence of this kind of recognition has thus far yielded negative results. vii) Our colleague, Dr. H. Claman, has searched for evidence of associative help from Ia-specific T_h cells in the generation of *H-2D*-specific T$_c$ cells *in vivo*, so far with negative results (and indeed with evidence of suppression possibly resulting from accelerated loss of the Ia-bearing antigenic cells). In the face of this conflicting evidence, we feel that a search for associative help in the generation of T$_c$ cells, using a more favorable system, is called for.

The responses which we have chosen to investigate have been mainly antibody responses to the murine allo-antigens Thy-1, *H-2K*, and *H-2D*. The reason for selecting these antigens are i) they are well-defined, individual molecules; ii) there is no ambiguity about the effector cells involved, and iii) inbred strains of mouse are now available which enable these antigens to be combined in cell surface assemblies with a variety of other antigens. Furthermore, these responses can be examined conveniently either by well-established, serological techniques, or in terms of plaque-forming cells (PFC).

The principle questions which we have sought to answer in these responses are i) is intra- or inter-molecular help required? ii) Insofar as intermolecular help is required, how many different molecules are effective and can they be ranked in order of effectiveness? iii) What are the kinetics of generation of help, and do they differ significantly from one helper molecule to another? iv) What are the rules of dual recognition between helper and Ia molecules? v) What happens to an immune system which has been exposed to molecules which are potential antigens but which cannot generate a response because they lack help? vi) How does associative inhibition occur? and vii) granted that strains differ in respect of these questions, is this heterogeneity under control of the *Ir-I* (Ia) loci?

Systems and Techniques

We have employed the following three systems:

i)   Cell transfers into 600 R sub-lethally irradiated hosts. This system has been described previously (*10, 11*). It involves the use of a B cell source which has received multiple immunisations against Thy-1, *H-2K*, or *H-2D*, a T cell source which has received one or two immunisations, anti-Thy-1 plus guinea pig complement treatment to deplete the B cells of T cells (recently we have begun to use the anti-Thy-1 products of hybridomas (*3*) for this purpose), and antigen in the form of 2,000 R irradiated thymocytes or spleen cells. The response is read after 9 days in terms of cytotoxic serum antibody titre, using a single-step assay for anti-Thy-1 and a two-step assay for anti-*H-2K* or *H-2D*. Under these conditions, the former response is largely IgM and the latter largely IgG, as judged by resistance to 2-mercaptoethanol and gel filtration.

ii)   Primary, at the 7-day peak, or secondary, at 3–4 days non-transferred responses to Thy-1 or *H-2D*. These are read in terms of undeveloped plaque-forming cells per spleen (*9*) although we have recently had encouraging results with a developing serum (IgM rabbit anti-mouse IgG). The distinct kinetics of the secondary response enables the effects of priming to be clearly observed.

iii)   The *in vitro* response to Thy-1 (*9*). Antigen released from cells will drive this response, while antigen on viable cells is inhibitory. In comparison with the *in vivo* responses, this response appears to be less T-dependent and manifests less associative control.

Associative Help

Clear evidence of associative help has been found in all the *in vivo* systems which have been adequately studied. Thus i) AKR/Cum×CBA (Thy-1.2) mice make little primary anti-Thy-1.1 response to AKR cells (Thy-1.1), or to a mixture of these cells with B10.Br cells (Thy-1.2). They do make a good response to (AKR×B10.Br)F$_1$ cells. AKR/Cum and AKR are highly congenic strains differing at Thy-1; B10.Br differs from AKR and CBA for many minor allo-antigens and all strains are *H-2^k* (thus avoiding interference from MHC-incompatibility effects). The conclusion follows that the anti-Thy-1 primary response can be driven by inter-molecular, intra-structural help from minor alloantigens. Thus also ii) B10 (*K^{b}I^{b}D^b*) are poorly primed by B10.A (5R) cells (*K^{b}I^{b}D^d*) to make an anti-*D^d* response to B10.A (5R) cells. They are well primed in the same system by B10.A cells (*K^{k}I^{k}D^d*). It follows that priming of the anti-*D* can be driven by intermolecular help from Ia antigens. Thus again iii) in the secondary transfer system, CBA B cells primed against AKR (anti-Thy-1.1) plus CBA T cells primed against B10.Br make a poor anti-Thy-1.1 response against a mixture of CBA.Thy-1.1 and B10.Br cells (CBA.Thy-1.1 is a Thy-1 congenic strain synthesised by us). They make a good response against (CBA.Thy-1.1×B10.Br)F$_1$ cells. It follows that this anti-Thy-1 secondary response can be driven by intermolecular, intrastructural help. And thus again, iv) again in this secondary transfer system, A.TH B cells (*K^{s}I^{s}D^d*) primed against A (*K^{k}I^{k}D^d*) plus unprimed A.TH T cells make a poor anti-*K^k* response against CBA cells, but make a good response if A.TH T cells primed against A.TL (*K^{s}I^{k}D^d*) are added. It follows that this anti-*K^k* secondary response can be driven by intermolecular help.

Thus far we have found no real evidence of inter-structural help, *i.e.*, help of the AEF-mediated type. No doubt this is a consequence of having picked conditions which minimise this kind of effect—avoiding graft-*versus*-host reactions, using moderate cell doses, *etc.*

Helper Antigens

Genetic analysis has been applied to helper antigens in two situations. In the primary and non-transfer secondary anti-Thy-1 system just mentioned, AKR mice have been immunised with mice of the CBA → AKR/Cum backcross. Just two or three "minor" alloantigens appear to determine help in this situation.

In the secondary transfer anti-Thy-1 system, also as mentioned, (B6×B10. D2) F$_1$ B cells (*H-2$^{b/d}$*) primed anti-Thy-1.1 have been helped by syngeneic T cells primed against C×B (BALB×B6) inbred recombinant cells or against B6.BALB H-minor cells (*H-7^c*, *H-25^c*, *H-37^c*). Challenge was with BALB.Thy-1.1 cells (BALB.Thy-1.1 is another locally synthesised Thy-1 congenic strain). Under these conditions all combinations of or individual minor alloantigens tested appeared to determine help.

Although we have no direct evidence, perhaps this difference can be attributed to the effect of priming in the generation of help. The priming employed in this second group of experiments may have lowered the threshold at which help could be detected.

A third group of experiments tested viral antigens. In the Thy-1 primary response, Sendai virus, vaccinia virus, and herpesvirus simplex type I can all provide help.

Thus, for example, AKR cells infected with Sendai generated an anti-Thy-1.1 primary PFC response in (AKR/Cum × CBA)F₁ hosts which had been primed with Sendai. Both anti-viral priming and viral infection of the Thy-1.1-bearing cells were necessary to obtain the full response, although in the Sendai system treatment of the cells with β-propiolactone-inactivated virus was also effective (as in the generation of T_c cells, Ref. 8). None of the viruses tested failed to generate help; we would expect this ability to be confined to viruses controlling cell surface antigens.

Latent Help

Mention has already been made of the 5R → B10 combination, in which an isolated H-2D-end can generate a substantial secondary response if and only if priming has been carried out with intermolecular help, e.g., from Ia antigens. A similar phenomenon has been observed with Thy-1, where this antigen in isolation (i.e., in the AKR/Cum ⇌ AKR combination) can generate a serological secondary but not a primary response. Several explanations of this phenomenon, which we call latent help, are possible. They have been discussed previously (14). We favour the hypothesis that H-2D or Thy-1 can enter the immune system slowly through the reprocessing route, and possibly only when the cell on which they are brought is subjected to immunological attack on other antigens. At any rate, our hypothesis is that only when they do enter through this route can they generate specific helper cells.

The Kinetics of Help

Kinetics of the generation of help have been examined in some detail in contrasting systems. One is with minor alloantigens priming for the Thy-1 response (using the PFC, non-transfer system); here priming follows kinetics not obviously different from those obtained with bovine serum albumin or other conventional strong soluble antigens, with a short latent period, a peak at 1–2 weeks, and a slow decline. Another is with Ia priming for anti-H-2K responses (using the serological, transfer system), where similar kinetics are observed. A third is with H-2K-specific help (itself obtained with help from Ia) for the same anti-H-2K responses; here priming occurs relatively slowly, reaching a maximum after about five weekly injections (13). This difference can be explained in terms of the slow development of latent help.

Dual Recognition

Macrophage reprocessing can be explored from another angle, by determining whether priming generates T cells which recognise helper antigens in association with donor or host Ia molecules. One such experimental design has been described previously (2). In other very similar transfer experiments performed in collaboraton with Dr. M. Cherry of the Jackson Laboratory we have enquired whether (CBA × B10)F₁ cells (H-2k/b, Thy-1.2) primed with either AKR cells (H-2k, Thy-1.1) or AK × L17 (H-2b, Thy-1.1)., express a preference for boosting with either H-2k or H-2b cells in generating an anti-Thy-1.1 secondary response. No such preference could be found, from which we conclude that under these conditions of hyperimmunisation host reprocessing predominates. Nevertheless, in other experiments involving one-shot priming against minor alloantigens, MHC-determined restrictions have been detected. We do not yet understand the factors which control the extent of reprocessing, but believe that this should provide a fertile field of investigation.

Inhibition

We have investigated inhibition in four superficially unconnected areas. i) Inhibition of the *in vitro* response by antigen in the form of intact cells has already been referred to. ii) An incompatible MHC on the immunogen can inhibit the anti-Thy-1 response, not only in secondary transfers (*11*) but also in the primary response driven by intermolecular help. Incompatibility at the K or D ends is sufficient for inhibition and the effect does not occur among cells which are tolerant of the incompatible MHC. The effect may be provisionally interpreted as intra-structural, inter-molecular antigen competition, and may perhaps be mediated through premature removal of the associated Thy-1 antigen. iii) Single-shot priming for the anti-Thy-1 response occurs with a biphasic dose-response curve: 10^7 cells regularly prime less effectively than 10^6 or 5×10^7. The drop at 10^7 cells does not occur after cyclophosphamide treatment, and can therefore tentatively be attributed to the action of T_s cells. iv) Inhibition of the IgG response has been observed as a consequence of immunisation with isolated *H-2* or AgB antigens lacking Ia incompatibility (*20, 22*). Although we have had some difficulty in extending these results to other MHC alleles in the mouse, our studies suggest that this kind of inhibition is not mediated by suppressor cells.

Immune Response Genes

The need for intermolecular help in generating a primary anti-Thy-1 response can be examined in mice of various MHC types by immunising F_1 hybrids of the AKR/Cum strain with AKR cells. Data obtained in this way suggest that an *H-2* allele controls the need for intermolecular help. This control maps on the *K-IA* region. Comparable *Ir-I* control, but in a somewhat different system, has been observed previously (*21*).

Implications

These findings provide the basis of a new theory of self-tolerance and auto-immunity (*2, 13*). The essence of this theory is that self-macromolecules on the surface of Ia$^-$ cells will not attract the attention of T_h cells unless they are reprocessed. Consequently, to the extent that reprocessing of cell surface is limited, this provides a non-acquired, genetically-programmed mechanism of self-tolerance. Inappropriate reprocessing may be an important cause of auto-immune disease.

More importantly, these findings, together with others of a similar nature, provide a rational strategy for cancer immunotherapy. It should be possible, as our understanding of intermolecular help grows, to design molecules suitable for insertion into the membranes of cancer cells to function as helper antigens. This idea is, of course, the central theme of the present symposium and has long been pursued by Kobayashi and his colleagues (7).

The main obstacles in pursuing this idea are, firstly, our relatively poor understanding of the associative control of cellular immunity. This deficiency has been discussed above, and is clearly open to remedy. A far more serious obstacle is the lack of well-defined tumour-specific antigens to serve as targets for manipulation. So many false hopes of immunotherapy have been raised that the subject is now under a cloud. The best hopes at the moment, in our view, come from i) the better definition of idiotypic, tumour-specific antigens in certain human tumours, particularly melanoma (*16*), ii) the increasing evidence of viral antigens on some tumours, particularly nasopharyngeal carcinoma (*6*), iii) the possibility that intervention of the type proposed may itself reveal tumour-specific antigen which would otherwise escape notice, and iv) the evidence that non-specific helper activity can in fact do just this for T_c responses *in vitro* (*12, 17, 23*).

REFERENCES

1. Al-Adra, A. R., and Pilarski, L. M. Antigen-specific suppression of cytotoxic T cell responses in mice. I. Suppressor T cells are not cytotoxic cells. *Eur. J. Immunol.*, **8**, 504–511 (1978).

2. Clark, E. A., Lake, P., Mitchison, N. A., and Nakashima, I. *In* "Cytotoxic Cell Interaction and Immunostimulation," ed. by G. Reithmuller, P. Wernet, and G. Cudkowitz (1978). Academic Press, New York, in press.

3. Clark, E. A., Lake, P., Mitchison, N. A., and Winchester, G. *In* "Proc. 4th European Immunol. Meeting, Budapest," (1978), in press.

4. Feldmann, M., Baltz, M., Erb, P., Howie, S., Kontiainen, S., Woody, J., and Zvaifler, N. A comparison of *I*-region associated factors involved in antibody production. *Prog. Immunol.*, **3**, 331–337 (1978).

5. Feldmann, M., Kilburn, D., and Levy, J. T-T interaction in the generation of helper cells *in vitro. Nature*, **256**, 741–743 (1975).

6. Ho, H. C., Ng, M. H., and Kwan, H. C. IgA antibodies to Epstein Barr viral capsid antigens in saliva of nasopharyngeal carcinoma patients. *Br. J. Cancer*, **35**, 888–892 (1977).

7. Kobayashi, H., Kodama, T., and Gotohda, E. "Xenogenisation of Tumour Cells," pp. 1–124 (1977). Hokkaido University School of Medicine Publ., Sapporo.

8. Koszinowski, U., Gething, M. J., and Waterfield, M. T cell cytotoxicity in the absence of viral protein synthesis in target cells. *Nature*, **267**, 160–163 (1977).

9. Lake, P. Antibody response induced *in vitro* to the cell surface alloantigen Thy-1. *Nature*, **262**, 297–298 (1976).

10. Lake, P. and Mitchison, N. A. Associative control of the immune response to cell surface antigens. *Immunol. Commun.*, **5**, 795–805 (1976).

11. Lake, P. and Mitchison, N. A. Regulatory mechanisms in the immune response to cell surface antigens. *Cold Spring Harbor Symp. Quant. Biol.*, **41**, 589–595 (1977).

12. Lee, S. K. and Oliver, R.T.D. Autologous leukaemia-specific T cell mediated lymphocytotoxicity in patients with acute myelogenous leukaemia. *J. Exp. Med.*, **147**, 912–922 (1978).

13. Mitchison, N. A. *In* "Clinics in Rheumatic Diseases," ed. N. Zvaifler (1978). W. B. Saunders, Eastbourne, in press.

14. Mitchison, N. A. and Lake, P. *In* "ICN-UCLA Symp. Immune System-Immune System: Genetics and Regulation," ed. E. Sercarz, L. A. Herzenberg, and C. F. Fox, pp. 555–558 (1978). Academic Press, New York.

15. Schendel, D. J., Alter, B. J., and Bach, F. H. Involvement of LD and SD region differences in MLC and CML: A three cell experiment. *Trans. Proc.*, **5**, 1651–1653 (1973).

16. Shiku, H. *In* "Manipulation of the Immune Response in Cancer," ed. N. A. Mitchison and M. Landy (1978). Academic Press, London, in press.

17. Sondel, P. M., O'Brien, C., Porter, L., Schlossman, S. F., and Chess, L. Cell mediated destruction of human leukaemic cells by MHC identical lymphocytes: Requirement for a proliferative trigger *in vitro*. *J. Immunol.*, **117**, 2197–2203 (1976).

18. Sprent, J. Restricted helper function of F_1 hybrid T cells positively selected to heterologous erythrocytes in irradiated parental strains of mice. II. Evidence for restrictions affecting helper cell induction and T-B collaboration, both mapping to the *K*-end of the *H-2* complex. *J. Exp. Med.*, **147**, 1159–1174 (1978).

19. Vogt, P. and Simpson, E. *In vitro* evidence from anti-hapten antibody responses for T helper and suppressor cells directed against major histocompatibility antigens in the mouse. I. Participation of *I* region determinants in induction of T helper cells. *Eur. J. Immunol.*, (1978), in press.

20. Welsh, K. I., Burgos, H., and Batchelor, J. R. The immune response to allogeneic rat platelets: Ag-B antigens in matrix form lacking *Ia*. *Eur. J. Immunol.*, **7**, 267–272 (1977).

21. Wernet, D. and Lilly, F. Genetic regulation of the antibody responses to *H-2D^b* alloantigens in mice. I. Differences in activation of helper T cells in C57BL/10 and BALB/c congenic strains. *J. Exp. Med.*, **141**, 573–583 (1975).

22. Wernet, D. and Lilly, F. Genetic regulation of the antibody responses to *H-2D^b* alloantigens in mice. III. Inhibition of the IgG response to non-congenic cells by pre-immunisation with congenic cells. *J. Exp. Med.*, **144**, 654–661 (1976).

23. Zarling, J. M., Reich, P. C., McKeough, M., and Bach, F. H. Generation of cytotoxic lymphocytes *in vitro* against autologous human leukaemia cells. *Nature*, **262**, 691–693 (1976).

24. Zinkernagel, R. M., Callahan, G. N., Althage, A., Cooper, S., Streilein, J. W., and Klein, J. The lymphoreticular system in triggering virus plus self-specific cytotoxic T cell: Evidence for T help. *J. Exp. Med.*, **147**, 897–911 (1978).

DIFFERENTIAL RECOGNITION BY CYTOTOXIC AND SUPPRESSOR T CELLS IN THE IMMUNE RESPONSE AGAINST SYNGENEIC TUMORS

Tomio TADA,[*1,*2] Shigeyoshi FUJIMOTO,[*1] Katsumi YAMAUCHI,[*1] and Masanori SHIMIZU[*1]

Laboratories for Immunology, School of Medicine, Chiba University

Evidence is presented that cytotoxic and suppressor T cells in syngeneic tumor immunity recognize different antigenic structures on the same tumor cells. This was first demonstrated by the fact that cytotoxic T cells generated by two methylcholanthrene-induced sarcomas of the A/J mouse origin (SaI and S1509a) showed considerable cross-reactivity in their cytotoxic effect on both sarcomas, whereas suppressor T cells induced by these two tumor cell lines displayed a very strict individual specificity for the corresponding tumors. In addition, soluble tumor extracts (STE) of these two sarcomas could induce suppressor T cells having the same individual specificities while being unable to generate cytotoxic T cells. STE, if present in excess, could inhibit the effect of suppressor T cells but not that of cytotoxic T cells. Thus, cytotoxic T cells are thought to recognize not only the solubilizable tumor antigens but also other structures possessed by live syngeneic tumor cells, possibly self antigens.

This postulate was supported by the following experiments. Rous sarcoma virus (RSV)-induced sarcomas were produced in various B10 congenic and recombinant mice. The cells were transplanted into strains sharing either the *H-2K* or *H-2D* locus (or none) with the tumor. After secondary rejection of the immunizing tumor, mice were then challenged with the syngeneic tumor. Successful tumor immunity was obtained only if the immunizing tumor and recipient shared the *H-2K* or *H-2D* locus, while immunization with an *H-2* incompatible tumor was unable to induce immunity against the syngeneic tumor. This indicates that cytotoxic effector T cells recognize self *H-2* antigens together with tumor antigens encoded by the viral genome. Modification of *H-2* antigens may provide a useful means for the so-called xenogenization.

The immune response is a series of complex cellular events in which various types of lymphoid cells interact with each other. Tumor immunity is no exception. It has been shown that the generation, as well as the final effect of cytotoxic T cells against a syngeneic tumor is regulated by other cell types, namely, suppressor, amplifier T cells, and probably macrophages (*6, 7, 12*).

Presence of the tumor-specific suppressor T cells in the tumor-bearing host (TBH)

[*1] Inohana 1-8-1, Chiba 280, Japan (多田富雄, 藤本重義, 山内克己, 清水正法).

[*2] Present address: Department of Immunology, Faculty of Medicine, University of Tokyo, Hongo 7-3-1, Bunkyo-ku, Tokyo 113, Japan.

is especially pertinent to the understanding of the apparent unresponsiveness of the host against the growing tumor. Fujimoto *et al.* (*4, 5*) demonstrated that the transfer of splenic T cells from a TBH suppressed the acquired tumor immunity in the recipient that had been induced by active immunization with the homologous tumor. Such a suppressive activity of T cells was recently demonstrated in an *in vitro* system as well (*6*). Since the mitomycin C (MMC)-treated tumor cells could induce a strong immunological resistance against the secondarily implanted tumor in syngeneic animals, they undoubtedly possess tumor-specific antigen recognizable by cytotoxic T cells. How, then, could the growing tumor escape from this host defense mechanism and result in the activation of an entirely different pathway leading to the generation of suppressor T cells?

We have been engaged in the analysis of the recognition system of cytotoxic and suppressor T cells in tumor immunity during the past few years, and have asked the question whether the cytotoxic and suppressor T cells could be activated by the same tumor-specific antigen. The question is, in fact, deeply concerned with the immune response to cell-surface antigen in general, and points to the role of major histocompatibility (MHC) antigens in the activation of protective immunity against cancer. Here we report the evidence which indicates that cytotoxic and suppressor T cells recognize different structural moieties present on the same tumor cells. The conditions under which cytotoxic and suppressor T cells are preferentially activated also are determined. The results will be discussed in the light of the concept of dual and single recognition of cell surface antigens by T cells.

Specificity of Cytotoxic and Suppressor T Cells

Fujimoto *et al.* (*3*) demonstrated that cytotoxic T cells generated by two methylcholanthrene-induced sarcomas of the A/J mouse origin (SaI and S1509a) showed a considerable cross-reactivity when tested in reciprocal combinations, whereas suppressor T cells induced by these two tumor cell lines displayed a very strict individual specificity for the corresponding tumors. Such a disparity in the specificity of cytotoxic and suppressor T cells was also demonstrated *in vitro* by the following two procedures (*6*).

A/J mice were immunized intraperitoneally with 10^6 MMC-treated tumor cells. Spleen cells were harvested 14 days after the immunization, and were reactivated *in vitro* by culturing the cells with MMC-treated homologous tumor for 5 days in the ratio of 300 : 1. The cytotoxic activity of the *in vitro* activated T cells was assayed by ^{51}Cr-release from target tumor cells during the 16-hr co-cultivation. The target to lymphocyte ratio was usually 1 : 20 or 1 : 40.

By this procedure we were able to demonstrate that the spleen cells from A/J mice immunized with SaI could equally kill S1509a, and that those immune to S1509a were capable of killing SaI. However, this cytotoxicity was proved to be specific for these two closely-related tumors, since other syngeneic and allogeneic tumor cells such as anaplastic carcinoma AC15091A and lymphoma L1117 of the A/J mouse origin, and EL-4 of C57BL/6, were not killed by the same spleen cells. Thus, it is clear that SaI and S1509a share cross-reactive determinants recognizable by the same cytotoxic T cells, and that the observed cytotoxic effect is directed at tumor antigen(s) possessed

TABLE I. Analysis of Specificity of Syngeneic Cytotoxic and Suppressor T Cells against Three Methylcholanthrene-induced Sarcomas of A/J Origin

Cyotoxic T cell generated by	Target	Suppressor T cell generated by	Result of cytotoxic killing
SaI	SaI	Not added	Yes
SaI	S1509a	Not added	Yes
SaI	S713a	Not added	No
S1509a	SaI	Not added	Yes
S1509a	S1509a	Not added	Yes
S1509a	S713a	Not added	No
SaI	SaI	SaI	No (suppressed)
SaI	S1509a	SaI	Yes (not suppressed)
SaI	S1509a	S1509a	No (suppressed)
SaI	SaI	S1509a	Yes (not suppressed)
S1509a	S1509a	S1509a	No (suppressed)
S1509a	SaI	S1509a	Yes (not suppressed)
S1509a	SaI	SaI	No (suppressed)

by these two tumors but not at antigens adsorbed to the cell membrane, *e.g.*, components of fetal calf serum. In fact, the same cross-resistance had been observed by an *in vivo* transplantation experiment (*3*). The effector cell in this syngeneic tumor immunity was determined to be a T cell by sensitivity to anti-Thy-1 antiserum (*6*).

The activity of suppressor T cells was detected by a method described elsewhere (*6*). In brief, spleen cells from A/J mice bearing the growing tumor were co-cultured with a mixture of radiolabeled target tumor and cytotoxic T cells. A control culture consisted of the tumor and cytotoxic T cells together with normal spleen cells instead of cells from the TBH. In general, the same number of spleen cells from the TBH to the cytotoxic cells almost completely inhibited cytotoxicity of the latter, provided the spleen cells were derived from mice carrying the tumor which is homologous to the *in vitro* target of the cytotoxic killing. An important point is that no inhibition of cytotoxicity was induced if the suppressor cell was obtained from animals bearing the cross-reactive tumor.

Thus, the following rule was derived from the experiment (Table I): Cytotoxic T cells activated with either one of the tumors, *i.e.*, SaI or S1509a, could kill both tumors to an equal degree. However, suppressor T cells generated by SaI could suppress the cytotoxic killing of SaI but not S1509a, and those generated by S1509a could suppress the killing of S1509a but not SaI regardless of the original stimulation of cytotoxic T cells by either sarcoma line.

The suppressor T cell heretofore mentioned conforms to all the criteria of the antigen-specific suppressor T cell which have been established in other experimental systems: The cell has strict antigen specificity, and suppresses the effect of a cytotoxic T cell in the presence of relevant tumor cells. It has been determined that the suppressor T cell in our system is killed by anti-Ia antisera having *I-J* subregion specificity (*6*) and by anti-Lyt-2,3 antiserum (manuscript in preparation). It is radiosensitive, present in the spleen and thymus, and is relatively short-lived (*5*). It is, therefore, probable that such a suppressor T cell plays an important role in the apparent loss of active resistance against growing tumors in the TBH.

Activation and Neutralization of Suppressor T Cell by a Soluble Tumor Cell Extract

Further evidence that suppressor and cytotoxic T cells recognize different antigenic moieties of the cell surface membrane was obtained by the following observation. We immunized A/J mice with 3M KCl extract of S1509a (14). With varying doses of antigen and immunization regimens, the extract was not able to prime animals to produce cytotoxic T cells. Conversely, spleen cells from animals immunized with the soluble tumor extract (STE) were found to possess a strong suppressive activity for the *in vitro* activated cytotoxic T cells. The specificity of the STE-induced suppressor T cell was identical to that derived from S1509a-bearing animals.

It has been shown that *in vitro* ^{51}Cr-release from S1509a by cytotoxic T cells was always inhibited by an excess of live cold tumor cells; not only by the homologous tumor (S1509a) but also by the cross-reactive tumor (SaI). In contrast, STE from S1509a could not neutralize this cytotoxicity even at a dose of 1.5 mg/ml. On the other hand, if STE was added to the mixture of S1509a, the cytotoxic and suppressor T cells (1: 40: 40), it could inhibit the suppressive effect exerted by the latter cell type resulting in the effective killing of the target cells (Table II). This indicates that STE is able to neutralize the suppressor T cell but not cytotoxic T cell.

These results indicate that (1) STE preferentially activates the suppressor T cell while lacking the ability to induce the cytotoxic T cell, (2) live attenuated tumor cells are required for the activation of the cytotoxic T cell, and (3) STE cannot inhibit the cytotoxic T cell but does neutralize the suppressor T cell. Hence, it is concluded that the cytotoxic T cell is only generated under conditions where the tumor-specific antigen is presented on the live tumor cell membrane to the precursor of the cytotoxic T cell, and that STE solubilized from the cell membrane preferentially stimulates the suppressor T cell, but not the cytotoxic T cell. This conclusion is consistent with previous reports which indicated that antigen-specific suppressor T cells can directly bind antigen, and that this antigen specificity is similar to that of an antibody (8, 13).

TABLE II. Evidence for Recognition of Different Antigenic Moieties on Tumor Cell Membrane by Cytotoxic and Suppressor T Cells[a]

Cytotoxic T cell	Suppressor T cell	Inhibitor	Result of cytotoxic killing
+	—	—	Yes
+	—	Live S1509a	No (inhibition)
+	—	Live SaI	No (inhibition)
+	—	STE from S1509a	Yes (no inhibition)
+	+	—	No (suppression)
+	+	STE from S1509a	Yes (no suppression)
+	+	STE from SaI	No (suppression)

[a] Cytotoxic killing was inhibited by live tumor cells but not STE the latter of which could effectively inhibit the activity of suppressor T cell.

Attribute of Major Histocompatibility Complex to the Structure Recognized by Cytotoxic T Cells

The above experiments suggest that the suppressor T cell recognizes tumor antigens which are unique to the individual tumor, and that such antigens are extractable from the tumor cell membrane without destruction of antigenic determinants. In clear contrast, in order to induce the cytotoxic T cell, it is essential to immunize animals with live attenuated tumor cells whose antigenic properties are destroyed by chemical extraction. Thus, these two cell types determining the tumor resistance are likely to recognize different antigenic structures on the same target cells.

What then, may be attributed to the difference in structure of the cell membrane which is differentially recognized by these two cell types? It has been reported by Zinkernagel and Doherty (2, 15) and Shearer et al. (9, 10) that cytotoxic T cells against virus-infected cells and chemically-modified cells recognize not only viral and chemical antigens but also a 'self' determinant coded for by MHC genes. To test whether MHC products would differentiate to the structure recognized by the cytotoxic T cells in syngeneic tumor immunity, the following experiments were carried out.

Fibrosarcomas were induced in various strains of B10 congenic and recombinant mice by injection of Rous sarcoma virus (RSV) of the Schmidt-Ruppin strain maintained in the chicken. After cloning and establishing cell lines, 10^5 tumor cells were transplanted subcutaneously in congenic strains sharing either the *H-2K*, *H-2D* locus or none with the tumor cells. The transplanted tumor was usually rejected within 2 weeks. Once the rejection had become apparent, the mice were challenged with an entirely *H-2* compatible RSV tumor (*i.e.*, the tumor derived from this strain), and the ratio of the take as well as growth of the tumor was measured.

Although not all the established fibrosarcomas are immunogenic to induce acquired immunity in the syngeneic host even after surgical removal of the tumor, some selected cell lines were capable of inducing resistance against a secondary implant of the syngeneic tumor. By certain combinations of the immunizing and challenging tumors having restricted identity at either the *K* or *D* end, we were able to examine the contribution of *H-2* antigens in the generation of cytotoxic T cells.

One such experiment is depicted in Table III. In this experiment, C57BL/6 (*H-2^b^*) mice were primarily immunized by implantation of tumors derived from mice sharing either the *K* end [B10.A(5R)], *D* end [B10.A(4R)], or none (B10.BR). After rejection of the tumor, animals were challenged with *H-2* compatible B10 (*H-2^b^*)

TABLE III. Associative Recognition of RSV-induced Tumor Antigens with MHC Products[a] by T Cells

Recipient	Immunizing tumor	Challenging tumor	Take of tumor
C57BL/6J (*bbbbbb*)	—	B10 (*bbbbbb*)	6/6
C57BL/6J (*bbbbbb*)	B10.A (5R) (*bbbkkdd*)	B10 (*bbbbbb*)	1/5
C57BL/6J (*bbbbbb*)	B10.A (4R) (*kkbbbbb*)	B10 (*bbbbbb*)	1/5
C57BL/6J (*bbbbbb*)	B10.BR (*kkkkkk*)	B10 (*bbbbbb*)	4/4

[a] *H-2* haplotypes of *K*, *I-A*, *I-B*, *I-J*, *I-E*, *I-C*, and *D* regions are indicated in parentheses. Underlined are the portions identical to those of the challenging tumor.

tumor. As shown in Table III, tumors from B10.A(5R) and B10.A(4R), which share either the *K* or *D* end of the *H-2* complex with the challenging tumor (B10), could induce resistance in C57BL/6 mice against a secondary implant of *H-2* compatible B10 tumor. However, the immunization of C57BL/6 mice with the B10.BR tumor, which is entirely *H-2* histocompatible to B10, was not able to induce resistance against the B10 tumor. In experiments using other combinations of fibrosarcomas, it was generally observed that successful immunity was achieved only if the immunizing and challenging tumors share the same *H-2K* or *H-2D* locus in the host whose *H-2* complex is identical to that of the challenging tumor. If the *H-2* antigens of the first and second tumors are entirely different, in no case was the successful induction of tumor resistance detected. These results indicate that cytotoxic effector cells recognize the "self" antigen coded for by the *H-2K* or *H-2D* locus which are perhaps associated on the cell membrance with the tumor antigens encoded by the viral genome.

COMMENT

Our present concept of the multicellular mechanism of tumor immunity is especially concerned with the interaction and balance between cytotoxic and suppressor T cells. The present results indicate that these functionally distinct cell types are generated under different conditions in which they are forced to recognize different antigenic moieties on the same tumor cell membrane. Probably the recognition of self

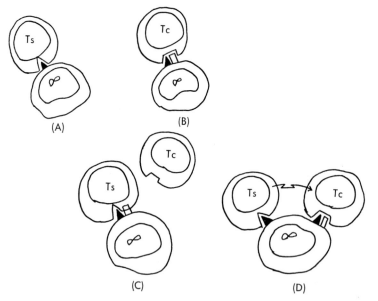

FIG. 1. Models for interactions between cytotoxic (Tc), suppressor (Ts) and target tumor cells. In (A) Ts recognizes tumor antigen unique to the individual tumor, and in (B) Tc recognizes tumor antigen in association with 'self' major histocompatibility antigen (□). Ts would simply occupy the reactive site for Tc blocking the interaction between Tc and Target (C). In the model (D), Ts and Tc recognize different antigenic determinants on the same cell, and then Ts directly inactivates Tc.

H-2 antigen which is associated with tumor-specific antigen is can be attributed to the cross-resistance of animals against related tumors, whereas the individual tumor antigen preferentially activates the suppressor T cell. The evidence for such a postulate has been discussed above.

The question remains as to how the suppressor T cell inhibits the effect of the cytotoxic T cell. A hypothetical scheme is presented in Fig. 1. If one were to admit that cytotoxic and suppressor T cells recognize different moieties of membrane antigen (*i.e.*, tumor antigen+self by the cytotoxic T cell, and tumor antigen alone by the suppressor T cell), the simplest explanation is that the suppressor T cell having a high affinity for the antigen inhibits the reaction of the cytotoxic T cell to the corresponding antigenic site by steric hindrance. The second possibility is that the suppressor and cytotoxic T cells would interact directly by close approximation to these antigens on the same target cell. Although our knowledge on the cellular mechanism of T cell-mediated suppression is still very limitted, such an interaction between the suppressor T cell and other cell types *via* the antigen has been reported in other experimental systems (*1, 11*). No formal proof for these possibilities has been presented as yet. However, if such a postulate holds true, one important approach to xenogenization of tumor cells may be an attempt to modify the *H-2*-associated-tumor specific antigen by chemicals and viruses.

Acknowledgment

We are grateful to Dr. T. Kuwata of the Department of Microbiology, School of Medicine, Chiba University for providing us with the RSV tumor of the chicken. We wish to acknowledge our thanks to Mr. Hidenori Takahashi and to Ms. Yoko Yamaguchi for their technical and secretarial assistance.

REFERENCES

1. Basten, A., Miller, J.F.A.P., and Johnson, P. T cell-dependent suppression of an anti-hapten antibody response. *Transplant. Rev.*, **26**, 130–169 (1975).
2. Doherty, P. C., Blanden, R. V., and Zinkernagel, R. M. Specificity of virus-immune effector T cells for H-2K or H-2D compatible interactions: Implications for H-antigen diversity. *Transplant. Rev.*, **29**, 89–124 (1976).
3. Fujimoto, S., Greene, M. I., and Sehon, A. H. Immunosuppressor T cells and their factors in tumor-bearing hosts. *In* "Suppressor Cells in Immunity," ed. S. K. Singhal and W.R.St.C. Sinclair, pp. 136–148 (1975). The University of Western Ontario Press, Ontario.
4. Fujimoto, S., Greene, M. I., and Sehon, A. H. Regulation of the immune response to tumor antigens. I. Immunosuppressor cells in tumor bearing host. *J. Immunol.*, **116**, 791–799 (1976).
5. Fujimoto, S., Greene, M. I., and Sehon, A. H. Regulation of the immune response to tumor antigens. II. The nature of immunosuppressor cells in tumor bearing host. *J. Immunol.*, **116**, 800–806 (1976).
6. Fujimoto, S., Matsuzawa, T., Nakagawa, K., and Tada, T. Cellular interaction between cytotoxic and suppressor T cells against syngeneic tumors in the mouse. *Cell Immunol.*, **38**, 378–387 (1978).
7. Glaser, M., Kirchner, H., Holden, H. T., and Herberman, R. B. Inhibition of cell-

mediated cytotoxicity against tumor-associated antigens by suppressor cells from tumor-bearing mice. *J. Natl. Cancer Inst.*, **56**, 865–867 (1976).

8. Okumura, K., Takemori, T., Tokuhisa, T., and Tada, T. Specific enrichment of the suppressor T cell bearing *I-J* determinants: Parallel functional and serological characterizations. *J. Exp. Med.*, **146**, 1234–1245 (1977).

9. Shearer, G. M., Rehn, T. G., and Garbarino, C. A. Cell-mediated lympholysis of trinitrophenyl-modified autologous lymphocytes. *J. Exp. Med.*, **141**, 1348–1363 (1975).

10. Shearer, G. M., Rehn, T. G., and Verhulst, A.M.S. Role of the murine major histocompatibility complex in specificity of *in vitro* T-cell-mediated lympholysis against chemically-modified autologous lymphocytes. *Transplant. Rev.*, **29**, 222–248 (1976).

11. Tada, T. Regulation of the antibody response by T cell products determined by different *I* subregions. *In* "Immune System: Genetics and Regulation," ed. E. Sercarz, L. A. Herzenberg, and C. F. Fox, pp. 345–361 (1977). Academic Press, New York.

12. Takei, F., Levery, J. G., and Kilburn, D. G. *In vitro* induction of cytotoxicity against syngeneic mastocytoma and its suppression by spleen and thymus cells from tumor-bearing mice. *J. Immunol.*, **116**, 288–293 (1976).

13. Taniguchi, M. and Miller, J.F.A.P. Enrichment of specific suppressor T cells and characterization of their surface markers. *J. Exp. Med.*, **146**, 1450–1454 (1977).

14. Yamauchi, K., Fujimoto, S., and Tada, T. Differential activation of cytotoxic and suppressor T cells against syngeneic tumor in the mouse. *J. Immunol.* submitted.

15. Zinkernagel, R. M. and Doherty, P. C. *H-2* compatibility requirement for T cell mediated lysis of targets cells infected with lymphocytic choriomeningitis virus. *J. Exp. Med.*, **141**, 1427–1436 (1975).

RECOGNITION OF RSV-INDUCED TUMOR CELLS IN SYNGENEIC MICE AND SEMISYNGENEIC RECIPROCAL HYBRID MICE[*1]

Takato O. Yoshida, Soichi Haraguchi, Hideki Miyamoto, and Tetsumichi Matsuo

*Department of Microbiology, Hamamatsu University School of Medicine[*2]*

The immunogenetic control of the growth of virus nonproducing tumor cells induced by the Schmidt-Ruppin strain of Rous sarcoma virus in inbred mice was investigated in syngeneic, F_1 hybrid semisyngeneic and H-2 identical allogeneic mice. The data of recognition (blastogenesis) *in vitro* and the resistance (transplantability, survival period, and rejection) of F_1 hybrid semisyngeneic mice against BALB/cCr sarcoma cells, C-SA-1M (derived from male mouse) and C-SA-9F (derived from female mouse) suggested that reciprocal semisyngeneic mice, $H-2^{d/k}$, $(C \times C3)F_1$, $(C \times B10BR)F_1$; $H-2^{k/d}$, $(C3 \times C)F_1$, $(B10BR \times C)F_1$; $H-2^{d/b}$, CBF_1; $H-2^{b/d}$, BCF_1 showed high resistance; $H-2^{d/a}$, $(C \times B10A)F_1$ showed a moderate resistance; and $H-2^{d/d}$, CDF_1, DCF_1, $(C \times B10D2)F_1$, $(B10D2 \times C)F_1$ showed a low resistance. Further evidence in reciprocal F_1 hybrid mice suggested that even if reciprocal semisyngeneic F_1 hybrid mice were the same at gene level, the phenotypic resistance of the mice to the transplantation of parental tumor cells was markedly different. This may be related to maternal inheritance. The role of H-Y antigen on the surface of tumor cells related to the immunological xenogenization of tumor cells may be very important in the future according to preliminary pioneer studies.

The immune recognition and resistance against tumor cells related to the mechanisms responsible for immune recognition and the control of subsequent effector cell functions are topics among tumor immunologists who are beginning to investigate them at the level of the gene (*6*).

The immune recognition of antigens has been investigated as playing an important role in the restriction of the major histocompatibility complex (MHC) during the processing and/or presentation of antigen to T and B lymphocytes together with marcophages (*4, 5, 10–11, 24*).

It was quite an important observation in the tumor immunology field that cytotoxic T cell target recognition elicited by viral infection (*25, 26*), chemically-modified tumor cells (*13*) and male cells (H-Y carrier cells) (*15*) has been observed to include certain genetic restriction, that is, T lymphocytes initially recognize antigens together

---

[*1] This study was presented at the 36th and 37th Annual Meetings of the Japanese Cancer Association, and was supported by a Grant-in-Aid for Cancer Research from the Ministry of Education, Science and Culture, Japan.

[*2] Handa-cho 3600, Hamamatsu 431-31, Japan (吉田孝人, 原口惣一, 宮本秀樹, 松尾哲道).

with MHC membrane components on the antigen-presenting cell (dual or single recognition).

In this paper, we report the investigation on the immunogenetic control of growth of virus nonproducing tumor cells induced by the Schmidt-Ruppin strain of Rous sarcoma virus (RSV) in inbred mice in syngeneic, semisyngeneic, H-2 congenic, H-2 recombinant, and H-2 identical allogeneic mice, that is 1) to BALB/cCr tumors, C-SA-1M (derived from a male mouse) and C-SA-9F (derived from a female mouse), semi-syngeneic H-2^{k}F$_1$ hybrid mice and H-2^b F$_1$ hybrid mice showed high resistance, semi-syngeneic H-2^{a}F$_1$ hybrid mice showed a moderate resistance, and semisyngeneic H-2^{d}F$_1$ hybrid mice showed a low resistance; 2) in reciprocal semisyngeneic mice, different resistance to the transplantation of parental tumor cells existed; 3) in the syngeneic system, female mice primed with male tumor cells showed a strong resistance against the transplantation of female tumor cells.

Inbred Mice and F$_1$ Hybrid Mice

Both female and male inbred mice, BALB/cCr, DBA/2Cr, C3H/He, C57BL/6Cr, and reciprocal F$_1$ hybrid female and male mice,
(C57BL/6×BALB/c)F$_1$ hybrid (BC)F$_1$ mice (H-2^b×H-2^d),
(BALB/c×C57BL/6)F$_1$ hybrid (CB)F$_1$ mice (H-2^d×H-2^b),
(C57BL/6×DBA/2)F$_1$ hybrid (BD)F$_1$ mice (H-2^b×H-2^d),
(DBA/2×C57BL/6)F$_1$ hybrid (DB)F$_1$ mice (H-2^d×H-2^b),
(BALB/c×DBA/2)F$_1$ hybrid (CD)F$_1$ mice (H-2^d×H-2^d), and
(DBA/2×BALB/c)F$_1$ hybrid (DC)F$_1$ mice (H-2^d×H-2^d),
were purchased from Shizuoka Agricultural Cooperative Association for Laboratory Animals, Hamamatsu, Shizuoka, and C57BL/10Sn(B10)(H-2^b), B10A/SgSn(H-2$^{k/d}$), B10A(5R)/SgSn(H-2$^{b/a}$), B10BR/SgSn(H-2^k) congenic and recombinant inbred mice, and reciprocal F$_1$ hybrid female and male mice,
(BALB/c×B10D2)F$_1$ hybrid (C×B10D2)F$_1$ mice (H-2^d×H-2^d),
(B10D2×BALB/c)F$_1$ hybrid (B10D2×C)F$_1$ mice (H-2^d×H-2^d),
(BALB/c×B10A)F$_1$ hybrid (C×B10A)F$_1$ mice (H-2^d×H-2$^{k/d}$),
(BALB/c×B10)F$_1$ hybrid (C×B10)F$_1$ mice (H-2^d×H-2^b),
(B10×BALB/c)F$_1$ hybrid (B10×C)F$_1$ mice (H-2^b×H-2^d),
(BALB/c×C3H/He)F$_1$ hybrid (C×C3)F$_1$ mice (H-2^d×H-2^k),
(C3H/He×BALB/c)F$_1$ hybrid (C3×C)F$_1$ mice (H-2^k×H-2^d),
(BALB/c×B10BR)F$_1$ hybrid (C×B10BR)F$_1$ mice (H-2^d×H-2^k),
(B10BR×BALB/c)F$_1$ hybrid (B10BR×C)F$_1$ mice (H-2^k×H-2^d),
(C3H/He×B10BR)F$_1$ hybrid (C3×B10BR)F$_1$ mice (H-2^k×H-2^k),
(C3H/He×B10)F$_1$ hybrid (C3×B10)F$_1$ mice (H-2^k×H-2^b), and
(B10×C3H/He)F$_1$ hybrid (B10×C3)F$_1$ mice (H-2^b×H-2^k),
were made in our laboratory.

Tumors and Cultured Cell Lines

Subcutaneous tumors, C-SA-1M in male BALB/cCr, C-SA-9F in female BALB/cCr, BD-SA-2M in male BDF$_1$, BD-SA-3F in female BDF$_1$, and B10BR-SA-1M in male B10BR were induced by RSV (Schmidt-Ruppin strain) (7, 23) ,and were maintained in each inbred strain mouse.

The cultured cell lines were established from C-SA-1M and C-SA-9F tumors and were maintained in medium-199 supplemented with 5 or 10% fetal calf serum (FCS), penicillin and streptomycin, and/or RPMI-1640 medium supplemented with 5% FCS, penicillin and streptomycin.

The cultured cell lines from RSV-induced tumors in B10 congenic mice kindly supplied by S. Fujimoto, Department of Immunology, Chiba University, were S908-(D2) established from the tumor of a male B10D2 mouse, S826(BA) established from the tumor of a female B10A mouse, and S623(BR) established from the tumor of a female B10BR mouse. They were maintained in RPMI-1640 supplemented with 5% FCS, penicillin and streptomycin.

A tumor cell suspension, 1×10^6 cells/ml in RPMI-1640 from a solid tumor, was prepared after the digestion of minced tumor tissue within 0.25% trypsin and hyaluronidase (3,000 unit/ml) phosphate buffered saline (PBS), and tumor cells were washed several times with RPMI-1640 medium.

A tumor cell suspension from cultured cells was prepared after the trypsinization

TABLE I. Take and Growth of RSV-induced Tumors in Syngeneic, Semisyngeneic and H-2 Identical Allogeneic Mice

Recipient mice	H-2	BALB/c tumor cells (1×10^5/mouse s.c.)							
		C-SA-1M		C-SA-9F		C-Br-1M		C-Br-2F	
		M	F	M	F	M	F	M	F
BALB/c	d	10/10[a]	7/10	5/5	5/5	5/5	5/5	5/5	5/5
DBA/2	d	1/9	3/10	4/5	3/3	3/5	4/5	5/5	4/5
B10D2	d	0/3	0/5	0/5	0/5	0/5	0/3		
CDF₁	d/d	10/10	6/10	5/5	5/5	5/5	5/5	5/5	5/5
DCF₁	d/d	6/6	5/10	6/6	5/5	5/5	5/5	3/3	3/3
(C×B10D2)F₁	d/d	4/4	4/4			5/5	2/2		
(B10D2×C)F₁	d/d	3/4	4/4			2/2	2/2		
(C×B10A)F₁	d/a	4/4	2/5	5/5	5/5	5/5	4/4		
(B10A×C)F₁	a/d			5/5	5/5	5/5	5/5		
(B10A(5R)×C)F₁	i5/c	4/4	4/4			3/3	6/6		
CBF₁	d/b	8/9	4/10	5/5	4/5	5/5	5/5		
BCF₁	b/d	4/5	1/5	6/6	5/5	6/6	4/5		
(C×B10)F₁	d/b	5/5	3/10	3/3	4/5	5/5	5/5	3/3	3/3
(B10×C)F₁	b/d	5/9	8/10	5/5	4/5	6/6	5/5	5/5	5/5
CC3F₁	d/k	1/1	2/2						
C3CF₁	k/d	5/5	3/5	3/6	2/6	5/5	6/7		
(C×B10BR)F₁	d/k	9/9	8/9	5/5	3/6	6/6	5/5		
(B10BR×C)F₁	k/d	9/9	3/9	5/5	5/5		10/10		
DBF₁	d/b	5/8	3/6	4/5	3/5	4/4	6/6		
BDF₁	b/d	5/10	3/10	1/5	3/5	4/5	4/5		

[a] $\dfrac{\text{No. of tumor take and growth mice}}{\text{No. of tested mice}}$

M, male ; F, female.

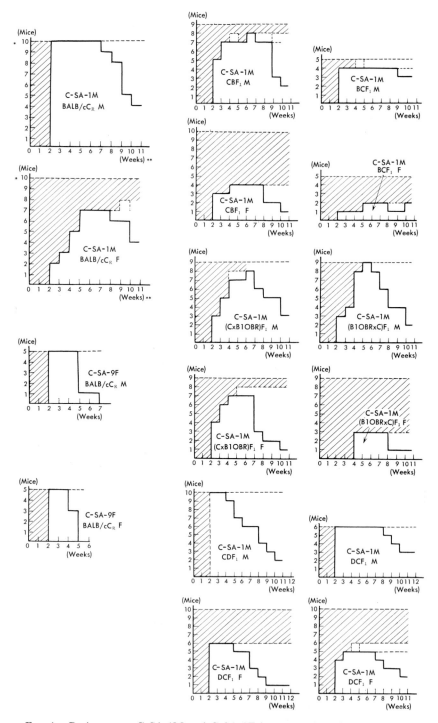

FIG. 1. Resistance to C-SA-1M and C-SA-9F in syngeneic and reciprocal F_1 hybrid semisyngeneic mice

    * No. of tumor taking and bearing mice.   ** Survival times.

of monolayer cultured cells with 0.25% trypsin-PBS solution, and was washed with RPMI-1640 medium. The viable cell number per ml was finally adjusted to a suitable cell number.

Transplantability of Mouse RSV-induced Tumors in Syngeneic, F_1 Hybrid Semisyngeneic and H-2 Identical Allogeneic Mice

An inoculation dose of 1×10^5 cells/0.1 ml was subcutaneously injected into mice, and the development and growth of tumors observed are listed in Table I and Fig. 1.

The take and the growth of the male BALB/cCr subcutaneous tumor, C-SA-1M, was slightly inhibited in male semisyngeneic mice, $(B10D2 \times C)F_1$, CBF_1, BCF_1, $(B10 \times C)F_1$; and was markedly inhibited in female syngeneic mice, BALB/cCr mice, and female semisyngeneic reciprocal F_1 hybrid mice, CDF_1, DCF_1, $(C \times B10A)F_1$, CBF_1, BCF_1, $(C \times B10)F_1$, $(B10 \times C)F_1$, $(C \times C3)F_1$, $(C3 \times C)F_1$, $(C \times B10BR)F_1$, and $(B10BR \times C)F_1$, compared with the female BALB/cCr tumor, C-SA-9F.

A female BALB/cCr subcutaneous tumor, C-SA-9F, was markedly inhibited in male and female $(C3 \times C)F_1$ and $(C \times B10BR)F_1$ hybrid semisyngeneic mice.

Both BALB/cCr brain tumors, C-Br-1M (derived from a male mouse) and C-Br-2F (derived from a female mouse), took and grew better than subcutaneous tumors in syngeneic and semisyngeneic mice.

In H-2^d identical allogeneic DBA/2Cr mice, the take and growth of BALB/cCr tumors, C-SA-9F, C-Br-1M, and C-Br-2F were slightly inhibited except C-SA-1M, and in H-2^d identical allogeneic B10D2 mice the above four tumors were completely inhibited.

Recognition of Tumor Cell Membrane-associated Antigens (TMAA) as Measured by Blastogenesis of Spleen cells

Figure 2 shows the immunological recognition of lymphocytes against BALB/cCr tumors, C-SA-1M and C-SA-9F expressed as the radioactivity of ^{3}H-TdR incorporation per 5×10^5 spleen cells of syngeneic, semisyngeneic, and H-2 identical allogeneic mice based on the blastogenesis of lymphocytes to react to TMAA. The blastogenesis was performed by spleen cells mixed with mitomycin-treated tumor cells cultured for 4 days in 5% CO_2 in an incubator at 37°. At the same time, the method of microassay for cell-mediated immunity (MCI) was applied to the cytotoxic activity of the spleen cells.

Syngeneic BALB/cCr and H-2^d identical semisyngeneic CDF_1 and DCF_1 mice spleen cells showed very low reactivity, less than 1×10^1 cpm of ^{3}H-TdR incorporation/ 5×10^5 spleen cells against C-SA-9F and $2–4 \times 10^2$ cpm of ^{3}H-TdR incorporation/ 5×10^5 spleen cells against C-SA-1M.

In the reciprocal semisyngeneic mice, (H-2$^{d/b}$, H-2$^{b/d}$; and H-2$^{d/k}$, H-2$^{k/d}$) spleen cells showed a relatively high reactivity, average about 3×10^2 cpm of ^{3}H-TdR incorporation/5×10^5 spleen cells, against C-SA-9F, and showed a relatively very high reactivity, average of about 12×10^2 cpm of ^{3}H-TdR incorporation/5×10^5 spleen cells, against C-SA-1M.

The H-2^d identical allogeneic DBA/2 and B10D2 mice, and H-2^d identical semi-

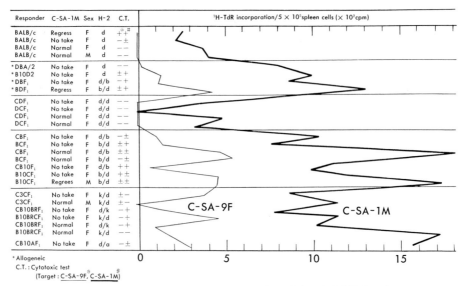

FIG. 2.   Recognition and resistance to male and female BALB/c mice

allogeneic BDF$_1$ and DBF$_1$ mice showed a very similar reactivity against C-SA-9F and C-SA-1M, as compared with the reciprocal semisyngeneic mice (H-2$^{d/b}$, H-2$^{b/d}$; and H-2$^{d/k}$, H-2$^{k/d}$).

Figures 3 and 4 show the blastogenesis of spleen cells derived from syngeneic, semisyngeneic, F$_1$ hybrid and H-2 identical allogeneic mice to various mitomycin-treated tissue culture tumor cells.

All these data suggested that C-SA-1M and S623 (BR) tumor cells were highly antigenic among the RSV-induced tumor cultured cell lines maintained in our laboratory.

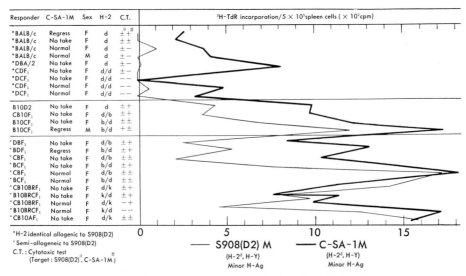

FIG. 3.   Recognition and resistance to BALB/c and B10D2 male tumors

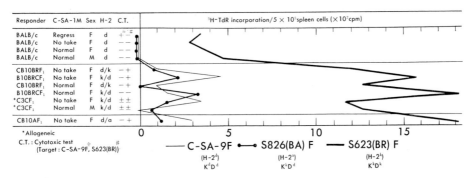

FIG. 4. Recognition and resistance to BALB/c, B10A, and B10BR female tumors

TABLE II. Recognition and Resistance to C-SA-1M (TMAA, H-Y)
and C-SA-9F (TMAA)

High resistance	$C \times C3$ F_1	$C3 \times C$ F_1	$H-2^k$
	$C \times B10BR$ F_1	$B10BR \times C$ F_1	
	CB F_1	BC F_1	$H-2^b$
	$CB10$ F_1	$B10C$ F_1	
Moderate resistance	$C \times B10A$ F_1		$H-2^a$
Low resistance	CD F_1	DC F_1	$H-2^d$
	$C \times B10D2$ F_1	$B10D2 \times C$ F_1	

Recognition: Blastogenesis
Resistance: Transplantability
Survival time
Rejection

The data of recognition (blastogenesis) and resistance (transplantability, survival time, and rejection) of semisyngeneic mice against C-SA-1M (possessing TMAA and H-Y antigen) and C-SA-9F (possessing TMAA) suggested that reciprocal semisyngeneic mice H-2$^{d/k}$, $(C \times C3)F_1$, $(C \times B10BR)F_1$; H-2$^{k/d}$, $(C3 \times C)F_1$, $(B10BR \times C)F_1$; H-2$^{d/b}$, CBF_1; H-2$^{d/b}$, BCF_1 showed a high resistance; H-2$^{d/a}$, $(C \times B10A)F_1$ showed a moderate resistance, and H-2$^{d/d}$, CDF_1, DCF_1, $(C \times B10D2)F_1$, $(B10D2 \times C)F_1$ showed a low resistance (Table II).

Different Resistance to Transplantation of Parental Mouse RSV-induced Tumors in Reciprocal F_1 Hybrid Mice

The recognition (blastogenesis) and the resistance (no take and/or rejection) to C-SA-1M (BALB/cCr, male) and S623(BR) (B10BR, female) tumor cells in reciprocal semisyngeneic F_1 hybrid mice appears in Table III. $(B10BR \times C)F_1$ hybrid mice showed a significantly higher resistance (67%) to C-SA-1M than $(C \times B10BR)F_1$ hybrid mice (11%), BCF_1 hybrid mice also showed a significant resistance (80%) to C-SA-1M as compared with CBF_1 hybrid mice. $(C \times B10BR)F_1$ hybrid mice showed significantly high resistance to S623(BR) tumor cells, and $(C3 \times B10)F_1$ hybrid mice also showed a significant high resistance as compared with reverse F_1 hybrid mice.

These data suggest that even if reciprocal semisyngeneic F_1 hybrid mice are

TABLE III.　Recognition and Resistance to RSV-Induced Tumor Cells
in Reciprocal Semisyngeneic F_1 Mice

Tumors	Reciprocal semisyngeneic recipients		Resistance no take and/or rejection (%)	Blastogenesis stimulation index		
BALB/c C-SA-1M	C×B10BR F_1	F	1/9[a] (11)	Primed Normal	11.32 4.31	15.6
	B10BR×C F_1	F	6/9 (67)	Primed Normal	9.87 6.59	16.4
	CB F_1	F	6/10 (60)	Primed Normal	4.36 3.78	8.11
	BC F_1	F	4/5 (80)	Primed Normal	16.98 6.61	23.6
B10BR S623(BR) F	**C**×B10BR F_1	F	6/6 (100)	Primed Normal	17.12 5.15	22.2
	C×B10BR F_1	M	4/6 (67)	Primed Normal	N.D.	
	B10BR×C F_1	F	2/4 (50)	Primed Normal	13.24 8.61	21.8
	B10BR×C F_1	M	1/7 (14)	N.D.		
	C3×B10 F_1	F	3/3 (100)	N.D.		
	C3×B10 F_1	M	1/4 (25)	N.D.		
	B10×C3 F_1	F	2/5 (40)	N.D.		
	B10×C3 F_1	M	2/7 (29)	N.D.		

[a] $\dfrac{\text{No. of tumor no take and/or rejection mice}}{\text{No. of tested mice}}$

( ) % resistance.　　N.D., not done.

theoretically the same at the gene level, phenotypical resistance to parental tumor cell transplantation is markedly different based on maternal inheritance.

Immunological Xenogenization of Tumor Cells Induced by H-Y Antigen

　　Figure 5 illustrates that female BDF_1 mice are very strongly immunized with 1×10^6 male BDF_1 raw tumor cells (H-Y, TMAA and histocompatibility antigens positive) and showed resistance to the transplantation of 1×10^5 cells and 5×10^5 cells of female BDF_1 tumor cells (TMAA and histocompatibility antigens positive) in the syngeneic system, in contrast to the immunization method according to the ligation technique of growing female tumors in female and male recipient BDF_1 mice, and of growing male tumors in male recipient BDF_1 mice.

　　It is suggested that male tumor cells possess male antigen H-Y, TMAA, and histocompatibility antigens; female tumor cells possess TMAA and histocompatibility antigens checked by the membrane immunofluorescence technique using highly immunized anti-H-Y antiserum and anti-TMAA antiserum; transplantation experiments yield the same information.

　　Evidence suggested that the H-Y antigen on the surface of male tumor cells induces the immunological xenogenization of tumor cells in female animals.

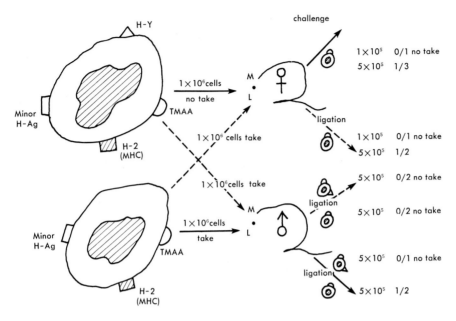

FIG. 5. RSV-induced BDF₁ male and female tumors in syngeneic system

DISCUSSION

Sjögren's group (*3, 16*) and Yamamoto's group (*8*) reported immunity to the virus nonproducing mouse tumors induced by RSV in the syngeneic system.

We have intensively investigated the immunogenetic control of the growth of virus nonproducing tumor cells induced by the Schmidt-Ruppin strain of RSV in syngeneic and F_1 hybrid semisyngeneic mice, and the blastogenesis of spleen cells primed with tumor cells *in vivo* and normal spleen cells as the recognition of TMAA, and cytotoxicity of the above spleen cells as resistance against tumor growth. The experimental results of the recognition (blastogenesis) and cytotoxicity *in vitro*, and the resistance (transplantability, survival time, and rejection) of semisyngeneic mice *in vivo* against C-SA-1M (TMAA, H-Y) and C-SA-9F (TMAA) have suggested that reciprocal semisyngeneic mice H-2$^{d/k}$, (C×C3)F_1, (C×B10BR)F_1; H-2$^{k/d}$, (C3×C)F_1, (B10BR×C)F_1; H-2$^{d/b}$, CBF$_1$; H-2$^{b/d}$, BCF$_1$ showed a high resistance; H-2$^{d/a}$, (C× B10A)F_1 showed moderate resistance; and H-2$^{d/d}$, CDF$_1$, DCF$_1$, (C×B10D2)F_1, (B10D2×C)F_1 showed low resistance. Further evidence of the resistance *in vivo* was quite interesting in reciprocal semisyngeneic F_1 mice (Tables I and III, Fig. 1), that is, (B10BR×C)F_1 and (C3×C)F_1 mice showed a stronger resistance than (C×B10BR)-F_1 and (C×C3)F_1 mice, and also BCF$_1$ mice showed a stronger resistance than CBF$_1$ against the growth of C-SA-1M tumor cells. It is conceivable that maternal inheritance (the mother is an influence on the embryo in the uterus, with fertilized nuclear DNA influenced by the ova-cytoplasmic factors, and milk factors in relation to the infant (*9, 19, 20, 22*)) is very important in cancer immunology, especially in human cancer immunology.

As to the helper T cells in F_1 hybrid mice, there are both parental H-2 helper T cell subpopulations, which have an immunological response against antigens based on H-2 restriction of macrophages, helper T cell and B cell interaction (17). Further interesting evidence is that, female C57BL/6 bone marrow cell chimeras in (C57BL/6 × CBA/J)F_1 sensitized with H-Y of C57BL/6 were able to recognize both C57BL/6 (H-2^b) and CBA/J (H-2^k) male cells (21). Therefore, if different H-2 cytotoxic T cell subpopulations exist in F_1 hybrid mice relating to maternal inheritance, it is conceivable that they may be sensitized to lyse the tumor cells derived from one parent over the H-2 restriction, and different reciprocal F_1 hybrid resistance may be easily understood.

The role of the H-Y antigen on the surface of tumor cells in relation to immunological xenogenization of tumor cells must be studied in the futurebased on our preliminary pioneer work.

Acknowledgment

The authors wish to thank Prof. T. Yamamoto for his cooperation in supplying the Schmidt-Ruppin strain of Rous sarcoma virus to induce mouse tumor cells, and for many instructive discussions during the course of present studies. We express great appreciation to Dr. M. Yazaki, Dr. M. Sugimoto, Mr. Y. Mizuno, and Mr. M. Maruyama for their great help during the experiments.

REFERENCES

1. Haraguchi, S., Yoshida, T. O., Miyamoto, T., Kotake, S., Matsuo, T., Ogino, T., and Sugimoto, K. Mechanisms of immune responsiveness to tumor cell membrane associated antigen (TMAA). I. Genetic control of immune responsiveness to RSV-induced tumor in BALB/cCr and F_1 hybrid of BALB/cCr. *Proc. Jpn. Cancer Assoc., 36th Annu. Meet.*, p. 68 (1977).
2. Haraguchi, S., Yoshida, T. O., Miyamoto, H., Matsuo, T., Ogino, T., Sugimoto, K. and Yazaki, M. Mechanisms of immune responsiveness to tumor cell membrane associated antigens (TMAA). II. Recognition of RSV-induced male and female tumor cells in syngeneic and semi-syngeneic mice. *Proc. Jpn. Cancer Assoc., 37th Annu. Meet.*, p. 63 (1978).
3. Jonsson, N. and Sjögren, H. O. Further studies on specific transplantation antigens in Rous sarcoma of mice. *J. Exp. Med.*, **122**, 403–421 (1965).
4. Katz, D. H., Hamaoka, T., Dorf, M. E., and Benacerraf, B. Cell interactions between histoincompatible T and B lymphocytes. The H-2 gene complex determines successful physiologic lymphocyte interactions. *Proc. Natl. Acad. Sci. U.S.*, **70**, 2624–2628 (1973).
5. Katz, D. H., Hamaoka, T., Dorf, M. E., and Benacerraf, B. Cell interactions between histoincompatible T and B lymphocytes. II. Failure of physiologic cooperative interactions between T and B lymphocytes from allogeneic donor strains in humoral response to hapten-protein conjugates. *J. Exp. Med.*, **137**, 1405–1418 (1973).
6. Klein, G. and Klein, E. Immune surveillance against virus-induced tumors and non-rejectability of spontaneous tumors: Contrasting consequences of host *versus* tumor evolution. *Proc. Natl. Acad. Sci. U.S.*, **74**, 2121–2125 (1977).
7. Kumanishi, T. Brain tumors induced with Rous sarcoma virus, Schmidt-Ruppin strain. I. Induction of brain tumors in adult mice Rous chicken sarcoma cells. *Jpn. J. Exp. Med.*, **37**, 461–474 (1967).
8. Kumanishi, T. and Yamamoto, T. Brain tumors induced with Rous sarcoma virus,

Schmidt-Ruppin strain. II. Rous tumor specific transplantation antigen in subcutaneously passaged mouse brain tumors. *Jpn. J. Exp. Med.*, **40**, 79–86 (1970).

9. Morse, III, H. C., Harrison, M. R., and Asofsky, R. Graft-*vs.*-host reactions in reciprocal hybrid mice. I. Dissociation of T-cell activities in the mixed lymphocyte reaction and two graft-*vs.*-host assays. *J. Exp. Med.*, **139**, 721–731 (1974).

10. Paul, W. E. and Benacerraf, B. Functional specificity of thymus-dependent lymphocytes. *Science*, **195**, 1293–1300 (1977).

11. Pierce, C. W., Kapp, J. A., and Benacerraf, B. Regulation by the H-2 gene complex of macrophage-lymphoid cell interactions in secondary antibody responses *in vitro*. *J. Exp. Med.*, **144**, 371–381 (1976).

12. Rosenthal, A. S. and Shevach, E. M. The function of macrophages in antigen recognition by guinea pig T lymphocytes. I. Requirement for histocompatible macrophages and lymphocytes. *J. Exp. Med.*, **138**, 1194–1212 (1973).

13. Shearer, G. M., Rhen, T. G., and Garbarino, C. A. Cell-mediated lympholysis of trinitrophenylmodified autologous lymphocytes: Effector cell specificity to modified cell surface components controlled by the H-2K and H-2D serological regions of the major histocompatibility complex. *J. Exp. Med.*, **141**, 1348–1364 (1975).

14. Shevach, E. M. and Rosenthal, A. S. The function of macrophages in antigen recognition by guinea pig T lymphocytes. II. Role of the macrophage in the regulation of the immune response. *J. Exp. Med.*, **138**, 1213–1229 (1973).

15. Simpson, E. and Gordon, R. Responsiveness to HY antigen Ir gene complementation and target cell specificity. *Immunol. Rev.*, **35**, 59–75 (1977).

16. Sjögren, H. O. and Jonsson, N. Resistance against isotransplantation of mouse tumors induced by Rous sarcoma virus. *Exp. Cell. Res.*, **32**, 618–621 (1963).

17. Swierkosz, J. E., Rock, K., Marrack, P., and Kappler, J. W. The role of H-2-linked genes in helper T-cell function. II. Isolation on antigen-pulsed macrophages of two separate populations of F_1 helper T cells each specific for antigen and one set of parental H-2 products. *J. Exp. Med.*, **147**, 554–570 (1978).

18. Takasugi, M. and Klein, E. The methodology of microassay for cell-mediated immunity (MCI). *In* "*In Vitro* Methods in Cell-Mediated Immunity," ed. by B. R. Bloom and P. R. Glad, pp. 415–422 (1971). Academic Press, New York.

19. Uphoff, D. E. Maternal modification of antigen recognition in the ova-transfer substrain RIIIeB. *J. Natl. Cancer Inst.*, **48**, 517–522 (1972).

20. Uphoff, D. E. Maternal modification of tissue antigenicity and the histocompatibility-2 (H-2) locus. *J. Natl. Cancer Inst.*, **45**, 1035–1037 (1970).

21. Von Boehmer, H., Haas, W., and Pohlit, H. Cytotoxic T cells recognize male antigen and H-2 as distinct entities. *J. Exp. Med.*, **147**, 1291–1295 (1978).

22. Wakasugi, N. Studies on fertility of DDK Mice: Reciprocal crosses between DDK and C57BL/6J strains and experimental transplantation of the ovary. *J. Reprod. Fert.*, **33**, 283–291 (1973).

23. Yamamoto, T. and Takeuchi, M. Studies on Rous sarcoma virus in mice. I. Establishment of an ascites sarcoma induced by Schmidt-Ruppin strain of Rous sarcoma virus in C3H/He mouse. *Jpn. J. Exp. Med.*, **37**, 37–50 (1967).

24. Yoshida, T. O., Haraguchi, S., Miyamoto, H., Matsuo, T., Ogino, T., Sugimoto, K., and Yazaki, M. Mechansims of immune responsiveness to tumor cell membrane-associated antigens (TMAA). III. RSV-induced tumor-*vs.*-host reaction in reciprocal hybrid mice. *Proc. Jpn. Cancer Assoc., 37th Annu. Meet.*, p. 77 (1978).

25. Zinkernagel, R. M., Adler, B., and Althage, A. The question of derepression of H-2

specificities in virus-infected cells: Failure to detect specific alloreactive T cells after systemic virus infection or alloantigens detectable by alloreactive T cells on virus-infected target cells. *Immunogenetics*, **5**, 367–378 (1977).

26. Zinkernagel, R. M. and Doherty, P. C. H-2 compatibility requirement for T-cell-mediated lysis of target cells infected with lymphocytic choriomeningitis virus: Different cytotoxic T-cell specificities are associated with structures coded from H-2K or H-2D. *J. Exp. Med.*, **141**, 1427–1436 (1975).

GENETIC REGULATION OF IMMUNE RESPONSE
TO TNP-MODIFIED CELLS

Gene M. Shearer, Anne-Marie Schmitt-Verhulst,
Carla B. Pettinelli, and Stephen Shaw

The Immunology Branch, National Cancer Institute*

T cell mediated cytotoxicity can be generated *in vitro* by culturing mouse spleen cells with trinitrobenzene sulfonate (TNBS)-modified syngeneic cells. The specificity of the effector cells generated is such that a) optimal lysis is detected when the responding, stimulating, and target cells share *H-2K* and/or *H-2D* haplotypes, and b) the stimulating and target cells must both be modified by the same agent. Further analysis of the specificity using cells modified a) with the trinitrophenyl (TNP) group separated from the cell surface by a tripeptide spacer, b) by non-covalent linkage with a TNP-fatty acid, or c) by preincubation with TNP-conjugated soluble proteins suggests that the antigenic moiety recognized involves more than TNP. TNP-specific, *H-2*-restricted cytotoxic responses can also be generated by culturing spleen cells with TNP-conjugated proteins such as bovine serum albumin. Multiple, *H-2*-linked immune response genes control the level of cytotoxicity generated against TNP in association with *H-2D* region products when that response is generated against either TNBS-modified cells or TNP-conjugated proteins. Cultures of human T-lymphocytes also generate cytotoxic responses against TNBS-modified human cells. Investigation of specificity indicates that human T cells can recognize TNP in association with a) determinants widely shared among humans, b) polymorphic HLA-A and -B locus associated determinants, and c) polymorphic HLA-linked determinants distinct from HLA-A and -B. Lymphocytes from all donors tested ($>30/30$) generated strong secondary cytotoxic responses to TNP-modified autologous cells. However, the same TNP-modified self antigens which elicited a strong response from one donor's lymphocytes did not necessarily elicit a comparable response from another donor's lymphocytes. These results raise the possibility that *Ir* genes control response to TNP in association with human self-determinants. The possibility of using TNP-modified tumor cells for enhancing immunity to the unmodified tumor has been discussed.

Cell mediated lympholysis (CML) effected by T-lymphocytes is generally considered to be an immune mechanism which could be relevant for surveillance against spontaneously arising tumors. Until recently, the majority of CML reactions were demonstrated against alloantigens, principally those coded for by genes mapping in the serologically detectable regions of the major histocompatibility complex (MHC).

---

* Bethesda, Maryland 20014, U.S.A.

Although of interest as a model for graft rejection, allogeneic CML provided no evidence for the relevance of cytotoxic cells nor of the MHC in host defenses against neoplastically transformed cells. Recent findings indicate that a) CML reactions could be generated against autologous virus-infected or chemically modified cells, and b) self structures controlled by genes mapping in or near the serologically detectable regions of the MHC were recognized in association with viral determinants (4, 23) or haptens (14, 19–21) on the cell surface. These findings suggest that immune responses to infection and tumors may include generation of cytotoxic T cells and that the MHC may play a crucial role in control of these responses. The objective of this article is to briefly review a number of parameters characteristic of *in vitro* generated T cell-mediated cytotoxic responses against trinitrophenyl (TNP)-modified murine and human cells, and to speculate about the possible immunological effects of chemically modified tumor cells. Although the majority of studies presented at the symposium are concerned with tumor cell models, most of the work reported with TNP-modified cytotoxicity has involved sensitization of cytotoxic precursors with modified normal cells, and lysis by effectors of modified tumor or mitogen-stimulated lymphocyte targets. Nevertheless, it is possible that a) insights gained from studies of the CML response to TNP-modified self may also apply to immune responses against neoplasms or b) that the cytotoxic reactions obtained against TNP-modified cells could provide a practical approach for enhancing immunity to weak tumor-associated antigens.

T Cell Mediated Cytotoxicity to TNP-modified Cells

Exposure of mouse spleen cells or human peripheral blood leucocytes to chemically reactive trinitrobenzene sulfonate (TNBS) for short time periods (10 min) results in covalent linkage of the TNP moiety to ε-amino groups of the lysines of cell surface proteins. Such TNP-modified cells can serve as efficient stimulators of syngeneic or autologous lymphocytes for the generation of primary and secondary cytotoxic responses (12, 19–21) as well as proliferative responses (12). Cells treated with TNBS in an identical manner can be used as efficient targets for lysis by cytotoxic effectors or as blockers of TNP-specific cytotoxic reactions.

MHC Restriction

The earliest studies involving CML to TNP-modified syngeneic cells suggested that the effectors recognized not only the TNP-moiety, but also self components coded for by genes mapping in the murine *H-2* complex (19). Mapping studies indicated that the cytotoxic effectors preferentially lysed TNP-modified target cells which expressed the same haplotype as the responding and stimulating cell populations at *H-2K* and/or *H-2D* (5, 20, 21). The general pattern of cytotoxic specificity for self components and for the haptenic moiety is summarized in Table I. It has also been reported that a weak but significant cytotoxic response can be generated against TNP in association with syngeneic *H-2I* region products (2, 22). Similar patterns of *H-2* restriction have been observed in the virus-infected (4, 23) and weak transplantation antigen (1) cytotoxic responses.

It was noted, however, that the *H-2* restriction for TNP cytotoxicity was not

TABLE I. Summary of Specificity Requirements in CML Reactions
Generated by Modified Autologous Cells

Responding cells	Stimulating cells	Target cells	Lysis of target by effector cells
A	A-M	A	—
		A-M	++
		B-M	±[a]
		A-m	—
	A-m	A-m	++
		A-M	—
(A×B) F$_1$	A-M	A-M	++
		B-M	±[a]
		(A×B) F$_1$-M	++
	B-M	B-M	++
		A-M	±

[a] Except if A and B share *K* and/or *D H-2* regions.
M and m indicate two distinct modifying agents.

TABLE II. Types of Crossreactive TNP CML

Type of stimulation	Responding cells	Stimulating cells	Target cells	Lysis detected
Modified self	A	A-TNP	A	— —
			A-TNP	###
			B-TNP	+
			C-TNP	+
			D-TNP	+
Allogeneic	A	B	B	###
			B-TNP	###
			A	— —
			A-TNP	++

absolute; lysis of TNP-modified *H-2*-unrelated targets which did not appear to be *H-2* restricted was observed by effectors generated by two types of stimulation (*3, 10, 20*) (Table II). First, it was observed that stimulation with TNP-modified syngeneic cells resulted in effectors which preferentially lysed modified *H-2*-matched targets, but which also lysed modified allogeneic targets to some extent (*3, 20*). By limiting dilution analysis of the cytotoxic precursors stimulated by TNP-modified syngeneic cells, it was estimated that approximately 40% of the clones activated lysed TNP-modified allogeneic targets (R. G. Miller, personal communication). Second, stimulation with unmodified allogeneic cells generated effectors which lysed TNP-modified targets syngeneic with the effector cells (*21, 10*). These two types of "cross-reactive" TNP-CML have been extensively studied by other investigators (*3, 10*).

Studies of the self determinants recognized in association with TNP by human cytotoxic T-lymphocytes suggest a quantitatively similar pattern of specificity (*17, 18*). Human cytotoxic T-effectors generated by primary and secondary *in vitro* stimulation with TNP-modified autologous cells recognized TNP in association with several different classes of determinants a) HLA-A and/or HLA-B locus-associated determinants, b) HLA-linked determinants which were not HLA-A nor HLA-B locus

TABLE III. Classes of Self Determinants Recognized in Association with TNP

Mouse	Human
I. *H-2K* and/or *H-2D* region (60–95%)	HLA-A and/or HLA-B locus associated (20–80%)
II. *H-2 I* region (-5%)	HLA-linked, but not HLA-A or HLA-B (5–30%)
III. Shared determinants (<40%)	Shared determinants (20–80%)

products, and c) determinants shared by leucocytes from all humans tested (*18*). A comparison of these self determinants recognized in association with TNP is shown for mouse and human lymphocytes in Table III.

Immune Response Genes

The MHC region is also involved in the control of the murine cytotoxic response to TNP-self by *H-2*-linked immune response (*Ir*) genes (*14, 15, 21*). At least two genes control the magnitude of the cytotoxic response to TNP in association with *H-2D* coded products without affecting the CML response to TNP in association with *H-2K* products. Weak responsiveness is associated with the *k* haplotype, and F_1 hybrids between weak responders and strong responders such as mice expressing either *b* or *d* alleles in the relevant regions are strong responders. One of these genes maps to the left of the *I-A* subregion, either in the *K* region or outside of *H-2*; the other gene lies between the *I-A* and *I-J* subregions. An unusual feature of this type of *Ir* gene control is that the specificity is not associated with a particular *H-2D* allele. Thus, TNP-specific cytotoxic responses of lymphocytes from *H-2*-recombinant donors expressing the *k* haplotype in the *K* and part of the *I* region are weak responders against TNP in association with self determinants expressing *d*, *b*, or *k* alleles at *H-2D*. It is not known whether this apparent lack of "specificity" with respect to the *Ir* gene control of the self determinants recognized represents a cluster of distinct and specific *Ir* genes, or whether single genes regulate the function of self recognition in association with *H-2D*, irrespective of the *H-2D* allele involved. Although it remains to be determined whether *Ir* genes control the TNP-self cytotoxic responses of human lymphocytes, differences observed in the magnitude of the three types of self components (see previous section) recognized in association with TNP suggest such genetic influences (*18*). Furthermore, differences recently observed in the proliferative responses of human lymphocytes to TNP-self among individual donors suggest HLA-linked *Ir* gene control (*16*).

Hapten Specificity

One potential advantage offered by the *in vitro* chemically modified syngeneic CML response is that this system can be utilized to investigate the fine specificity of the haptenic moiety. Effector cells generated by sensitization against TNP-modified syngeneic cells did not lyse *H-2*-matched target cells modified with TNP separated from the cell surface by a β-alanylglycylglycyl tripeptide spacer (*11*). Furthermore, mouse T-effector cells generated against TNP-modified syngeneic cells did not lyse DNP-modified, *H-2*-matched targets and *vice versa* (*6*). The same degree of exquisite specificity for the haptenic or modifying agent has been observed for human T-ef-fectors against TNP- and dinitrophenyl (DNP)-modified autologous cells (S. Shaw, unpublished data).

Mode of Cell Modification with TNP

Cell surfaces can be modified by the TNP group in different ways. For example, TNP-modification of cell surfaces can be performed with TNBS, which covalently links the TNP group to cell surface lysines, or with TNP-fatty acids such as TNP-stearoyldextran (TSD), which can be inserted into the lipid bilayer of the cell membrane and binds to cells by non-covalent forces (9). Mouse spleen cells modified with these two reagents were compared for their ability to a) sensitize syngeneic spleen cells for cytotoxic effector generations, b) serve as lysable targets for TNP-specific cytotoxicity, and c) act as blocking cells of TNP-specific lysis by effector cells. In none of these three experimental protocols did TSD-modified cells serve as sensitizing immunogens or as target antigens for TNP-specific cytotoxic responses (9). This contrasts with cells modified with TNBS, which served as good stimulating, target, and blocking cells for TNP-specific CML reactions. These findings raised the possibility that a covalent or at least a stable linkage with cell surface proteins is necessary for immunological function (9).

More recent studies indicate that covalent linkage of TNP to the cell surface is not a prerequisite for immune function. Mouse spleen cells can generate TNP-specific, H-2-restricted effector T cells when cultured with TNP-conjugated soluble proteins such as bovine serum albumin (BSA), bovine γ-globulin, ovalbumin, or mouse serum albumin (13). All those characteristics of H-2 restriction, Ir gene, control, and "cross-reactivity" observed for cells modified by TNBS were also observed for cells cultured with TNP-conjugated proteins. Cells preincubated with TNP-conjugated proteins serve both as good stimulators and effective targets for TNP-specific, H-2-restricted cytotoxicity. Targets preincubated with TNP conjugated to one protein are efficiently lysed by effectors generated by sensitization with cells treated with TNP conjugated to another protein, suggesting that the soluble protein is not involved in the immune response. Three mechanisms have been considered which could account for the generation of such effector cells by TNP-conjugated proetins (13). These include a) covalent linkage of activated TNP groups from the soluble proteins to cell surface components, b) macrophage processing of the soluble conjugates and presentation to the responding lymphocytes in association with H-2-coded self structures, or c) hydrophobic interaction of the TNP-protein to cell surfaces. Results obtained from sodium dodecyl sulfate gel patterns indicating that cell-bound TNP was still linked to bovine serum albumin (BSA) and not to serologically detectable H-2-coded products and the finding that phagocytic-depleted cells could interact with the soluble TNP-conjugated proteins and still function as H-2 restricted targets and stimulating cells seem not to favor the first two proposed mechanisms.

A summary of the various ways TNP can interact with cell surfaces and the functional assessment of such cells in TNP-specific, H-2 restricted CML reactions is shown in Table IV. The results observed in the TNP-conjugated proteins appear to contradict those obtained with TSD- or the TNP-tripeptide-modified cells. As noted above,

TABLE IV. Summary of the Ways TNP can Interact with Cell Surfaces and Functional
Assessment of Such Cells in TNP-Specific, *H-2*-Restricted CML

Modifying agent	Type of modification	Will such modified cells serve as:		
		Stimulators?	Targets?	Reference
TNBS	Covalent linkage	Yes	Yes	(*19*)
TNP-stearyl-dextran	Non-covalent (lipophilic)	No	No	(*9*)
TNP-conjugated proteins	Non-covalent (possibly hydrophobic)	Yes	Yes	(*13*)

results of the TSD experiments suggested that the TNP groups had to be linked to
the cell surface in a covalent or at least stable manner (*9*). Results of the TNP-tripeptide
spacer experiments indicated that TNP coupled directly to the cell surface is antigenically distinct from TNP separated from the cell by the spacer (*11*). All of these
findings can be resolved if it is assumed that TNP is an incomplete hapten or antigenic
determinant, and that the T cell receptor recognizes TNP plus some adjacent structures. These results can be interpreted either by a model requiring a single receptor
on T cells specific for an antigenic moiety formed by the association of TNP groups
and *H-2*-coded proteins, or by a dual receptor model in which a receptor would be
specific for TNP plus adjacent structures on the cell surface and the second one would
interact with unmodified *H-2*-coded products.

Possible Role of TNP-modified Cells in Tumor Immunity

Thus far, a brief summary has been presented indicating a number of the characteristics typical of T cell-mediated cytotoxic reactions by mouse and human leucocytes.
It may be worth considering here whether TNP-modification of tumor cells expressing
weak tumor-associated antigens could have any potential for enhancing cellular immunity to syngeneic or autologous tumors. It was noted above that TNP-conjugated
proteins might interact with cell surfaces by hydrophobic forces, and the possibility
has been considered that TNP-modified cells may interact with other cells in non-
specific ways. To examine whether TNP-modified cells can enhance the response to
other presumably unrelated antigens, spleen cells from normal mice were sensitized
in vitro with suboptimal number of unmodified or TNP-modified allogeneic cells.
The cytotoxic effectors generated were assayed on unmodified targets *H-2* matched
with the allogeneic stimulators. The results, summarized in Fig. 1, illustrate that effector
activity was not generated by sensitization with suboptimal number of unmodified
allogeneic stimulators. However, effectors were generated which lysed unmodified
allogeneic targets when sensitized with the same number of TNP-modified allogeneic
cells. The optimal concentration of TNBS for modification of allogeneic stimulators
to show this effect was 0.5 mM. At least two possible mechanisms could account for
this enhanced cytotoxic response a) non-specific enhanced interaction between cytotoxic
precursors and stimulating cells or b) the introduction of a second immunological
signal by TNP, which results in more effective activation of clones against the weak
antigen. It remains to be established whether TNP-modification of stimulator cells

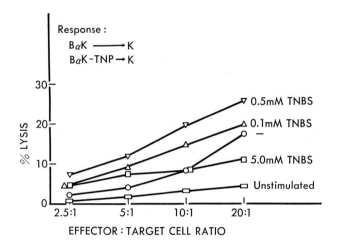

FIG. 1. Effect of TNP-modification of stimulator cells on a suboptimal *in vitro* generated allogeneic cell-mediated cytotoxic response

C57BL/10 responder mouse spleen cells (7×10^6) were cultured for 5 days with 2×10^4 (suboptimal number) irradiated (2,000R) B10.BR stimulating cells which were either unmodified (○) or modified with 5.0 mM (□), 0.5 mM (▽), or 0.1 mM (△) TNBS. Lysis by unstimulated cultures indicated by (▭). Cytotoxic activity was assayed on ^{51}Cr-labeled, unmodified *H-2^k* tumor target cells.

can result in enhanced effector activity in systems such as minor transplantation or tumor-associated antigens.

In this context, it is noteworthy that immunization against TNP-modified tumor cells has been reported to result in enhanced immunity to the tumors themselves. Galili *et al.* (*7*) have reported that immunization with TNP-modified, syngeneic tumor cells resulted in enhanced immunity to subsequent challenge with the same tumor which was unmodified. Gillette *et al.* (*8*) have recently observed that mice immunized with TNP-modified allogeneic lymphoma cells were resistant to subsequent challenge with an unmodified syngeneic lymphoma. The immunological mechanism involved in such studies remain to be resolved, and the findings in the two reports need to be confirmed. Such studies, however, raise the possibility that enhanced immunity against a syngeneic or autologous tumor could occur by immunization with TNP-modified, allogeneic tumor cells expressing the same tumor-associated or viral antigens. The introduction of a foreign antigenic determinant which might be relevant for enhancing tumor-specific immune responses could also be approached by viral infection. Chemical modification might be a more practical and ethical approach, since TNP is non-infectious, is generally not immunosuppressive, and can be administered *in vivo* or used to modify cells *in vitro*.

REFERENCES

1. Bevan, M. J. Interaction antigens detected by cytotoxic T cells with the major histocompatibility complex as modifier. *Nature*, **256**, 419–421 (1975).
2. Billings, P., Burakoff, S., Dorf, M. E., and Benacerraf, B. Cytotoxic T lymphocytes

induced against allogeneic *I*-region determinants react with *Ia* molecules or trinitrophenylconjugated syngeneic target cells. *J. Exp. Med.*, **146**, 623–628 (1977).

3. Burakoff, S. J., Germain, R. N., and Benacerraf, B. Cross-reactive lysis of trinitrophenyl (TNP)-derivatized H-2 incompatible target cells by cytotoxic T lymphocytes generated against syngeneic TNP spleen cells. *J. Exp. Med.*, **144**, 1609–1619 (1976).

4. Doherty, P. C., Blanden, R. V., and Zinkernagel, R. M. Specificity of virus-immune effector T cells for H-2K or H-2D compatible interaction: Implications for H-antigen diversity. *Transplant. Rev.*, **29**, 89–123 (1976).

5. Forman, J. The specificity of thymus derived T-cells in cell-mediated cytotoxic reactions. *Transplant. Rev.*, **29**, 146–163 (1976).

6. Forman, J. Cytotoxic T cells distinguish between trinitrophenyl- and dinitrophenyl-modified syngeneic cells. *J. Exp. Med.*, **146**, 600–605 (1977).

7. Galili, N., Naor, D., Asjo, B., and Klein, G. Induction of immune responsiveness in a genetically low responsive tumour-host combination by chemical modification of the immunogen. *Eur. J. Immunol.*, **6**, 473–476 (1976).

8. Gillette, R. W., Berringer, D. C., and Wunderlich, D. A. Resistance to syngeneic lymphoma cells caused by immunization with chemically modified allogeneic lymphoma cells in mice. *J. Natl. Cancer Inst.*, in press.

9. Henkart, P. A., Schmitt-Verhulst, A.-M., and Shearer, G. M. Specificity of cytotoxic effector cells directed against trinitrobenzene sulfonate-modified syngeneic cells. Failure to recognize cell surface-bound trinitrophenyl dextran. *J. Exp. Med.*, **146**, 1068–1078 (1977).

10. Lemmonier, F., Burakoff, S. J., Germain, R. N., and Benacerraf, B. Cytotoxic thymus-derived lymphocytes specific for allogeneic stimulator cells crossreact with chemically modified syngeneic cells. *Proc. Natl. Acad. Sci. U.S.*, **74**, 1229–1233 (1977).

11. Rehn, T. G., Inman, J. K., and Shearer, G. M. Cell-mediated lympholysis to *H-2*-matched target cells modified with a series of nitrophenyl compounds. *J. Exp. Med.*, **144**, 1134–1136 (1976).

12. Schmitt-Verhulst, A.-M., Garbarino, C. A., and Shearer, G. M. H-2 homology requirements for secondary cell-mediated lympholysis and mixed lymphocyte reactions to TNP-modified syngeneic lymphocytes. *J. Immunol.*, **118**, 1420–1427 (1977).

13. Schmitt-Verhulst, A.-M., Pettinelli, C. B., Henkart, P. A., Lunney, J. K., and Shearer, G. M. H-2-restricted cytotoxic effectors generated *in vitro* by the addition of trinitrophenyl-conjugated soluble proteins. *J. Exp. Med.*, **147**, 352–368 (1978).

14. Schmitt-Verhulst, A.-M., Sachs, D. H., and Shearer, G. M. Cell-mediated lympholysis of trinitrophenyl-modified autologous lymphocytes. Confirmation of genetic control of response to trinitrophenyl-modified H-2 antigens by the use of anti-*H-2* and anti-*Ia* antibodies. *J. Exp. Med.*, **143**, 211–213 (1976).

15. Schmitt-Verhulst, A.-M. and Shearer, G. M. Multiple *H-2*-linked immune response gene control of *H-2D*-associated T-cell-mediated lympholysis to trinitrophenyl-modified autologous cells: *Ir*-like genes mapping to the left of *I-A* and within the I region. *J. Exp. Med.*, **144**, 1701–1706 (1976).

16. Seldin, M. F. and Rich, R. R. Human immune responses to hapten-conjugated cells. I. Primary and secondary proliferative responses *in vitro*. *J. Exp. Med.*, in press.

17. Shaw, S., Nelson, D. L., and Shearer, G. M. Human cytotoxic response *in vitro* to trinitrophenyl-modified autologous cells. I. T-cell recognition of TNP in association with widely shared antigens. *J. Immunol.*, in press.

18. Shaw, S. and Shearer, G. M. Human cytotoxic response *in vitro* to trinitrophenyl-modified autologous cells. II. Diversity of self determinants recognized in association with TNP. *J. Immunol.*, in press.

19. Shearer, G. M. Cell-mediated cytotoxicity to trinitrophenyl-modified syngeneic lymphocytes. *Eur. J. Immunol.*, **4**, 527–533 (1974).

20. Shearer, G. M., Rehn, T. G., and Garbarino, C. B. Cell-mediated lympholysis of trinitrophenyl-modified autologous lymphocytes. Effector cell specificity to modified cell surface components controlled by the *H-2K* and *H-2D* serological regions of the murine major histocompatibility complex. *J. Exp. Med.*, **141**, 1348–1364 (1975).

21. Shearer, G. M., Rehn, T. G., and Schmitt-Verhulst, A.-M. Role of the murine major histocompatibility complex in the specificity of *in vitro* T cell-mediated lympholysis against chemically-modified autologous lymphocytes. *Transplant. Rev.*, **29**, 222–248 (1976).

22. Wagner, H., Starzinski-Powitz, A., Jung, H., and Rollinghoff, M. Induction of *I* region-restricted hapten-specific cytotoxic T lymphocytes. *J. Immunol.*, **119**, 1365–1368 (1977).

23. Zinkernagel, R. M. and Doherty, P. C. Restriction of an *in vitro* T-cell mediated cytotoxicity in lymphocytic choriomeningitis within a syngeneic or semi-allogeneic system. *Nature*, **248**, 701–702 (1974).

XENOGENIZATION
BY CELL HYBRIDIZATION

GANN Monograph on Cancer Research 23, 1979

ANTIGENIC EXPRESSION IN SOMATIC HYBRIDS AND THE USE OF CELL FUSION IN TUMOR XENOGENIZATION

George KLEIN

*Department of Tumor Biology, Karolinska Institutet**

The evidence has been reviewed on antigenic expression in somatic cell hybrids. Genetically determined antigens, such as *H-2*, *HLA*, and β_2-microglobulin show a codominant (autonomous) expression, with one exception: Hybrids produced by fusing the virtually *H-2*-negative Ehrlich ascites tumor with other cells. In this case, the antigenic expression of the partner is suppressed but can reappear after chromosome losses. Fusion of β_2-microglobulin and HLA negative cells (Daudi) with microglobulin-positive mouse or human cells leads to a reexpression of the missing HLA. Another situation of minor histocompatibility complex (MHC) antigen reexpression concerns the TA3/Hauschka ascites tumor, low in *H-2* antigens, where fusion with normal fibroblast partners of a different *H-2* specificity leads to full reexpression of the minimally expressed $H-2^a$.

Antigens and other markers related to differentiation are usually suppressed when expressor cells of a given lineage are fused with non-expressor cells of a different lineage. In contrast, when expressor and non-expressor cells of the same lineage are fused, co-dominant expression appears to be the rule, like in the genetically determined antigen systems.

Virally determined and tumor-associated antigens show a whole range of behavior. This has been discussed for polyoma T antigen and tumor specific transplantation antigen (TSTA), Epstein-Barr virus (EBV)-associated antigens, and murine C-type virus-determined antigens.

The usefulness, or otherwise, of somatic hybrids as an approach to xenogenization, *i.e.*, augmentation of tumor immunogenicity, has been discussed. Examples will be given for both positive and negative findings. It appears that while certain somatic hybrids can show an increased immunogenicity, this is by no means the rule and the relevant variables are not yet understood.

Induction of Tumor Rejection in the Low-responsive YAC Lymphoma Strain A Host Combination by Immunization with Somatic Cell Hybrids

Inoculation of the Moloney virus (MLV) induced YAC lymphoma of strain A origin (*29*) induces both antibodies and rejection response against the MLV-induced surface antigen (MCSA) in certain semisyngeneic F_1 hybrid mice (*e.g.*, A×C57B1,

* S-104 01 Stockholm 60, Sweden.

A×C57leaden, A×CBA). It is poorly immunogeneic in the syngeneic strain, A and some other F_1 hybrids (*e.g.*, A×ASW, A×ACA) (*12, 29, 45*). The spleen cell population of certain unmanipulated F_1 hybrids is cytotoxic to cultured YAC cells *in vitro* (*17*), a phenomenon that is designated as the "natural killer" (NK) cell activity. Spleen cells of other F_1 hybrids and of the syngeneic A host have only weak or no activity in the NK test. NK cell activity was found to be correlated with resistance against the inoculation of a small number (10^3–10^4) of YAC cells (*18*). Back-cross tests indicated that both effects (cytotoxicity and resistance) were under genetic control, with a relatively strong *H-2* linked resistance factor (*37*). The induction of serumantibody was also found to be under the influence of a major dominant gene. This was not identical with the gene(s) regulating NK-cell activity, however, and was not linked to *H-2* (*45*).

We have proposed (*19*) that *Ir* or *Ir*-like genes play an important role in the immunity against tumor-associated antigens. According to this view, the strong immune surveillance mechanisms that were demonstrated to operate against many of the virus induced tumors, have evolved through the selection of the natural host species for *Ir* gene-mediated rejection responses, directed against antigens associated with potential neoplastic cells induced by the virus. As a rule, the efficiency of the resistance is proportional to the ubiquitousness of the virus. Polyoma in mice, Feline leukemia virus (FeLV) in cats, *Herpes saimiri* in the squirrel monkey, and Epstein-Barr virus (EBV) in man can be quoted as examples (*28*).

In contrast, the evidence for immune surveillance against chemically induced or spontaneous tumors is weak or non-existent (*14, 19*). This may be attributed to the absence of comparable host selection, rather than the absence of tumor-specific or tumor-associated membrane changes, potentially capable of eliciting a rejection response on the appropriate genetic background.

If this view is correct, mobilization of rejection responses against tumor associated membrane changes becomes a problem of overcoming genetic unresponsiveness, rather than correcting the breakdown of an immune response that may never have existed. The problem is somewhat analogous to the overcoming of genetic unresponsiveness in fundamental immunology, although with some important differences. Immunologists usually depart from a well-defined immune response, search for the rare unresponsive individual, explore the genetics and the mechanism of unresponsiveness, and seek to overcome it by administering the unrecognized moiety after chemical coupling to, or together with, a well recognized antigen (for reviews, see Refs. *3* and *39*). In the case of the spontaneous or chemically induced tumor we are dealing with the mirror image of this situation. The natural history of most tumors reflects a multistep evolution, designated by the generic name "tumor progression" (*10*). The successive selection for increasing independence from growth restricting mechanisms involves, in all probability, selection for non-immunogenic and/or non-rejectable tumor cells. As a consequence, we may have to face a wide variety of neoplasm-associated membrane changes that have been preselected for non-recognition (or no rejection, in spite of recognition) in the given host, and we shall have to deal with the problem of inducing efficient responses in spite of this situation.

Antigenic modification of the tumor cell is one of the possible ways to overcome unresponsiveness and induce rejection. Hapten coupling is one possibility. In a previous study (*12*), we have found that immunization with TNP-coupled YAC cells can induce at least some humoral antibody response and the rejection of relatively small cell number in the low-responsive strain A host. Another approach would be the "xenogenization" of the established tumor, by superinfection with another, highly antigenic virus, as performed in other tumor systems (*31, 33, 41*).

A third possibility is to introduce the poorly recognized tumor antigen into a somatic cell hybrid by fusing the target tumor cell with a highly antigenic (allogeneic or xenogeneic) partner. Several authros have shown that both virally and chemically induced, tumor-associated antigens can be expressed on somatic cell hybrids of this type (*1, 6, 7, 16, 24, 27, 32*). Watkins and Chen (*42*) concluded that hybrid cells are more immunogenic than the parental tumor cell whereas Satya Murthy *et al.* (*38*) found no increase in immunogenicity. Both groups used interspecies hybrids, but different tumor-partner cell combinations.

The purpose of the present study was to explore the feasibility of overcoming host unresponsiveness in the genetically and antigenically well defined YAC-strain A system. Compared to the previous studies this system appeared to offer the following advantages:

1) A relatively strong virus-induced tumor-associated transplantation antigen (MCSA) can be demonstrated on the target YAC cell;

2) F_1 hybrid hosts of certain genotypes can respond to this tumor, whereas the syngeneic A strain and some other F_1 hybrids do not respond well; responsiveness can be thus directly related to host genetics;

3) Successful attempts to overcome the low responsiveness of the syngeneic hosts may have a direct bearing on the question of how to mobilize host responses against an existent, but normally poorly recognized tumor-associated antigen.

1) Cell lines and mice

Table I summarizes the origin and characteristics of the cells and hybrids used in the present study. All hybrids were maintained as monolayer cultures on RPMI-1640 medium, with 10% fetal calf serum. The tumor lines were maintained by serial intraperitoneal passage of ascitic fluid in the syngeneic host. For all *in vivo* rejection tests and most of the experiments concerned with antibody formation after immunization, strain A/Sn mice were used. In some antibody tests, $(A \times C57\text{1eaden})F_1$ hybrid mice were included for comparison.

2) Experimental design

The mice were immunized with 6,000 rad irradiated cells at biweekly intervals. Each immunizing inoculation contained about 5×10^6 cells. The cells used for immunization are listed in Table I. Two weeks after the fifth and last immunization all mice were bled for anti-MCSA antibody titration. One day later they received 400 R wholebody X-irradiation and were immediately thereafter challenged with live YAC cells, given subcutaneously. Wholebody irradiation was considered necessary as in previous studies (*26*), to distinguish between an established immunity, resistant to 400 R, and a non-specific boostering of the primary immune response (sensitive to 400 R). Tumor growth was followed by caliper measurements, twice weekly.

TABLE I. List of Cell Lines

Moloney virus-induced lymphoma line	Genotype	Hybridized with	Known antigens introduced by partner cell
YAC	$H\text{-}2^a$	A9[1]	$H\text{-}2^k$, L virion L cell
YAC	$H\text{-}2^a$	A9HT[2]	— ,, —
YACIR[3]	$H\text{-}2^a$	A9[1]	— ,, —[4]
YACIR	$H\text{-}2^a$	A9HT[2]	— ,, —[4]
YACIR	$H\text{-}2^a$	MSWBS[5]	$H\text{-}2^s$, MC-TSTA
YACIR	$H\text{-}2^a$	Normal CBA T6T6 fibroblast	$H\text{-}2^k$
YBA	$H\text{-}2^k$ (CBA)	—	—
YBB	$H\text{-}2^k$ (CBA)	—	—
YALB	(A × C571eaden) F$_1$, $H\text{-}2^a H\text{-}2^b$	—	—
YA7C	(A × C57B1) F$_1$, $H\text{-}2^a H\text{-}2^b$	—	—

[1] Low malignant L cell subline.
[2] High malignant L cell subline.
[3] Immunoresistant subline of YAC, with reduced MCSA concentration.
[4] In the YAC/A9 and YACIR/A9 hybrids, the characteristic high MCSA concentration of YAC was reestablished (7).
[5] Ascitic form of methylcholanthrene induced sarcoma (20).

In certain experiments, immunized mice were followed by regular weekly bleedings for cytotoxic antibodies, in parallel with tumor size measurements.

Cytotoxicity tests were performed as described elsewhere (45).

3) Results

Groups of 3 strain A mice were immunized with irradiated cells of the syngeneic Moloney lymphoma YAC, or the allogeneic (CBA-derived) Moloney lymphoma YBA, or similarly irradiated somatic cell hybrids of the types YACIR/A9 and YACIR/A9HT, respectively. Two weeks after the last immunization, all the mice were irradiated with 400 R and challenged with 10^2, 10^3, or 10^4 viable YAC cells in parallel with untreated controls. Both YACIR/A9 and YACIR/a9HT induced protection whereas immunization with YAC cells had only minimal effect and YBA cells had no detectable effect.

From groups of 10 A mice immunized with irradiated cells, equal amounts of sera were pooled for each group and tested for cytotoxicity against YAC target cells. Neither YAC nor YBA induced detectable antibodies (titer 2) whereas the somatic hybrids and the (A × C57B1)F$_1$ lymphoma YA7C induced significant antibody titers.

With some of the cells (A × C571eaden)F$_1$ mice were also immunized. In this case, antibodies appeared earlier and reached higher titers than in A mice. Moreover, the radiated YAC cells were also capable of inducing antibody formation in this F$_1$ hybrid.

The immunity against subcutaneously grafted YAC cells varied according to the cell used for immunization. Figure 1 summarizes all experiments that were carried out with the same design, in 2 or 3 parallel series for each immunizing hybrid-target cell combination. YAC had a slight immunizing effect only. Immunization with YACIR/A9HT was most efficient, detectable both by an increased incidence of rejection with all three cell doses, increased survival time of the tumor-bearing animals, and the highest antibody levels. The latter was found both in the syngeneic A mice and in the (A × C571eaden)F$_1$ hybrid (compare legend to Fig. 1).

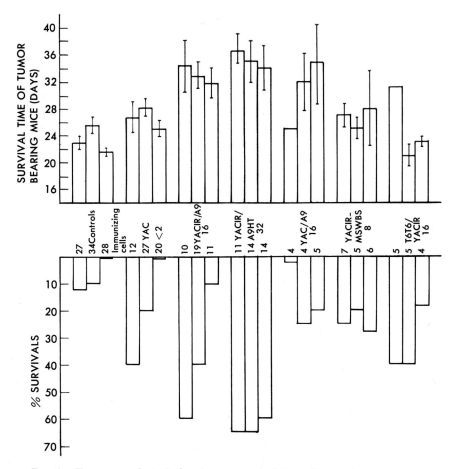

FIG. 1. Frequency of survival and mean survival time of tumor-bearing mice, after immunization with heavily irradiated YAC cells or various somatic cell hybrids as indicated

For each group, the three columns show the results after the inoculation of 10^2, 10^3, and 10^4 viable YAC cells to strain A mice that have been preimmunized with the cells indicated. All hosts were irradiated with 400R prior to the viable inoculum. The figures in the middle, under each immunizing cell, designate the mean antibody titers in strain A mice, as measured by cytotoxic tests. After immunization by the identical schedule, the mean antibody titers induced in (A× C57 leaden) F_1 mice were 32 for YAC, 64 for YACIR/A9, and 256 for the YACIR/A9HT immunization group. The figures at the foot of the columns indicate the number of mice used for each experiment.

Lower degrees of immunization were achieved with other somatic cell hybrids. They appeared to be immunogenic, to some extent at least, as reflected both by rejection and by antibody titers, but appeared to be intermediate between the low immunogenic YAC and the relatively highly immunogenic YACIR/A9HT.

In addition to the somatic hybrids, allogeneic MLV lymphomas were also tested (not shown on the curves). Immunization with irradiated cells of the MLV-induced YBB lymphoma of CBA origin, YALB lymphoma of (A×C57leaden)F_1 origin, or

YA7C lymphoma of $(A \times C57Bl)F_1$ origin had no discernible protective effect against 10^2, 10^3, or 10^4 YAC cells in strain A mice.

4)   Conclusions

Somatic cell hybrids, derived from the fusion of YAC with an unrelated normal or malignant mouse cell that introduced new, genetically or virally determined antigens, were immunogenic in strain A mice, as reflected both by the rejection and the cytotoxicity tests. In this strain, YAC cells are either non-immunogenic or induce only very low levels of antibodies and rejection responses. All somatic cell hybrids were efficient, although to a variable degree. YACIR/A9HT was the most immunogenic hybrid, both by humoral antibody formation and graft resistance. Other somatic hybrids were intermediate. Allogeneic Moloney lymphomas did not induce detectable rejection responses, although they did induce variable antibody levels.

The mechanism that determines the variation in the ability of different hybrids to induce rejection reactions is unknown. Since hybrids derived from basically similar partner cell combinations (e.g., YAC/A9, as compared to YACIR/A9 and YACIR/A9HT) showed differences in this respect, it must be assumed that their antigen expression or presentation was different. Somatic cell hybrids were indeed found to vary in their antigen expression (7, 20, 21). Further studies will be performed to establish whether the relevant parameter can be pinpointed as one of the serologically detectable (e.g., MCSA antigens) or other phenotypic or karyotypic properties.

Recent studies have shown that the YAC lymphoma is uniquely susceptible to the NK cell that can mediate resistance against *small* inocula in non-preimmunized mice of certain genetic constitutions (17, 18, 37). In contrast, YAC cells show little or no susceptibility to semisyngeneic $(A \times C57BL)F_1$ T cells in MLV- or MSV-immunized syngeneic mice, although these T cells were highly cytotoxic for the Rauscher virus-induced lymphoma line (RBL) (2). This suggests a difference in the susceptibility of different cell lines induced by the same or antigenically closely related viruses to different immune effectors. The ability of YACIR/A9HT and other somatic hybrids to induce an efficient anti-YAC rejection in syngeneic A mice deserves further study with regard to the effector mechanisms involved.

Viewed in a more general context, antigenic modification of tumor cells by somatic cell hybridization appears to be one of the potentially rewarding pathways that can render a relatively non-immunogenic tumor highly immunogenic. The existence of "universal fuser"-cells, e.g., cell lines unable to grow on HAT but sensitive to ouabain (36), makes this approach eminently practical, since a single cell line that carries the appropriate markers can be readily fused with *any* murine or human tumor cell. The selection of universal fusers that are outstanding in rejection-induction experiments of the type described in this paper appears as an important task for the future.

Antigenic Expression in Somatic Hybrids

1)   H-2 antigen losses

We have previously shown that *H-2* antigenic loss variants can be selected from heterozygous tumors, induced in F_1 hybrid hosts with two different *H-2* complexes. Loss of one antigen complex, achieved after passage through one parental strain, is permanent and irreversible also when the cell is returned to the original F_1 hybrid host (25). Recently, we have found by banding analysis (43) that such variants arise by sub-chromosomal changes, since they carry both normal 17 chromosomes of the original hybrid. In spite of intense efforts, we have never been able to select "zero" variants that would have lost both parental isoantigen complexes (4). This was taken to suggest that one H-2 complex is essential for the life of the cell, perhaps for the integrity of the cell membrane.

Similar isoantigenic variants can be selected from somatic cell hybrids, derived from the fusion of two tumor cells carrying different H-2 complexes. In this case, isoantigenic variant formation was equally permanent and irreversible as in the hybrid tumors. Zero variants could not be established. In one combination, derived from the fusion of the TA3Ha ascites carcinoma with the MSWBS sarcoma, the cytogenetical and serological situation was exceptionally favorable. The $H-2^a$ carrying 17 chromosomes derived from TA3Ha had a normal, telocentric morphology, whereas MSWBS carried two translocated 17 chromosomes, readily distinguishable from each other and from the two normal elements introduced from TA3Ha. Selection of the two reciprocal, parent compatible variants showed that the H-2 isoantigen losses were due to chromosome elimination. In each variant, the 17 chromosomes derived from the opposite parental strain were eliminated while the 17 chromosomes of the selective parent were maintained (44). Analogous findings were made on the Moloney lymphoma/methylcholanthrene sarcoma hybrid, YACIR/MSWBS (5). In the latter case, variant selection was achieved by the usual in vivo selection and also by serial in vitro exposure to isoantiserum and complement.

Since selection could be made to act on the H-2 carrying 17 chromosomes of each parent, the TA3Ha/MSWBS hybrid allowed a study of the question whether the tumor-specific (TSTA-type) antigen derived from the methylcholanthrene-induced MSWBS sarcoma was a modified form of H-2, as suggested (15, 35, 40), or due to some H-2-linked determinant. As described elsewhere in detail (27), this was not the case because both the $H-2^s$ and the $H-2^a$ loss variants were still immunogenic, i.e., were capable of immunizing ASW mice against the syngeneic MSWBS sarcoma, although the immunogenicity of all variants was quantitatively reduced.

Symmetric, parent-compatible variants could be selected from all tumor/tumor hybrids tested. One interesting asymmetry has been noted in one tumor/normal cell hybrid, derived from the crossing of TA3Ha ascites tumor cells ($H-2^a$) with the normal, diploid ACA fibroblast ($H-2^f$). Whereas strain A compatible variants that have lost the normal fibroblast-derived $H-2^f$ complex could be readily selected by passage in the A strain, we have been unable to obtain any $H-2^a$ negative variant by selection in the parental ACA strain (11, 22). Since the latter strain is otherwise highly efficient in selecting $H-2^a$ loss variants from $H-2^a$ $H-2^f$ heterozygous tumors, there is no reason to assume that the asymmetry was due to the inefficiency of the selective system. All TA3Ha/tumor hybrids readily gave rise to symmetrical variants. It is therefore possible that the asymmetry of the TA3Ha/fibroblast hybrid has some other and more interesting reason. It is conceivable that the 17 chromosome of the TA3/Ha cell may carry some determinant essential for the malignant behavior of this particular carcinoma cell. This hypothesis is presently being tested by producing other TA3Ha/normal cell hybrids and testing them in a similar way. Also, we are attempting to select the "missing" *H-2ᵃ* negative variants from TA3Ha/ACA *in vitro*, by repeated exposure to isoantiserum and complement. If successful, the *in vitro* selected variants will be tested for malignancy.

It has to be stressed that this interpretation does not imply any generalization concerning the possible role of 17-chromosome for malignant behavior in general. We know that symmetrical variants *can* be selected from SEWA/T6T6 fibroblast hybrids, where the tumor parent is a polyoma-induced sarcoma, or from A9HT/C57BL lymphocyte hybrids, where A9HT is an *in vitro* transformed sarcoma line. There is no reason, however, why malignancy determinant(s) could not be localized on different chromosomes, particularly in tumors of diverse etiology. Recent developments in tumor cytogenetics actually suggest that specific chromosomal changes occur in tumors of different etiologies.

2) *Epigenetic changes in antigen expression*

In addition to the complete and permanent antigen losses from heterozygous cell described above, quantitative decrease of antigen expression, rather than complete antigen loss, can be encountered as well, *e.g.*, in the so-called "nonspecific," *i.e.*, widely homotransplantable, tumors. This is probably a more frequent reason for the development of "immunoresistance" than complete antigenic loss.

In the course of our hybrid studies, we have encountered two different types of reduced antigen expression. One is characteristic of the long-transplanted, allogeneic Ehrlich carcinoma. On fusion, this tumor suppresses the antigen expression of the allogeneic partner cell (*23*). This suppression can afflict genetically and virally determined antigens and cell type specific antigens as well. Following chromosome loss from the somatic hybrid, full antigen expression can reappear (*13*). A very different *H-2* antigen reduction is encountered in the TA3Ha line, an ascites carcinoma of strain A origin. In this case, fusion of TA3Ha with allogeneic fibroblasts has led to the full reappearance of the high *H-2ᵃ* expression characteristic for the original TA3St line. If the antigen suppression of the Ehrlich tumor was dominant in the hybrid, the antigen suppression of the TA3Ha is therefore "recessive." This shows that decreased surface antigen expression and parallel immunoresistance can develop by at least two entirely different mechanisms.

A "recessive" decrease of antigen expression was noted in a virus induced, tumor-associated antigen system as well. The YAC-YACIR pair of sublines has been derived from the same original MLV-induced lymphoma. YAC has a high MCSA antigen expression and is sensitive to the cytotoxic effect of anti-Moloney antibodies in the presence of complement, whereas YACIR selected for immunoresistance has approximately 10 times less MCSA. When YACIR was fused with A9 cells, full antigen expression was reestablished, comparable to the parallel A9/YAC hybrid (*7*).

Analysis of the TA3Ha/ACA-derived hybrids revealed further details about the surface changes in the unusual TA3Ha variant (*11*, *12*). In addition to its low *H-2* antigen expression and its resistance to the cytotoxic action of anti-*H-2ᵃ* antibodies, compared to the original TA3St line, TA3Ha has a smooth surface while TA3St is rough. TA3Ha is inagglutinable by concanavalin A (con A) while TA3St agglutinates readily. It is tempting to attribute all these changes in surface phenotype to a single cellular change. However, the TA3Ha/ACA hybrids show a full reexpression of *H-2ᵃ*, as already mentioned, and revert to the rough, tuberous surface characteristic for TA3St, but they do *not* revert to con A agglutinability. It must there fore be concluded that the low antigen expression and the inagglutinability of TA3Ha by con A must be due to different cellular mechanisms. Perhaps even more remarkable was the fact that the full reexpression of *H-2ᵃ* in the TA3Ha/ACA hybrids was not paralleled by the reestablishment of high cytotoxic sensitivity. Only 4 of 12 independently selected segregants became sensitive to humoral cytotoxicity, whereas 8 remained resistant. This implies that while the importance of high antigen expression for cytotoxic sensitivity cannot be questioned, it is not the sole determinant and other membrane phenomena must play a role as well.

3) Viral expression

In the course of these studies, several situations were encountered where oncogenic or tumor-associated viruses were introduced into the hybrid line by one parental strain. A number of interesting interactions occurred, informative in relation to the cellular controls that influence viral expression. Some of the conclusions, described in detail in the papers quoted, are as follows:

   a) L cells carry a C-type virus, often called L virion. We found that the L virus is N-tropic. When Fv-$1ⁿFv$-$1ⁿ$ cells that produce this virus are fused with Fv-$1ᵇFv$-$1ᵇ$ or Fv-$1ᵇFv$-$1ⁿ$ cells, virus production is switched off (*8*). When chromosomes are lost in the course of serial passage, virus production may reappear again. This shows that the *Fv-1* gene, known to play a major role for the amplification of some C-type viruses, acts *via* an intracellular mechanism. This work also showed that virus production and virus-determined membrane antigen expression were independently controlled since the former could be switched off without any change in the expression of the latter.

   b) Virux populations obtained from somatic cell hybrids often show new combinations of characteristics, compared to the virus populations released by both parents (*9*), suggesting the occurrence of viral recombination and subsequent selection of the recombinant virus populations in the somatic hybrid.

   c) When two EBV genome-carrying cells, differing in their EBV inducibility, are fused with each other, the relatively more permissive condition is dominant over the less permissive, suggesting a positive control (*34*).

   d) When EBV-carrying human lymphoid cells are fused with mouse fibroblasts, surface immunoglobulins, EBV receptors, other human B-lymphocyte receptors, and EBV inducibility are completely suppressed, whereas the EBV-determined nuclear antigen (EBNA) is maintained in a fraction of the cell population (*30*). The percentage of EBNA-positive cells is directly related to the average number of EBV-genomes per cell. In the course of serial propagation of such interspecies hybrids, detectable EBV-genomes, and EBNA antigens are lost in parallel with each other. After complete loss, there is still a considerable number of human chromosomes present, suggesting that the viral genome is *not* associated with the majority of human chromosomes.

ADDENDA

Proposed by N. Kuzumaki: The basic idea of using hybrid cells for xenogenization of tumors is that foreign histocompatibility antigens introduced by cell fusion may have a cellular carrier effect that increases the host's response to the tumor-associated transplantation antigens. However, I would like to show you that in addition to such foreign histocompatibility antigens, we have to consider other antigens, for instance, endogenous virus-associated antigens as well. We have formed 2 hybrid cell lines between CBA mammary tumors and allogeneic C3H fibroblast subline A9HT by the inactivated Sendai virus-induced fusion. To compare the immunogenicity of the hybrid cells with parental cells, CBA mice were inoculated with irradiated parental and hybrid lines once each week for 3 weeks, and 7 days after the last immunization, the mice were irradiated, and then challenged with each mammary tumor (Table II). In SBfnHA system, even mice immunized with irradiated SBfnHA showed complete protection against this tumor, but mice immunized with irradiated hybrid cells: SBfnHA/A9HT did not show complete protection against the SBfnHA challenge. Allogeneic irradiated A9HT cells did not induce any immunity at all. In contrast, in SBfnHC system, CBA mice immunized with irradiated SBfnHC and irradiated al-

TABLE II. Comparison of Immunogenicity between Irradiated CBA Mammary Tumors and Their Hybrid Lines with a C3H Fibroblast Subline

Immunization[a]			Challenge[b]		
Cell line	Dose	Times	Cell line	Dose	Lethal growth (MSD)[c]
SBfnHA (CBA)	10^6	3	SBfnHA	10^4	0/2
SBfnHA (CBA)	10^6	3	SBfnHA	10^5	0/4
					0/6
SBfnHA/A9HT	10^6	3	SBfnHA	10^4	0/4
SBfnHA/A9HT	10^6	3	SBfnHA	10^5	5/8 (72)
					5/12
A9HT (C3H)	10^6	3	SBfnHA	10^4	2/2 (53)
A9HT (C3H)	10^6	3	SBfnHA	10^5	2/2 (45)
					4/4
None			SBfnHA	10^4	2/2 (54)
None			SBfnHA	10^5	3/3 (42)
					5/5
SBfnHC (CBA)	10^6	3	SBfnHC	5×10^2	3/4 (101)
SBfnHC (CBA)	10^6	3	SBfnHC	5×10^3	8/8 (59)
					11/12
SBfnHC/A9HT	10^6	3	SBfnHC	5×10^2	6/19 (136)
SBfnHC/A9HT	10^6	3	SBfnHC	5×10^3	7/8 (72)
					13/17
A9HT (C3H)	10^6	3	SBfnHC	5×10^2	3/4 (102)
A9HT (C3H)	10^6	3	SBfnHC	5×10^3	4/4 (47)
					7/8
None			SBfnHC	5×10^2	4/4 (99)
None			SBfnHC	5×10^3	4/4 (57)
					8/8

[a] Heavily irradiated (10,000 rad) cells were inoculated into CBA mice 3 times at weekly intervals.

[b] Challenge 8 days after final immunization. Hosts were irradiated with 400 rad 24 hr before tumor inoculation.

[c] Mean survival time in days.

logeneic A9HT did not show any protection against SBfnHC challenge, but some mice immunized with the hybrid cells: SBfnHC/A9HT rejected SBfnHC and other mice showed retardation of mean survival time. Both of CBA and C3H mice have H-2^k antigen, so A9HT has only minor histocompatibility difference. Do these foreing minor histocompatibility antigens play any role on changing immunogenicity of SBfnHC tumor, we don't know.

Table III shows sensitivity of parental and hybrid cell lines to anti-MuLV gp70, p30, MMTV gp52 sera, and anti-H-2^k serum. There is no change of H-2^k antigen expression between parental and hybrid lines. A9HT cells express very high gp70, p30, and gp52 antigens. High antigenic SBfnHA expresses high gp70 and considerable amount of p30 and gp52, while low antigenic SBfnHC expresses gp70 but does not show any p30 and gp52 expressions. On both hybrid cells, they express gp70, and in case of SBfnHC/A9HT, expression of gp70 is increased. But, surprisingly, they had no expression of p30 and gp52. To confirm these results of direct cytotoxicity tests, we performed absorption tests (Fig. 2). You can see both hybrid lines show similar absorb-

TABLE III. Sensitivity of Parental and Hybrid Cell Lines to Anti-MuLV gp 70, p 30, MMTV gp 52, Sera, and anti-H-2^k Serum by Micro-Cytotoxicity tests

Cell line	Cytotoxic titer[a] with			
	Anti-gp 70	Anti-p 30	Anti-gp 52	Anti-H-2^k
Parents				
SBfnHA	2,560	20	40	1,280
SBfnHC	320	—[b]	—	1,280
A9HT	10,240	2,560	80	2,560
Hybrids				
SBfnHA/A9HT	1,280	—	—	1,280
SBfnHC/A9HT	5,120	—	—	1,280

[a] Reciprocal of serum dilution producing more than 0.20 of cytotoxic index.

[b] No positive reaction at 1 : 10 serum dilution.

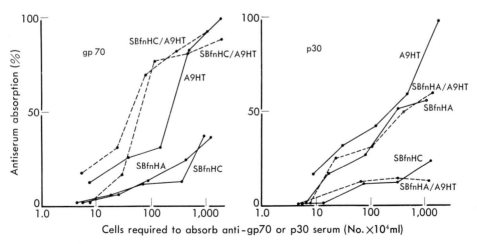

FIG. 2. Quantitative absorption assays using anti-MuLV gp70 and p30 sera and tested against a Moloney lymphoma: YBA cells

ing activity to anti-gp70 serum against a Moloney lymphoma: YBA as A9HT does, but the p30 expression of A9HT is suppressed on both hybrid lines, especially in SBfnHC/A9HT. We are interested in this selective suppression mechanism of p30 antigen. In addition, very lately, we found that a mouse mammary tumor has a serologically defined, individually distinct antigen unrelated to MTV (Kuzumaki and Klein, JNCI submitted). We are now doing experiments to know relationship between expression of such tumor specific antigens and rejection reaction of these hybrid cell lines.

Acknowledgment

The investigation was supported by Grant No. 2 RO1 CA 14054-06, awarded by the National Cancer Institute, DHEW.

REFERENCES

1. Barski, G., Blanchard, M. G., Youn, J. K., and Leon, B. Expression of malignancy in interspecies Chinese hamster X mouse cell. *J. Natl. Cancer Inst.*, **51**, 781–792 (1973).

2. Becker, S. and Klein, E. Decreased "natural" killer effect in tumor-bearing mice and its relation to the immunity against oncorna virus-determined cell surface antigens. *Eur. J. Immunol.*, **6**, 892–898 (1976).

3. Benacerraf, B. and McDevitt, H. O. Histocompatibility-linked immune response genes. *Science*, **175**, 273–279 (1972).

4. Bjaring, B. and Klein, G. Antigenic characterization of heterozygous mouse lymphomas after immunoselection *in vivo. J. Natl. Cancer Inst.*, **41**, 1411–1429 (1968).

5. Dalianis, T., Wiener, F., and Klein, G. Alloantigenic variant selection *in vitro* from a mouse lymphoma-sarcoma hybrid. *Immunogenetics*, **1**, 370–397 (1974).

6. Defendi, V., Ephrussi, B., and Koprowski, H. Expression of polyoma-niduced cellular antigen(s) in hybrid cells. *Nature*, **203**, 495–496 (1964).

7. Fenyö, E. M., Grundner, G., Klein, E., and Harris, H. Surface antigens and release of virus in hybrid cells produced by the fusion of A9 fibroblasts with Moloney lymphoma cells. *Exp. Cell Res.*, **68**, 323–331 (1971).

8. Fenyö, E. M., Grundner, G., Wiener, F., Klein, E., Klein, G., and Harris, H. The influence of the partner cell on the production of L virus and the expression of viral surface antigen in hybrid cells. *J. Exp. Med.*, **137**, 1240–1255 (1973).

9. Fenyö, E. M., Nazerian, K., and Klein, E. Characteristics of murine C-type viruses. II. The behaviour of viruses resident in various cell lines and their hybrids on BA1b/3T3 and mouse embryo fibroblast cultures. *Virology*, **59**, 574–579 (1974).

10. Foulds, L. The natural history of cancer. *J. Chronic Dis.*, **8**, 2–37 (1958).

11. Friberg, S., Klein, G., Wiener, F., and Harris, H. Hybrid cells derived from fusion of TA3-Ha ascites carcinoma with normal fibroblasts. II. Characterization of isoantigenic variant sublines. *J. Natl. Cancer Inst.*, **50**, 1269–1286 (1973).

12. Galili, N., Naor, D., Åsjö, B., and Klein, G. Induction of immune responsiveness in a genetically low-responsive tumor-host combination by chemical modification of the immunogen. *Eur. J. Immunol.*, **6**, 473–476 (1976).

13. Grundner, G., Fenyö, E. M., Klein, G., Klein, E., Bregula, U., and Harris, H. Surface antigen expression in malignant sublines derived from hybrid cells of low malignancy. *Exp. Cell Res.*, **68**, 315–322 (1971).

14. Hewitt, H. B., Blake, E. R., and Walder, A. S. A critique of the evidence for active

host defence against cancer, based on personal studies of 27 murine tumours of spontaneous origin. *Br. J. Cancer*, **33**, 241–259 (1976).

15. Heywood, G. R. and McKhann, C. F. Reciprocal relationship between normal transplantation antigens (H-2) and tumor-specific immunogenicity. *J. Exp. Med.*, **133**, 1171–1187 (1971).

16. Jami, J. and Rietz, E. Expression of tumor-specific antigen in mouse somatic cell hybrids. *Cancer Res.*, **33**, 2524–2528 (1973).

17. Kiessling, R., Klein, E., and Wigzell, H. "Natural" killer cells in the mouse. I. Cytotoxic cells with specificity for mouse Moloney leukemia cells. Specificity and distribution according to genotype. *Eur. J. Immunol.*, **5**, 112–117 (1975).

18. Kiessling, R., Petranyi, G., Klein, G., and Wigzell, H. Genetic variation of *in vitro* cytolytic activity and *in vivo* rejection potential of non-immunized semi-syngeneic mice against a mouse lymphoma line. *Int. J. Cancer*, **15**, 933–940 (1975).

19. Klein, G. Immunological surveillance against neoplasia. The Harvey Lectures, Academic Press, New York, 69, pp. 71–102 (1975).

20. Klein, G., Bregula, U., Wiener, F., and Harris, H. The analysis of malignancy by cell fusion. I. Hybrids between tumour cells and L cell derivatives. *J. Cell. Sci.*, **8**, 659–672 (1971).

21. Klein, G., Friberg, S., Jr., and Harris, H. Two kinds of antigen suppression in tumor cells revealed by cell fusion. *J. Exp. Med.*, **135**, 839–849 (1972).

22. Klein, G., Friberg, S., Wiener, F., and Harris, H. Hybrid cells derived from fusion of TA3Ha ascites carcinoma with normal fibroblasts. I. Malignancy, karyotype, and formation of isoantigenic variants. *J. Natl. Cancer Inst.*, **50**, 1259–1268 (1973).

23. Klein, G., Gars, U., and Harris, H. Isoantigenic expression in hybrid mouse cells. *Exp. Cell Res.*, **62**, 149–160 (1970).

24. Klein, G. and Harris, H. Expression of polyoma induced transplantation antigen in hybrid cell lines. *Nature New Biol.*, **237**, 163–164 (1972).

25. Klein, G. and Klein, E. Histocompatibility changes in tumors. *J. Cell. Comp. Physiol.*, **52** (*Suppl.* 1), 125–168 (1958).

26. Klein, G. and Klein, E. Antigenic properties of other experimental tumors. *Cold Spring Harbor Symp. Quant. Biol.*, **27**, 463–470 (1963).

27. Klein, G. and Klein, E. Are methylcholanthrene-induced sarcoma associated, rejection-inducing (TSTS) antigens, modified forms of H-2 or linked determinants? *Int. J. Cancer*, **15**, 879–887 (1975).

28. Klein, G. and Klein, E. Rejectability of virus-induced tumors and nonrejectability of spontaneous tumors: A lesson in contrasts. *Transplant. Proc.*, **9**, 1095–1104 (1977).

29. Klein, G., Klein, E., and Haughton, G. Variation of antigenic characteristics between different mouse lymphomas induced by the Moloney virus. *J. Natl. Cancer Inst.*, **36**, 607–621 (1966).

30. Klein, G., Wiener, F., Zech, L., zur Hausen, H., and Reedman, B. Segregation of the EBV-determined nuclear antigen (EBNA) in somatic cell hybrids derived from the fusion of a mouse fibroblast and a human Burkitt lymphoma line. *Int. J. Cancer*, **14**, 54–64 (1974).

31. Kobayashi, H., Sendo, F., Shirai, T., Kaji, H., Kodama, T., and Saito, H. Modification in growth of transplantable rat tumors exposed to Friend virus. *J. Natl. Cancer Inst.*, **42**, 413–419 (1969).

32. Liang, W. and Cohen, E. P. Resistance to murine luekemia in mice rejecting syngeneic somatic hybrid cells. *J. Immunol.*, **116**, 623–626 (1976).

33. Lindenmann, J. and Klein, P. A. Viral oncolyeses: Increased immunogenicity of host cell antigen associated with influenza virus. *J. Exp. Med.*, **126**, 93–108 (1967).

34. Nyormoi, O., Klein, G., Adams, A., and Dombos, L. Sensitivity to EBV superinfection and IUdR inducibility of hybrid cells formed between a sensitive and a relatively resistant Burkitt lymphoma cell line. *Int. J. Cancer*, **12**, 396–408 (1973).

35. Oth, D. and Barra, Y. Séparation de deux spécificités antigéniques tumorales différentes, chez deux variants iso-antigéniques obtenus á partir d'une tumeur induite chimiquement dans des hybrides F_1 (ACA×ABY). *C.R. Acad. Sci., Ser.*, **D278**, 177–180 (1974).

36. Ozer, H. L. and Jha, K. K. Malignancy and transformation: Expression in somatic cell hybrids and variants. *Adv. Cancer Res.*, **25**, 53–93 (1977).

37. Pétranyi, G. G., Kiessling, R., Povey, S., Klein, G., Herzenberg, I., and Wigzell, H. The genetic control of natural killer cell activity and its association with *in vivo* resistance against a Moloney lymphoma isograft. *Immunogenetics*, **3**, 15–28 (1976).

38. Satya Murthy, M., Belehradek, J., and Barski, G. Interspecies mouse X akodon urichi somatic cell hybrids: Comparative immunogenicity of parental and hybrid cells. *Eur. J. Cancer*, **12**, 33–39 (1976).

39. Shearer, G. M., Mozes, E., and Sela, M. Cellular basis of the genetic control of immune responses. *In* "Progress in Immunology," ed. D. B. Amos, 509 pp. (1971). Academic Press, New York.

40. Smith, R. T. and Landy, M. The immunobiology of the tumor host relationship. *Proc. Int. Symp. Tumor Immunol.*, Milano (1974).

41. Svet-Moldavsky, G. J. and Hamburg, V. P. An approach to the immunological treatment of tumors by artificial hetergenization. *In* "Specific Tumor Antigens," 323 pp. (1967). UICC Monogr. Series 2, Munksgaard, Copenhagen.

42. Watkins, J. F. and Chen, L. Immunization of mice against Ehrlich ascites tumors using a hamster/Ehrlich ⧻ ascites tumor hybrid cell line. *Nature*, **223**, 1018–1022 (1969).

43. Wiener, F., Dalianis, T., and Klein, G. Cytogenic studies on H-2 alloantigenic loss variants selected from heterozygous tumors. *Immunogenetics*, **2**, 63–72 (1975).

44. Wiener, F., Dalianis, T., Klein, G., and Harris, H. Cytogenetic studies on the mechanism of formation of isoantigenic variants in somatic cell hybrids. I. Banding analyses of isoantigenic variant sublines derived from the fusion of TA3Ha carcinoma with MSWBS sarcoma cells. *J. Natl. Cancer Inst.*, **52**, 1779–1795 (1974).

45. Åsjö, B., Kiessling, R., Klein, G., and Povey, S. Genetic variation in antibody response and natural killer cell activity against a Moloney virus-induced lymphoma (YAC). *Eur. J. Immunol.*, **8**, 554–558 (1977).

GANN Monograph on Cancer Research 23, 1979

ANTIGENIC EXPRESSION ON MOUSE HYBRID CELLS

Takehiko TACHIBANA and Toshio DEI

*Department of Immunology, Research Institute for Tuberculosis,
and Cancer, Tohoku University**

In general, hybrid cells codominantly express the major histocom-patibility antigens of the parental cells. However, when L cells are fused with Ehrlich ascitic tumor cells, it has been found that the expression of the H-2 antigen being introduced into the somatic cell hybrids by the L cells is largely reduced.

Similar suppression of the H-2 antigenic expression was also ob-served in hybrids between L cells and FM3A ascitic tumor cells as well as in hybrids of the L cells with spontaneous mammary carcinoma (SMCA) cells. FM3A ascitic tumor cells were derived from a SMCA of C3H/He mouse and serially passaged through a syngeneic host. FM3A cells carrying hypotetraploid chromosomes are nonspecific tumor cells by reducing the expression of the H-2 antigen, but concomitantly express mouse mammary tumor-specific surface antigen (MM antigen) which is lacking in SMCA cells. The inverse relationship between the suppression of the H-2 antigen and the expression of the MM antigen was observed in both hybrids, indicating induction of the MM antigen with simultaneous reduction of the H-2 antigen contributed by both parental cells in the case of the L-SMCA hybrid. Thus, it is suggested that this suppression of the surface antigens of the partner is, in common, produced by mammary tumor cells (Ehrlich, FM3A, and SMCA cells).

The suppressive mechanism was discussed in relation to selective loss of chromosomes, behavior of cell growth *in vitro* and expression of the tumor surface antigen in hybrids.

It has been shown, in general, that the parental H-2 antigens on somatic cell hybrids of mice are codominantly expressed by cell fusion (*1, 11*). However, when L cells are fused with Ehrlich ascitic tumor cells, it has been observed that the ex-pression of H-2^k antigen, which is introduced into the hybrid cells by the L cells, is largely suppressed (*3, 4, 9*). At the same time, it has also been observed that other virally-or chemically-induced tumor cells which are fused with the L cells fully express the H-2 antigens introduced by the parent cells (*4*). Thus, the suppression of H-2^k antigens in L-Ehrlich hybrid cells has been considered to be due to a specific effect produced by Ehrlich tumor cells.

The Ehrlich tumor has been maintained by continuous serial passage in many histoincompatible mice for a long time. Therefore, it was thought that the L-Ehrlich hybrid cells inherited the characteristics termed 'immunoresistance' of Ehrlich tumor cells which escape the homograft reaction by reducing the expression of histocom-

---

* Seiryo-machi 4-1, Sendai 980, Japan (橘　武彦, 出井敏雄).

patibility antigen. In L-Ehrlich hybrids, not only H-2 antigens but also the L-cell antigen, which is suggested to be an embryonic antigen (2), are suppressed. Therefore, it is conceivable that this suppression of antigenic expression would occur epigenetically.

The usefulness of somatic cell hybrids as a potent immunogen in active tumor immunity depends on the production of stable nonmalignant hybrid cells expressing the target surface antigens from parent cells. From this point of view, it would be valuable to see whether the eclipse phenomenon of the H-2 antigenic expression could be seen in a somatic cell hybrid formed between the L cells and other tumor cells than Ehrlich tumor cells.

Inverse Expression between H-2 Antigen and Tumor-specific Surface Antigen on FM3A Ascitic Mammary Tumor Cells

Nishioka and his colleagues (10) have shown that ascitic tumor cells derived from spontaneous mammary tumor cells of C3H/He mice express a tumor-specific surface antigen which is termed MM antigen, capable of inducing tumor rejection. A high level of antibody against MM antigen is obtained from C3H/He mice resistant to the ascitic tumor after repeated immunization with tumor cells treated with xenogeneic antiserum or an appropriate tumor antigen preparation, followed by challenges of the viable ascitic tumor cells. Irie *et al.* (6) have reported that hypotetraploid ascitic tumor cells express this antigen, while hyperdiploid ascitic tumor cells and spontaneous mammary tumor cells have much less or no MM antigen.

Three sublines of FM3A ascitic tumor cells, *i.e.*, FM3A #1, FM3A #2, and FM3A/R, derived from a spontaneous mammary tumor were selected during continous serial passage in syngeneic C3H/He mice. They have a different number of chromosomes and different expression of H-2 antigen and MM antigen, as shown in Table I.

TABLE I. Expression of the Surface Antigens in Hybrids of FM3A Sublines with L_{AG} Cells

Cells	Modal number or chromosomes		Relative expression of surface antigens[a]				
			Exp. 1		Exp. 2		
	Total	Bi-armed	H-2^k	MM	H-2^k	L cell	MM
Parents							
L_{AG}	58	16	100	—	100	100	—
FM3A #1	43	3	36	3	NT	NT	NT
FM3A #2	62	2	13	22	NT	NT	NT
FM3A/R	70	3	9	100	21	—	100
Hybrids							
L-FM3A #1	95	15	83	—	79	63	—
L-FM3A #2	95	9	13	70	17	—	41
L-FM3A/R	106	16	20	22	34	14	32

[a] The antigenic expression is denoted as the relative percent of the expression to that of the L_{AG} cells for the H-2^k and the L cell antigen, as well as to that of the FM3A/R tumor cells for the MM antigen. — means no detectable amount of antigen. Experiment 1 and 2 were done 6 months and 2 years after hybridization, respectively. NT, not tested.

In addition to confirmation of the above results obtained by Irie *et al.* (*6*), it was noted that the MM antigen is inversely expressed in relation to the H-2 antigen.

Antigenic Expression of the Somatic Cell Hybrids between the FM3A Tumor Cells and L Cells (*13*)

The three different FM3A tumor cells were fused with L_{AG} cells, an 8-azaguanine-resistant subline of the mouse L cells, by means of ultraviolet (UV)-irradiated Sendai viruses. The somatic cell hybrids were selected in the medium (HAT) devised by Littlefield (*8*). The FM3A tumor cells do not adhere to the glass surface. Thus, three different hybrid cells (L-FM3A#1, L-FM3A#2, and L-FM3A/R) were obtained by cell fusion between the L_{AG} cells and the three different FM3A tumor cell sublines.

The morphology of the hybrids in the culture can be divided into two types (Fig. 1). One type is seen in the L-FM3A#1 hybrid cells, similar to that of the L_{AG} cells. The cells grow in an extended, flat form, adhering to glass, and show contact inhibition of growth. The other type of cellular morphology is seen in the L-FM3A#2 and L-FM3A/R hybrids. In a sparse monolayer culture, they are highly dendritic, but in a confluent monolayer the cells become round pile up as they grow, showing no contact inhibition of growth.

The expression of surface antigens on the somatic cell hybrids and the parent cells was determined by an antibody absorption test. The antibody remaining after absorption was assayed by the mixed hemadsorption test (*14*). $(DBA/2 \times C57BL)F_1$ anti-C3H antiserum was used for the H-2^k antigen complex, C3H anti-MM antigen antiserum for MM antigen, and C3H anti-L cell antiserum for the L-cell antigen.

The antigenic expression was represented as the relative percent of the expression to that of the L_{AG} cells for both H-2^k and L-cell antigen as well as to that of the FM3A/R tumor cells for MM antigen, as shown in Table I. The L-FM3A#1 hybrid expressed the H-2^k antigen almost fully but no MM antigen, while in the L-FM3A#2 and L-FM3A/R hybrid the expression of the H-2^k antigen largely introduced by the

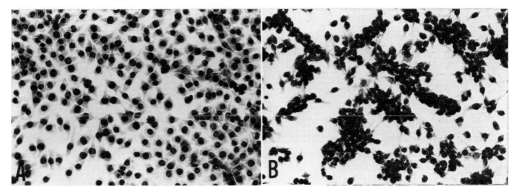

FIG. 1. The two types of cellular growth of the somatic cell hybrids *in vitro*. Stained by May-Grünwald-Giemsa.

A: Confluent monolayer of the L-FM3A #1 hybrids showing contact inhibition of growth.

B: Sparse monolayer of the L-FM3A/R hybrids showing clustered cell growth with loss of contact inhibition of growth.

L_{AG} cells to the hybrid was suppressed. Suppression of the MM antigen was also observed in the L-FM3A/R hybrids, while the expression of the MM antigen was enhanced in the L-FM3A#2 hybrids in comparison with the relevant parental tumor cells. An inverse relationship in the expression between the H-2^k antigens and the MM antigen seems to have been maintained in all of the hybrid cell lines. Taking account of the concomitant suppression of the L-cell antigen expression, it is possible that a suppressive effect similar to that seen in the L-Ehrlich hybrid cells will work on the H-2 antigenic expression of these two L-FM3A hybrid cells.

Antigenic Expression of the Somatic Cell Hybrids between Spontaneous Mammary Tumor Cells and L Cells (12)

Both Ehrlich and FM3A ascites tumor cells suppressed the surface antigen expression introduced by the L cells into the hybrids. These tumor cells commonly originate from mouse mammary tumor. Therefore, it was of interest to see if spontaneous tumor cells could suppress the H-2 antigenic expression and inversely express the MM antigen when fused with the L cells.

A free-cell suspension from spontaneous mammary tumor tissue was prepared by either trypsinization or treatment with collagenase. The former is called SAT and the latter, SAC. After preparing the free-cell suspension, SAT and SAC were immediately fused with 5-bromodeoxyuridine-resistant L cells (L_{BudR} cells) by using UV-irradiated Sendai virus. The somatic cell hybrids were selected and cloned in a HAT medium. This medium prevents the growth of the L_{BudR} cells. The tumor cells grow poorly *in vitro*.

As for the morphological features of cell growth *in vitro*, the hybrid clones could be divided into two types similar to those observed in the L-FM3A hybrids (see Photo 1): One type was characterized by a confluent monolayer with contact inhibition of growth. The other was characterized by scatterd cell growth having a tendency to roundness and to form clusters. The L-SAC-3 and L-SAC-7 hybrid clones belong to the former type, all the remaining hybrid clones belong to the latter type.

The karyotype of the parental tumor cells was analyzed with the primary transplant of tumor cells in a syngeneic C3H/He mouse. They were euploid, while the L_{BudR} cells were aneuploid, and the modal number of total chromosomes was 55, including 15 bi-armed ones. The karyotypes of the hybrid clones are summarized in Table II.

The deletion of chromosomes was outstanding particularly in the L-SAC-3 and L-SAC-7 hybrid clones though bi-armed chromosomes were relatively preserved. In contrast, the bi-armed chromosomes were markedly depleted in all other hybrid clones, albeit the total chromosome number being less depleted in these hybrid clones than in the above two hybrid clones.

It is clearly shown in Table II that the expression of the H-2^k antigen and the L-cell antigen was concomitantly suppressed in all the hybrid clones, except for the L-SAC-3 and L-SAC-7 clones having a characteristic morphology and karyotype readily distinguishable from those of the others. The amount of surface antigens is expressed relatively in Table II from the results of the antibody absorption test. The facts were very surprising in that the MM antigen, which was neither detected on the parental

TABLE II. Expression of Surface Antigens of Hybrid Clones of Spontaneous Mammary Carcinoma (SMCA) Cells with L_{BudR} Cells

Cells	Modal number of chromosomes		Relative expression of surface antgens[a]		
	Total	Bi-armed	H-2^k	L cell	MM
Parents					
SMCA	40	0	(卌)	(−)	(−)
L_{BudR}	55	15	125	55	—
Hybrids					
L-SAT-1	88	4	—	7	36
L-SAT-2	87	3	—	11	17
L-SAT-3	85	3	—	8	32
L-SAT-4	90	6	—	4	63
L-SAT-5	85	5	—	5	22
L-SAC-1	86	4	—	2	32
L-SAC-2	89	4	—	9	40
L-SAC-3	70	9	70	52	—
L-SAC-4	86	4	—	12	38
L-SAC-7	76	11	125	39	—

[a] 100 indicates 50% absorption of a given amount of antibody with 1×10^5 cells. — indicates no absorption of antiserum with 2×10^6 or 5×10^6 cells. SMCA cells were not tested by antibody absorption test simultaneously. The antigenic expression of SMCA cells was tested by the mixed hemadsorption test. (卌) strongly positive; (−) negative.

cells nor on normal cells of adult C3H/He mice, was induced and inversely expressed together with the suppression of the H-2 antigen in the majority of hybrids. There seems to be a correlation of H-2 antigen expression with the preservation of the bi-armed chromosomes presumably contributed by the L_{BudR} cells in the hybrids. *In vivo* growth of the hybrids in normal C3H/He mice, when 10^6 cells were inoculated intraperitoneally, does not correlate with the MM antigenic expression of the cells.

DISCUSSION

It has been demonstrated that expression of the histocompatibility antigen as well as the L-cell antigen which is contributed into hybrid cells by the L cells, was simultaneously reduced by cell fusion with the so-called nonspecific ascitic mammary tumor cells, irrespective of their serial passage through either an allogeneic or syngeneic host. However, the same suppression of both the H-2 and L-cell antigens was also observed in hybrids, when the free cells prepared from spontaneous mammary tumor tissue were fused with the L cells. Here, questions will arise regarding the H-2 expression of spontaneous mammary tumor cells or the nature of the parental cells of the hybrid, derived from tumor tissue, either malignant or nonmalignant. The amount of H-2 antigen expressed on the parent cells used in the cell hybridization was not measured directly. However, after several passages of the cells derived from the tumor tissue in *in vitro* cultivation, expression of the H-2^k antigen was clearly demonstrated by a mixed hemadsorption test although the quantity of H-2 antigen was uncertain. In separate experiments, however, a quantitative assay for H-2 antigen was made with free cell preparations made from several individual spontaneous mammary tumor tissues of

C3H/He mice by an antibody absorption test. All the cell preparations examined showed full H-2^k antigenic expression compared with that of normal lymphoid cells.

The MM antigen is found in ascitic mammary tumor cells carrying hypotetraploid chromosomes which had converted from a solid tumor mass after repeated transplantation in syngeneic C3H/He mice (5, 6). Immunoresistant Ehrlich ascites tumor cells also express the MM antigen (9). Considering the appearance of the MM antigen in the majority of hybrids, it may be argued that the parental cells made from spontaneous mammary tumor tissue for the cell hybridization of the L-SAT and L-SAC series are malignant cells. Of course, the possibility that these cells might have originated from the normal counterpart of mammary tumor tissue and that activation of the gene controlling the MM antigen might be induced by cell fusion may not be excluded. Regarding the origin of the parent cells derived from the tumor tissue for the L-SAC-3 and L-SAC-7 hybrid clones, it is uncertain whether the cells were derived from malignant or nonmalignant cells in the tumor tissue.

Thus, this suppression of the major histocompatibility antigen accompanying the expression of the MM antigen seems to be limited in the L-mammary tumor cell hybrids. In this connection it is of interest that the TA3/Ha ascites tumor, which originated from the mammary tumor of an A mouse and was low in H-2 antigen, expressed H-2^a antigen after cell fusion with an A.CA fibroblast (7).

The mechanism operating on suppression of the surface antigens is unknown. Further, it is unknown why there is an inverse relationship constantly present in the expression between the MM antigen and the H-2 antigen. Grundner et al. (3) found that full antigen expression reappeared following chromosome loss from the somatic hybrid, indicating the presence of chromosomes determining antigenic suppression. It would be very interesting if the gene loci coding the MM antigen are linked to the chromosomes determining H-2 antigenic suppression.

At present, it may be possible that the selective loss of the chromosomes and characteristic behavior of cell growth which is due to the alteration of cell membrane properties may be closely associated with antigen suppression.

The mechanism controlling this type of antigenic expression and suppression should be clarified for the application of somatic cell hybridization to tumor cell xenogenization.

Acknowledgment

This work was supported by a Grant-in-Aid for Cancer Research from the Ministry of Education, Science and Culture, Japan.

REFERENCES

1. Defendi, V., Ephrussi, B., Koprowski, H., and Yoshida, M. C. Properties of hybrids between polyoma-transformed and normal mouse cells. *Proc. Natl. Acad. Sci. U.S.*, **57**, 299–305 (1967).
2. Fenyö, E. M., Grundner, G., and Klein E. Virus-associated surface antigens on L cells and Moloney lymphoma cells. *J. Natl. Cancer Inst.*, **52**, 743–751 (1974).
3. Grundner, G., Fenyö, E. M., Klein, G., Klein, E., Bregula, U., and Harris, H. Surface antigen expression in malignant sublines derived from hybrid cells of low malignancy. *Exp. Cell Res.*, **68**, 315–322 (1971).

4. Harris, H., Miller, O. J., Klein, G., Worst, P., and Tachibana, T. Suppression of malignancy by cell fusion. *Nature*, **223**, 363–368 (1969).
5. Irie, R. F. Antigenic cross-reactivity between primary spontaneous mouse mammary tumors and their transplantable ascites tumors. *Cancer Res.*, **31**, 1682–1689 (1971).
6. Irie, R. F., Koyama, K., and Hino, S. Relation between the tumor-specific antigen and cytological characteristics in mouse mammary tumors. *J. Natl. Cancer Inst.*, **45**, 515–524 (1970).
7. Klein, G., Friberg, S., Jr., and Harris, H. Two kinds of antigen suppression in tumor cells revealed by cell fusion. *J. Exp. Med.*, **135**, 839–849 (1972).
8. Littlefield, J. The use of drug-resistant markers to study the hybridization of mouse fibroblasts. *Exp. Cell Res.*, **41**, 190–196 (1966).
9. Murayama-Okabayashi, F., Okada, Y., and Tachibana, T. A series of hybrid cells containing different ratios of parental chromosomes formed by two steps of artificial fusion. *Proc. Natl. Acad. Sci. U.S.*, **68**, 38–42 (1971).
10. Nishioka, K., Irie, R. F., Inoue, M., Chang, S., and Takeuchi, S. Immunological studies on mouse mammary tumors. I. Induction of resistance to tumor isograft in C3H/He mice. *Int. J. Cancer*, **4**, 121–129 (1969).
11. Spencer, R. A., Hauschka, T. S., Amos, D. B., and Ephrussi, B. Codominance of iso-antigens in somatic hybrids of murine cells grown *in vitro*. *J. Natl. Cancer Inst.*, **33**, 893–903 (1964).
12. Tachibana, T., Dei, T., and Makita, T. Cell fusion and expression of cell surface antigens. *Sym. Cell Biol.*, **26**, 77–84 (1974) (in Japanese).
13. Tachibana T., Dei, T., and Nori, C. Hybrids between malignant and normal cells: Their tumorigenicity, expression of surface antigens, and resistance-inducing ability. *Gann Monogr. Cancer Res.*, **16**, 183–193 (1974).
14. Tachibana, T., Worst, P., and Klein, E. Detection of cell surface antigens on monolayer cells. II. The application of mixed haemadsorption on a microscale. *Immunology*, **19**, 809–816 (1970).

GANN Monograph on Cancer Research 23, 1979

IMMUNE RESPONSES INDUCED BY INOCULATION OF HYBRID CELLS IN NORMAL AND TUMOR-BEARING MICE

Toshio Dei and Takehiko Tachibana

Department of Immunology, Research Institute for Tuberculosis and Cancer, Tohoku University*

Primary tumor cells induced by 3-methylcholanthrene in a C3H mouse were fused with 8-azaguanine-resistant L cells. Two types of hybrid cell clones were obtained; one was of the hybrid cells of two tumor cells with one L cell, the other was of one tumor cell with one L cell. Both hybrid cell lines expressed H-2^k antigen, the tumor cell antigen and L-cell antigen, and failed to produce a tumor in normal C3H mouse when as many as 10^6 cells were inoculated intraperitoneally (i.p.) or subcutaneously (s.c.). Normal C3H mice pretreated with inocula of viable hybrid cells showed resistance to the challenge of the parental tumor cells. It was seen by the Winn test that growth of the tumor cells was suppressed by splenic lymphoid cells from the resistant mice. This suppression of tumor growth was also observed by immune splenic lymphoid cells passed through a nylon fiber column, but not by immune splenic lymphoid cells treated with anti-Thy-1.2 antiserum and complement. On the other hand, when the hybrid cells were inoculated into mice bearing the parental tumor, tumor growth was seen to be enhanced. In these mice, cytotoxic T cells were also generated. In the sera of these mice collected at 5 weeks after tumor inoculation, antibody to the tumor cells and antigen-antibody complex were detected at a higher level than those of the tumor bearer. The sera of these mice blocked at the level of the target cells and also inhibited the reactivity of immune spleen cells in *in vitro* cellular cytotoxicity.

It is concluded that inoculation of viable hybrid cells can preferentially stimulate cellular immunity in the normal mouse but accelerates the humoral response in the tumor-bearer, resulting in the enhancement of tumor growth in the latter.

It has been reported that hybrid cells between tumor cells and normal cells are not able to grow in syngeneic normal mice but thereafter do make the mice resistant to the challenge of parental tumor cells in some cases (*5, 12, 17*). In the previous study, we observed that hybrid cells between FM3A tumor cells, ascitic mammary tumor cells, and L cells were more immunogenic than irradiated tumor cells. Normal mice pretreated with these hybrid cells could specifically reject the parental FM3A tumor cells (*19*). On the other hand, it was also observed that the repeated injection of hybrid cells into tumor-bearing mice brought about the enhancement of growth of tumor

---

* Seiryo-machi 4-1, Sendai 980, Japan (出井敏雄, 橘　武彦).

cells. It is important to know the mechanisms of such enhancement in terms of application of the tumor cell hybrid as an immunotherapeutic tool. However, ascitic mammary tumor cells are known to have rather particular properties such as preferential induction of antibody production (7, 16).

In order to determine whether this enhancement is generally observed, hybrid cells between methylcholanthrene-induced tumor cells in a C3H mice and L cells were used in this experiment. In this context, these hybrid cells could also induce the enhancement of tumor growth when inoculated into the tumor-bearing host, and this mechanism of enhancement was investigated.

Characteristics of Hybrid Cells

C3H mice were injected subcutaneously with 3-methylcholanthrene. About 2 months later the growing tumor was cut off and trypsinized. The free cells thus obtained were mixed and hybridized with 8-azaguanine-resistant L cells, using ultraviolet (UV)-irradiated HVJ (Sendai virus). After 2 weeks, several cell clones were grown and selected in the medium (HAT) devised by Littlefied (14). Two groups of hybrid clones were obtained after several repeated clonings. One group of hybrid cells named LMCT-

TABLE I. Chromosome Number of Hybrid Cells

| Cell line | Chromosome number | |
	Total	Metacentric
C3H MCT	40	0
L_{AG}	58 (52–60)[a]	16 (15–18)
LMCT-11	101 (100–114)	14 (9–14)
LMCT-12	112 (106–116)	11 (9–12)
LMCT-32	77 (70–78)	8 (6–9)
LMCT-34	80 (74–89)	10 (8–12)

[a] The range of chromosome number is shown in parenthesis.

TABLE II. Antigen Expression and Tumorigenicity of MCT Hybrid Cells

| Cells | Antigen expression[a] (%) | | | Tumorigenicity | | Resistance[b] |
	MCT	H-2^k	L cell	10^6 i.p.	10^6 s.c.	
L_{AG}	0	100	100	—	—	—
MCT	100	89.3	0	—	5/5[c]	—
LMCT-11	29.3	67.7	45.7	0/5	0/4	1/5[c]
LMCT-34	14.1	13.5	NT[d]	0/5	0/2	3/5

[a] Expression of surface antigens is denoted as the relative percent of the relevant antigenic expression of the parental cells by means of an antibody absorption test. Antisera used were C3H anti-MCT tumor surface antigen antiserum absorbed with L cells, A.BY×DBA/2 anti-CBA antiserum (anti-H-2^k), and C3H anti-L-cell antiserum.

[b] C3H mice were injected i.p. with hybrid cells three times with a 1-week interval, 2 weeks after the last injection, 10^7 tumor cells were challenged s.c., and observed for 2 months.

[c] No. of takes/No. of mice tested. The data were obtained 2 months after the inoculation of hybrid cells or challenging tumor.

[d] Not tested.

11 and LMCT-12 cells, piled up and lost contact inhibition of growth which is considered to be contributed to the hybrid cells by L cells. Another group of hybrid cells grew in a monolayer. They had some metacentric chromosomes of L cell origin and many telocentric chromosomes. The number of chromosomes of LMCT-11 and -12 cells was greater than the sum of those of the parental MCT tumor and L cell. However, the number of metacentric chromosomes of these hybrid cells was fewer than those of the L cell. Therefore, this group of hybrid cells might consist of two MCT tumor cells and one L cell. The other group of hybrid cells, LMCT-32 and -34 cells, were considered to consist of one tumor cell and one L cell (Table I).

The relative expression of surface antigens of hybrid cells was determined by an antibody absorption test. The hybrid cells expressed H-2^k antigen, L-cell antigen, and MCT tumor-specific antigen(s), but their levels were lower than those of the parental cells. One million of these hybrid cells could not grow in normal adult C3H mice when inoculated subcutaneously or intraperitoneally (Table II).

Induction of Tumor Resistance in a Normal Syngeneic Host by Inoculation of Hybrid Cells

C3H mice previously inoculated with hybrid cells could prevent growth of the parent MCT tumor cells. This resistance was induced more strongly by increasing the number of injections of hybrid cells. Four out of 5 mice receiving LMCT-11 cells and 2 out of 5 receiving LMCT-34 cells completely prevented growth of challenging tumor (Table II). Even though some of the mice had progressive tumors, the tumor growth was markedly suppressed compared with the control. The resistance to tumor induced by LMCT-11 cells was more effective than the one induced by LMCT-34 cells. A neutralization test (Winn test) showed that immune spleen cells from the mice receiving the hybrid cells three times with a 1-week interval, completely prevented growth of the admixed tumor cells (Table III). Among the spleen cells, a lymphocyte fraction passed through a nylon fiber column showed antitumor activity, but this activity was lost after treatment with anti-Thy-1.2 antiserum and complement. The same results were obtained when recipients immunologically crippled by 400 rad γ-irradiation from ^{60}Co were used. These results suggest that the cytotoxic T cells were

TABLE III. Characterization of Effector Cells

Treatment of spleen cells	Experiments[a]			
	1st	2nd	3rd	4th (400 rad)[c]
Normal	4/5[d]	4/4	5/5	10/10
Immune[b]	0/3	0/4	0/5	0/7
Immune-nylon fiber passed	0/3	0/4	—	0/4
Immune-a/Thy-1.2+C	—	3/3	5/5	4/4
Immune-C	—	0/2	0/3	0/3

[a] 10^7 immune spleen cells admixed with 10^6 tumor cells were injected into C3H mice subcutaneously.

[b] Spleen cells from mice injected with LMCT 11 cells three times.

[c] Recipients irradiated with 400 rad.

[d] No. of takes/No. of mice tested.

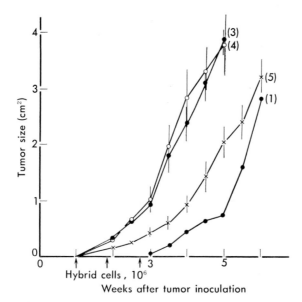

FIG. 1.   Enhancement of tumor growth by hybrid cells
    One million hybrid cells were injected three times with a 1-week interval from
1 week after the injection of 10^7 tumor cells into C3H mice. ● LMCT-11;
○ LMCT-34; × no hybrid cells injected. Vertial bars represent SE.

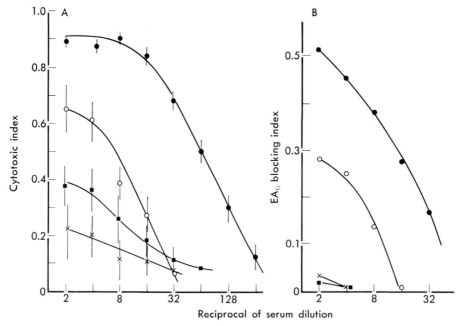

FIG. 2.   Cytotoxic antibodies and immune complexes in the sera
    (A) Cytotoxic antibodies against MCT tumor cells in the complement-de-
pendent microcytotoxicity test. (B) Blocking activity of the sera to the receptor
for IgG-Fc of Daudi cells. Daudi cells were pretreated with sera at 37° for 1 hr
and EA (sheep erythrocytes sensitized with rabbit IgG antibodies)-rosette formation of Daudi cells was tested. ● Serum from mice showing enhancement of
tumor growth; ○ serum from tumor-bearing mice; ■ serum from mice immunized with LMCT 11 hybrid cells, three times; × serum from normal mice.
Vertical bars represent SE.

generated by inoculation of the hybrid cells, and that they play a major role in the resistance against challenging tumors.

Enhancement of Tumor Growth in the Tumor-bearer by Inoculation of Hybrid Cells

When hybrid cells were injected three times with a 1-week interval from 1 week after the transplantation of tumor cells into syngeneic hosts, enhancement of tumor growth was observed. Among 8 mice inoculated with the hybrid cells, 7 showed enhancement of tumor growth (Fig. 1). Splenic lymphoid cells obtained from the mice bearing enhanced tumor growth at 5 weeks after tumor cell inoculation were also able to suppress the tumor growth in the Winn test. Nonadherent cells, which were obtained by a nylon fiber column, could suppress growth of tumor more strongly but suppressive activity was lost by pretreatment of the cells with anti-Thy-1.2 antiserum and complement. These results suggest that the cytotoxic T cells are also generated in mice showing enhancement of tumor growth.

One possibility concerning this enhancement is that the humoral antibodies and immune complexes generated will interfere with cell-mediated immunity and promote tumor growth. Cytotoxic antibodies against the MCT tumor cells were detected at higher levels in the serum of mice showing the enhancement phenomenon than those in the sera of tumor-bearing mice as well as in immune mice (Fig. 2A). The blocking test of EA (sheep erythrocytes sensitized with rabbit IgG antibodies) rosette formation of Daudi cells, carrying the receptor for the Fc part of IgG, was applied to detect soluble immune complexes in the sera. The sera were ultracentrifuged at 105,000 g for 1 hr to remove aggregated immunoglobulin prior to the test. Pretreatment of Daudi

TABLE IV. Effect of Sera on Cellular Cytotoxicity *in vitro*[a]

MCT cells	Immune spleen cells	Specific cytotoxicity[e] (%)		
Treated with		Exp. 1	Exp. 2	Exp. 3
—	—	38.5 ± 2.6[f]	41.9 ± 4.5	16.8 ± 4.0
NS[b]	—	NT[g]	34.7 ± 11.9 (17.2)[h]	16.7 ± 5.6 (0)
ES[c]	—	15.0 ± 8.1 (61.0)	$-7.8\pm17\cdot0$ (100)	16.9 ± 2.9 (0)
ES-1W[d]	—	NT	NT	-6.2 ± 11.0 (0)
—	NS[b]	NT	28.6 ± 2.2 (31.7)	25.1 ± 6.2 (100)
—	ES[c]	1.2 ± 1.7 (96.9)	13.4 ± 3.9 (68.0)	8.5 ± 6.9 (49.4)
—	ES-1W[d]	NT	NT	-18.2 ± 9.8 (100)

[a] 5×10^4 MCT tumor cells labeled with ^{3}H-uridine and 5×10^6 immune spleen cells were cultured in a microtiter plate, Falcon #3040. After 12 hr, cells were harvested with a multisample cell harvester onto glassfiber filters and counted by a liquid scintillation counter.

[b] Normal C3H mice serum.

[c] Serum from mice showing enhancement of tumor growth taken at 2 weeks after the last injection of LMCT-11 cells.

[d] Serum taken 1 week after the last injection of LMCT 11 cells.

[e] % of specific cytotoxicity $=\left(1-\dfrac{\text{test sample cpm-background}}{\text{control sample cpm-background}}\right)\times100.$

[f] S.E.

[g] Not tested.

[h] % of blocking or inhibition indicated in parentheses.

cells with these sera caused the blocking of EA rosette formation, indicating the presence of immune complexes in the sera. Sera of mice showing enhancement blocked the target cells and also inhibited immune spleen cells in *in vitro* cytotoxicity using ³H-uridine (*11*). The sera taken at an earlier stage of tumor development blocked and inhibited more strongly (Table IV). The factor which is present in these sera might interfere with the cytotoxic T cells and tumor growth might be enhanced.

Another possibility is that the generation of suppressor cells may enhance tumor growth. Splenic lymphoid cells of mice showing enhancement suppressed the growth of tumor in the Winn test. The treatment of lymphoid cells with anti-Thy-1.2 antiserum and complement abrogated this suppressive activity, and brought about a slight enhancement of tumor growth. However, splenic lymphoid cells pretreated with anti-Thy-1.2 antiserum and complement could not suppress the activity of killer T cells in the Winn test *in vivo* or in cellular cytotoxicity *in vitro*. Furthermore, the adherent lymphoid cells which were retained in the nylon fiber column did not enhance but suppressed the growth of tumor cells. These results suggest that the suppressor cells may not play an important role, if any, in this enhancement phenomenon.

DISCUSSION

Many investigators have tried to use somatic cell hybrids as immunoprotective agents and to introduce protective activity against parental tumor cells by the injection of somatic hybrid cells into normal mice (*5, 12, 17*). It would be of considerable interest if these somatic hybrid cells could be used as immunotherapeutic agents. We first used the hybrid cells between the FM3A tumor cell and L cell. The growth of FM3A tumor cells was enhanced by inoculation of the hybrid cells into the tumor bearer, but this phenomenon was thought to be peculiar to the tumor-cells, because it is well known that FM3A tumors could preferentially induce a humoral response to the host (*7, 16*).

In the present experiment, hybrid cells between methylcholanthrene-induced tumor cells and L cells were used, and a similar phenomenon was observed. Thus, the enhancement of tumor growth by injection of hybrid cells into the tumor-bearing host may be considered to be a more or less general phenomenon.

Although LMCT-11 cells could, and LMCT-34 cells could not grow in immunologically-deficient nude mice, these hybrid cells could not grow in syngeneic normal C3H mice and were very useful in prophylaxis. The difference in tumorigenicity between hybrid cells may be due to the difference in the number of tumor cells induced into hybrid cells. LMCT-11 cells contained two tumor cells, LMCT-34 cells contained one tumor cell. Splenic lymphoid cells of the mice which rejected hybrid cells could suppress tumor growth in the Winn test and this antitumor activity was completely lost by treatment with anti-Thy-1.2 antiserum and complement. Liang and Cohen (*13*) reported that the killing activity of spleen cells immunized with syngeneic hybrid cells was not completely lost by treatment with anti-Thy-1.2 antiserum and complement in *in vitro* cytotoxicity. The difference between the results of these studies might be due to the difference of tumor cells and the assay system used.

When hybrid cells were injected into tumor-bearing mice, tumor growth was enhanced. It has been reported that tumor-specific, cell-mediated immunity in the tumor-bearing animal may be interfered through the antigen released from tumor cells, antibodies, and antigen-antibody complexes (*1, 3, 4, 15*) and that the growth of tumor cells was enhanced by these humoral factors (*2, 10*).

It also has been reported that suppressor cells have inhibited tumor immunity in tumor-bearing animals. Specific T lymphocytes (*6*), suppressor B lymphocytes (*18*) through specific immune complexes (*9*), and the monocyte/macrophage series may exert a suppressive effect. Gabizon *et al.* (*8*) reported that spleen cells from tumor-bearing mice yielded specific inhibition of tumor growth in the early stage of tumor growth but spleen cells showed enhancement of tumor growth in the later stage of tumor growth in the Winn test.

In this study, antibodies against tumor cells and antigen-antibody complexes existed more abundantly in the sera of mice showing enhancement of tumor growth than in those of the tumor-bearer and immune mice. These sera of mice showing enhancement blocked the target cells and inhibited the immune spleen cells in cytotoxicity *in vitro*. Spleen cells from mice showing enhancement could suppress tumor growth in the Winn test *in vivo*. These results suggest that hybrid cells injected into the tumor-bearer stimulated humoral response and brought about the enhancement of tumor growth.

In summary, hybrid cells inoculated into normal mice stimulated cellular immunity and generated cytotoxic T cells but they also stimulated humoral immunity and accelerated the production of humoral antibodies and the immune complexes preexisting in the tumor-bearer. This means that an uncontrolled active immunotherapy to the tumor-bearer produces unfavorable effects on the tumor-bearing host.

Acknowledgment

This work was supported by Grants-in-Aid for Cancer Research from the Ministry of Education, Science and Culture and from the Ministry of Health and Welfare, Japan.

REFERENCES

1. Baldwin, R. W. Immune responses to tumor specific and embryonic antigens on chemically-induced tumours. *Progr. Immunol.*, **3**, 538–546 (1977).
2. Biddle, C. Stimulation of transplanted 3-methylcholanthrene induced sarcomas in mice by specific immune and by normal serum. *Int. J. Cancer*, **17**, 755–764 (1976).
3. Blair, P. B. and Lane, M. A. Serum factors in mammary neoplasia: Enhancement and antagonism of spleen cell activity *in vitro* detected by different methods of serum factor assay. *J. Immunol.*, **112**, 439–443 (1974).
4. Bowen, J. G., Robins, R. A., and Baldwin, R. W. Serum factors modifying cell mediated immunity to rat hepatoma D23 correlated with tumor growth. *Int. J. Cancer*, **15**, 640–650 (1975).
5. Favre, R., Carcassonne, Y., and Meyer, G. The use of hybrid cells in immunotherapy. *Oncology*, **34**, 84–86 (1977).
6. Fujimoto, S., Greene, M. E., and Sehon, A. H. Regulation of the immune response to tumor antigens. I. Immunosuppressor cells in tumor bearing hosts. *J. Immunol.*, **116**, 791–799 (1976).
7. Fujiwara, H., Hamaoka, T., Teshima, K., Aoki, H., and Kitagawa, M. Preferential generation of killer or helper T lymphocyte activity directed to the tumor associated transplantation antigens. *Immunology*, **31**, 239–248 (1976).
8. Gabizon, A., Small, M., and Trainin, N. Kinetics of the response of spleen cells from

tumor-bearing animals in an *in vivo* tumor neutralization assay. *Int. J. Cancer*, **18**, 813–819 (1976).

9. Gorcznski, R. M., Kilburn, D. G., Knight, R. A., Norbury, C., Parker, D. C., and Smith, J. B. Nonspecific and specific immunosuppression in tumor-bearing mice by soluble immune complexes. *Nature*, **254**, 141–143 (1975).

10. Harris, T. N., Harris, S., Henri, E. M., and Farber, M. B. Enhancement of growth of allogeneic mouse tumor by the IgG$_1$ fraction of alloantibody preparations. *J. Natl. Cancer Inst.*, **60**, 167–171 (1978).

11. Hashimoto, Y. and Sudo, H. Evaluation of cell damage in immune reactions by release of radioactivity from ³H-uridine labeled cells. *Gann*, **62**, 139–143 (1971).

12. Liang, W. and Cohen, E. P. Resistance to murine leukemia in mice rejecting syngeneic somatic hybrid cells. *J. Immunol.*, **116**, 623–636 (1976).

13. Liang, W. and Cohen, E. P. Activation of specific cellular immunity toward murine leukemia in mice rejecting syngeneic somatic hybrid cells. *J. Immunol.*, **119**, 1054–1060 (1977).

14. Littlefield, J. The use of drug-resistant makers to study the hybridization of mouse fibroblasts. *Exp. Cell Res.*, **41**, 190–196 (1966).

15. Nepom, J. T., Hellström, I., and Hellström, K. E. Antigen-specific purification of blocking factors from sera of mice with chemically induced tumors. *Proc. Natl. Acad. Sci. U.S.*, **74**, 4605–4609 (1977).

16. Nishioka, K., Irie, R. F., Inoue, M., Chang, S., and Takeuchi, S. Immunological studies on mouse mammary tumors. I. Induction of resistance to tumor isograft in C3H/He mice. *Int. J. Cancer*, **4**, 121–129 (1969).

17. Parkman, R. Tumor hybrid cells: An immunotherapeutic agent. *J. Natl. Cancer Inst.*, **52**, 1541 (1974).

18. Rudczynski, A. B. and Mortensen, R. F. Suppressor cells in mice with murine mammary tumor virus-induced mammary tumors. I. Inhibition of mitogen-induced lymphocyte stimulation. *J. Natl. Cancer Inst.*, **60**, 205–211 (1978).

19. Tachibana, T., Dei, T., and Nori, C. Hybrids between malignant and normal cells: Their tumorigenicity, expression of surface antigens, and resistance-inducing ability. *Gann Monogr. Cancer Res.*, **16**, 183–193 (1974).

LIPOSOMAL FUSION AS A MEANS OF INTRODUCING SURFACE ANTIGENS INTO LIVING CELL MEMBRANES

T. D. Heath, D. Robertson, M.S.C. Birbeck, and
A.J.S. Davies

Chester Beatty Research Institute, Institute of Cancer Research

The membranes of liposomes are equivalent in many respects to the phospholipid component of mammalian plasma membranes. The similarity may be enhanced when proteins are associated with the liposomes to form proteoliposomes. The proteins may be readily encapsulated within the liposomal membranes but it has also proved possible to covalently bind certain proteins to the outside surface of liposomes.

The method of binding will be reviewed and the possible applications of proteoliposomes will be considered. The emphasis will lie on the possibility of fusing proteoliposomes with mammalian cells in such a way that the protein component becomes an integral part of the cell membranes. A process of xenogenization of this kind could be useful not only for modification of the surface antigenicity of mammalian cells but also for studies of the turnover of cell surface glycoproteins.

When suspended in aqueous media, phospholipids spontaneously form lipid bilayers. For all pure phospholipid classes except phosphatidylethanolamine these bilayers become sealed vesicles known as liposomes (*4*). Liposomes can be formed from mixtures of phospholipids in which phosphatidylethanolamine may be included, and from phospholipids mixed with other lipid substances. Liposomes will only form when the lipid mixture used is above its solid-liquid crystalline phase transition temperature. They may be cooled below this temperature after their formation, the membranes then become more rigid and less permeable to low molecular weight solutes.

For convenience Poste and Papahadjopoulos (*30*) have distinguished three classes of liposomes as multilammellar large vesicles (MLV), small unilammellar vesicles (SUV), and large unilammellar vesicles (LUV). The multilammellar forms consist of concentric spheroidal structures with many phospholipid bilayers. The unilammellar forms have only one bilayer per liposome.

Several methods are available for the preparation of liposomes, the simplest involving the hydration and suspension of a thin film of phospholipid in an aqueous medium (*4*), which produces multilammellar liposomes of 1–2 μm in size. MLV may be reduced in size by sonication, which, if performed exhaustively, will produce SUV of 25 nm in diameter (*20*). Such small liposomes may also be produced without sonication by the method of Batzri and Korn (*5*) in which an ethanolic lipid solution is injected into an aqueous medium, or, alternatively, by dialysis of detergent-lipid mix-

Fulham Road, London SW3 6JB, U.K.

tures (35), which preferentially removes detergents because phospholipids have very low critical multimer concentrations.

Two methods have also been devised for producing LUV. The first (10) involves the injection of an etheral lipid solution into an aqueous medium at 60°, and in the second method 25 nm phosphatidylserine vesicles are fused with calcium ions to produce cochleate cyclinders which are transformed into the requisite liposomes by ethylenediamine tetraacetic acid (EDTA) treatment (29).

Liposomes possess several attributes which have made them of importance to biological science. Their phospholipid membranes are similar to the lipid portions of cell membranes, for which they act as a useful model. They are stable structures whose composition and size may readily be manipulated. Liposomal membranes are semipermeable and define two distinct aqueous compartments which allows the entrapment of water-soluble compounds. The study of membrane permeability to low molecular weight solutes is also possible using liposomes. In consequence, numerous studies have been performed with liposomes of which there are comprehensive reviews elsewhere (4, 30, 38). Here we shall select a few topics for discussion which are close to our particular interests.

Permeability of Liposomes

Liposomes have been used extensively to study the permeability of phospholipid bilayers to low molecular weight solutes (3). It has been shown that some solutes including glucose, sucrose, Na^+, K^+, and SO_4^{2-} are impermeant whereas solutes such as ethanediol, ethylurea, NH_4^+, and Ac^- are rapidly permeant, the latter two passing through the membrane as the unionised species. They have also been used to study the effects of pharmacological agents, believed to act on cell membranes. Substances such as anaesthetics (24), steroids (43), and lytic peptides (34) have been investigated, and we are currently looking at the effects of levamisole on liposome permeability, and have found that it accelerates the movement of chromate ions but not of glucose across liposome membranes.

Immunological Aspects of Liposomes

The lack of toxicity of many kinds of liposomes has led to the widespread notion that they may have uses as adjuvants given in combination with antigenic material which would otherwise be non-immunogenic. Kinsky and his colleagues for example have shown that injection into rabbits of a synthetic lipid antigen dinitrophenylcaproyl-phosphatidylethanolamine (DNP-cap-PE) incorporated into a liposome led to anti-DNP antibody production, whereas the substituted lipid alone was non-immunogenic (39). This seems to indicate that lipid antigens incorporated in lipid membrane are more immunogenic than in the free form but it gives little indication of the mechanism involved. The same investigators have shown (23) that liposomes with integrated haptens can be "lysed" by the action of specific anti-hapten antibody in the presence of complement. Such a result is clearly analogous to immune haemolysis and in addition to re-emphasising the close similarities between liposomal and plasma membranes it perhaps indicates that the position of a hapten in a lipid bilayer might indeed facilitate

TABLE I.   Immune Response to BSA in CBA/Lac Mice 20 μg or
20×20 μg Given in Various Adjuvants

Adjuvant	Primary response		Secondary response	
	Titre	p	Titre	p
CFA	1.92±0.1	<0.001	2.19±0.20	<0.001
Alum precipitate	0.59±0.25	<0.001	2.20±0.44	NS
9:1 PC: DCP liposomes	1.75±0.30	—	2.04±0.27	—

Titres were measured by Farr assay and expresed as $\log_{10}$ μg ^{125}I-BSA monomer bound per ml serum. PC, phosphatidyl choline; DCP, dicetyl phosphate.

its recognition. The alternative hypothesis that liposomes are dealt with by phagocytosis in a very different manner to free lipids and that this, rather than any unique positional effect is responsible for the heightened immune response, is tenable but less interesting.

From a totally different view point, liposomes can exert an adjuvant effect with protein antigens entrapped within them (1, 17). The results in Table I show that 10 μg soluble bovine serum albumin (BSA), which is incapable of eliciting an immune response in solution, will produce a response when given entrapped in liposomes. However, when compared to Freund's adjuvant or Alhydrogel, liposomes are seen not to be the most effective of adjuvants. Despite this, of the three adjuvant preparations mentioned, liposomes are at the present time the most acceptable for human immunisation.

Liposomes are a particularly poor adjuvant when administered intravenously, perhaps due to their rapid hepatic uptake (16). For example, 3 mg lipid given to an adult rat can be 80–90% cleared from the circulation within 30 min (16). After injection of liposomes, water- or lipid-soluble markers for them can be found in the liver and spleen, and have been shown in the liver to be localised in the lysosomes (15).

The fate of subcutaneously and intraperitoneally administered liposomes is less well documented although it is known that markers for the liposomes persist at the site of injection for several days (26). Whether in these circumstances the liposomes maintain their integrity seems uncertain.

The ability of liposomes to encapsulate water-soluble compounds has resulted in attempts to use them in vivo as carriers of therapeutic agents. Such attempts have been based on the possibility either that intravenously administered liposomes might be induced to home on specific cell targets (16) or that subcutaneously administered liposomes might act as depots which would slowly release entrapped drug (26). It has also been suggested that liposome-entrapped compounds might penetrate cells which the non-entrapped compound could not enter. Of the attempts made to use liposomes as therapeutic carriers the most successful to date have been in the treatment of visceral leishmanias (7) which is effective because the leishmanial parasites are found in liver and spleen cells which avidly take up intravenously injected liposomes, and in the alleviation of arthritic joint inflammation which is based on a depot effect of the liposomes, the steroid being slowly released at the site of injection (11).

Proteoliposomes

Some of the techniques developed for producing liposomes allow the simultaneous introduction of proteins into the phospholipid bilayer to form structures resembling cell membranes, and termed proteoliposomes *(33)*. The exact relationship of the protein to the phospholipids in proteoliposomes and the extent to which it can be compared to the protein-plasma membrane association in living cells has occupied the attentions of many workers. The approach has varied according to the properties of the protein in question. Membrane-bound enzymes such as mitochondrial enzymes *(13)* and microsomal enzymes *(12)* exhibit their catalytic activity when incorporated into proteoliposomes. Some enzymes *(35)* such as the (Na$^+$K$^+$)-dependent ATPase lose activity on extraction from their natural milieu but regain activity upon incorporation into liposomes.

The incorporation of membrane carrier proteins into liposomes has been shown to render the liposomes specifically permeable to the solute which the incorporated proteins are known to transport across cell membranes *(9)*. Proteoliposomes containing transport proteins which carry protons actively at the expense of ATP have been shown specifically to concentrate protons in the presence of ATP *(36)*. Glycophorin, the major sialoprotein of the erythrocyte, when it is incorporated into proteoliposomes, has been shown both to interact with lectins *(32)* and to give rise to the characteristic intramembranous granules of a transmembrane protein visualised with freeze fracture electron microscopy *(14)*. Influenza surface proteins have been incorporated into proteoliposomes and are sufficiently large to be visualised when negatively stained under the electron microscope. The term "virosome" has been coined for such viral protein-liposomal associations *(2)*. Two surface proteins are found on influenza virus, the haemagglutinin subunit which appears rod-shaped in the electron microscope, and the neuraminidase subunit which appears T-shaped. Morphological observations show unambiguously that the neuraminidase subunit is inserted into the virosome membrane in the same manner as it is inserted into the viral lipid envelope. The haemagglutinin appears also to be inserted in the virosome membrane in the correct manner although it could be upside down on strictly morphologic criteria. However, the haemagglutinin rod has one hydrophobic end which is normally inserted into the lipid envelope of the virus and which will almost certainly be similarly inserted into the liposomal membrane.

Liposome-cell Interactions In Vitro

It seems to be a characteristic of liposomal membranes that under certain circumstances they can interact one with another *(28)* or indeed with living cells. The exact mechanisms involved in this latter phenomenon are unclear but are currently attracting much attention. One important distinction that has been made is between these liposomal-cell interactions in which the outcome is dependent on the metabolic state of the cell in question and those in which it does not. For example Poste and Papahadjopoulos *(31)* have studied the interaction of liposomes with BALB/c 3T3 cells and found that fluid-negative, fluid-neutral, and solid-negative liposomes all interact with metabolically active cells. However, in the presence of Cytochalasin B or in the presence of sodium azide and deoxyglucose, which together completely block ATP synthesis, the uptake of fluid-neutral or solid-negative liposomes is 90% inhibited whereas the uptake of fluid-negative liposomes is only 20–30% inhibited. This suggests that the uptake of fluid-neutral or solid-negative liposomes is predominantly energy dependent and involves phagocytosis, leaving none of the liposomal material in the plasma membrane The uptake of fluid-negative liposomes, however, is largely energy independent and probably involves fusion of the liposomes with the cell plasma membrane, although lipid exchange or simple adhesion of the liposomes to the cells cannot be ruled out. Several other workers have similarly studied the interaction of liposomes with cells and the results conflict with those of Poste and Papahadjopoulos in various ways. Batzri and Korn (6) claim that solid 25 nm and fluid multilammellar liposomes fuse with cells. Pagano and Huang (18) have shown that neutral fluid 25 nm liposomes fuse with cells, whilst Martin and MacDonald (25) claim that only positively charged 20% lysolecithin liposomes will fuse with erythrocytes. Whilst further study is necessary it may well be that the differences observed are primarily due to the different properties of the cells used.

Weissmann et al. (42) have shown that for some lymphoid cell lines, liposome-cell fusion is promoted by putting lysolecithin in the cell membrane. The same workers (41) have also studied the endocytosis of liposomes by dogfish phagocytes and have found it to be promoted if the liposomes are opsonised by coating them with heat-aggregated isologous IgM. Pagano and Takeichi (27) have shown that "solid" liposomes will adhere to cells via a trypsin-labile protein. This process may be distinguished from fusion since the liposomes are released from the cells by trypsin treatment. Fusion and adhesion can also be distinguished in the manner described by Weinstein et al. (40) who have shown that fusion of liposomes that contain 6-carboxy fluorescein with cells results in whole cell fluorescence since the dye is released into the cytoplasm, whereas adhesion of 6CF laden liposomes to cells results in peripheral cell fluorescence.

Liposomal Fusion

Of the three types of liposome-cell interactions described, perhaps the most potentially useful is fusion since it results in the entry of water-soluble liposome contents into the cell cytoplasm (42) and opens up the possibility of inserting the liposome membrane into the cell membrane (18). Martin and MacDonald (25) have used liposome fusion with erythrocytes as a means of introducing a new antigenic determinant into the red-cell membrane. The antigen used was DNP-cap-PE and when introduced in this manner rendered the cells susceptible to lysis by anti-DNP antibodies and complement. Moreover, the antigen could be localized in the membrane with an anti-DNP ferritin conjugate. By fusion with liposomes a defined antigen may be introduced into the cell membrane, and we are interested in the possibility that liposomes might be used to xenogenise cells with protein antigens. As mentioned above, membrane proteins can be purified and incorporated into liposome membranes, and if such proteoliposomes were fused with cells a novel membrane protein might be incorporated into the cell membrane. Complementary to this approach and one which we shall consider here is the possibility that soluble proteins, if covalently linked to liposomes, might be introduced onto cells as "pseudo-membrane proteins" by fusion of the liposomes with the cell.

We felt that before attempting covalently to link a protein to a liposome consideration should be given to a number of factors the first being whether such a linking was likely to hold a protein at the liposome membrane or whether the phospholipid-protein complex would pull away from the membrane. This was approached by calculating the hydrophobic interaction in methylene group equivalents for glycophorin and for dipalmitoyllecithin. Glycophorin has 83 methylene groups equivalent and dipalmitoyllecithin has 32. Consequently, since glycophorin is a tightly bound membrane protein it seems likely that a soluble protein of molecular weight $\sim$50,000, if bound to 1–2 phospholipids in a liposome would remain membrane bound. Consideration was also given to how much protein one might reasonably expect to link to a liposome. This was approached by considering how much cytochrome c would be required completely to coat 25 nm liposomes. Cytochrome c is assumed to be a perfect sphere of diameter 3.1 nm (22) and cross sectional area of 7.55 nm^2. To completely coat a 25 nm liposome which has a surface area of 1,963 nm^2 would require 260 molecules and assuming cytochrome c has a molecular weight of 14,500 and that 1 μmol of lipid will produce 1.7×10^{14} liposomes then 1.4 mg cytochrome c would be required to coat 1 mg lipid as 25 nm liposomes. On this basis 1 mg protein/mg lipid is the goal which has been set for successful coupling.

The choice of conjugation method is also quite critical to this project. Many experimenters have conjugated proteins to other proteins or to cells using bifunctional reagents whose two reactive groups react simultaneously, which gives rise to a heterogeneous mixture of polymerisation products. Coupling methods have been devised in this department (37) in which the two reactive groups of the bifunctional reagent can be reacted separately, and we have aimed to use these methods in a manner which results in proteins combining only with liposomes, thereby eliminating heterogeneity of products. The choice of protein is also critical and in practice many proteins are unsuitable because they bind non-specifically to liposomes under the conditions used. The protein chosen was horseradish peroxidase (HRP) which has been linked to liposomes by the method of Nakane (21), normally used for preparation of antibody-HRP conjugates. HRP is treated with fluorodinitrobenzene to block the ϵ-amino groups of lysine and then with periodic acid to generate aldehydes on the carbohydrate portion of the molecule. The activated enzyme is then desalted on Sephadex G50 and then mixed with liposomes prepared from 2:1 phosphatidylcholine: phosphatidylethanolamine. At pH 9.5 the enzyme binds to the liposomes *via* an aldehyde amino reaction, and the coated liposomes are separated from the non-bound enzyme on Sepharose 6B. The level of non-specific binding of HRP is very low (Table II), but when linked as much as 400 μg/mg lipid has been bound to a 25 nm liposome preparation. The reaction is quite specific and any omission such as failure to raise the pH to 9.5 or the use of liposomes without primary amino groups on their membranes results in negligible binding. When bound to the exterior of a liposome the enzyme activity of HRP is totally non-latent, no further activity being revealed by disruption of the liposomes with detergent. A reduction in specific activity of the enzyme is observed when it is periodic acid treated and when it is exposed to pH 9.5. However, no specific inactiva-

TABLE II. Binding of HRP to Liposomes

Treatment	μg HRP/mg lipid
PC/PE liposomes+non-activated HRP	Nil[a]
PC liposomes+activate enzyme	0.66[a]
PC/PE liposomes+activated enzyme	412[b]

In all cases liposomes and enzyme were subjected to pH 9.5 for 2 hr and then treated with lysine. Phospholipid was measured per phosphorus and HRP by [a] enzyme activity (35) or [b] nitrogen content (11).

TABLE III. Specific Activity of HRP following the
Treatments Required for Coupling

	Specific activity (U/mg)
Untreated enzyme	758
Activated enzyme	633
Liposome-bound enzyme	342
Reacted but unbound enzyme	347

Enzyme activity was measured by the ABTS-H_2O_2 assay (35) and protein by nitrogen content (11).

tion of the enzyme is observed due to covalent linking to liposomes, since bound and non-bound enzymes have similar specific activity following treatment (Table III).

The fact that HRP may be visualised in both the optical and electron microscope has allowed the nature of the interaction of HRP-coated liposomes with cells to be examined. HRP-coated 25 nm liposomes have been injected into the peritonea of CBA/Lac mice and the mice killed and peritoneal washes taken at between 1 min and 24 hr after injection. The wash is then fixed, diamino benzidine (DAB) stained, and embedded, and examined in the optical microscope and under electron microscope. This simple approach has allowed a simultaneous examination of the interaction of these liposomes with several different cell types. It appears that mast cells and erythrocytes interact very little with HRP-coated liposomes, although a population of cells that could be lymphocytes or monocytes acquire a surface coat of HRP in 15 min which is still apparent at 1 hr but not at 6 hr. It seems likely that these cells are fusing with the liposomes but the degree of resolution does not allow a morphological distinction between fusion and surface adhesion of 25 nm particles. Macrophages rapidly become heavily labelled with 25 nm HRP liposomes. At 1–60 min surface labelling is apparent and at 5–60 min the cells contain densely labelled superficial phagocytic vesicles. At 6 hr the phagocytic vesicles have fused with lysosomes to produce large densely labelled secondary lysosomes and the HRP is still visible in these lysosomes 24 hr after injection. A comparable dose of soluble HRP does not produce any significant labelling of cells.

Protein-coated liposomes may therefore provide a means of introducing protein antigens into cell membranes. Whilst morphological studies have not conclusively demonstrated fusion it is hoped that cell agglutinability or anti-peroxidase antibody-complement lysis may demonstrate that a novel antigen has been functionally inserted into the cell membrane.

REFERENCES

1. Allison, A. C. and Gregoriadis, G. Liposomes as immunological adjuvants. *Nature*, **252**, 252 (1974).
2. Almeida, J. D., Brand, C. M., Edwards, D. C., and Heath, T. D. Formation of virosomes from influenza subunits and liposomes. *Lancet*, **ii**, 899–901 (1975).
3. Bangham, A. D., DeGier, J., and Greville, G. D. Osmotic properties and water permeability of phospholipid liquid crystals. *Chem. Phys. Lipids*, **1**, 225–246 (1967).
4. Bangham, A. D., Hill, M. W., and Miller, N.G.A. Preparation and use of liposomes as models of biological membranes. *Methods Memb. Biol.*, **1**, 1–68 (1974).
5. Batzri, S. and Korn, E. D. Single bilayer liposomes prepared without sonication. *Biochim. Biophys. Acta*, **298**, 1015–1019 (1973).
6. Batzri, S. and Korn, E. D. Interaction of phospholipid vesicles with cell. Endocytosis and fusion as alternate mechanisms for the uptake of lipid-soluble and water-soluble molecules. *J. Cell Biol.*, **66**, 621–634 (1975).
7. Black, C. D., Watson, G. J., and Ward, R. J. The use of Pentostam liposomes in the chemotherapy of experimental leishmaniasis. *Trans. Roy. Soc. Trop. Med. Hyg.*, **71**, 550–552 (1977).
8. Boehringer Mannheim routine assay sheet.
9. Crane, R. K., Malathi, P., and Preiser, H. Reconstitution of specific Na^+-dependent D-glucose transport in liposomes by triton X-100-extracted proteins from purified brush border membranes of rabbit kidney cortex. *FEBS Lett.*, **67**, 214–216 (1976).
10. Deamer, D. and Bangham, A. D. Large volume liposomes by an ether vaporization method. *Biochim. Biophys. Acta*, **443**, 629–634 (1976).
11. Dingle, J. T., Gordon, J. L., Hazelman, B. L., Knight, C. G., Page Thomas, D. P., Phillips, N. C., Shaw, I. H., Fildes, F.J.T., Oliver, J. E., Jones, G., Turner, E. H., and Lowe, J. S. Novel treatment for joint inflammation. *Nature*, **271**, 372–373 (1978).
12. Enoch, H. G., Fleming, P. J., and Strittmatter, P. Cytochrome b_5 and cytochrome b_5 reductase-phospholipid vesicles. Intervesicle protein transfer and orientation factors in protein interactions. *J. Biol. Chem.*, **252**, 5656–5660 (1977).
13. Eytan, G. D., Matheson, M. J., and Racker, E. Incorporation of mitochondrial membrane proteins into liposomes containing acitic phospholipids. *J. Biol. Chem.*, **251**, 6831–6837 (1976).
14. Grant, C.W.M. and McConnell, H. M. Glycophorin in lipid bilayers. *Proc. Natl. Acad. Sci. U.S.*, **71**, 4653–4657 (1974).
15. Gregoriadis, G. and Ryman, B. E. Lysosomal localization of β-fructofuranosidase-containing liposomes injected into rats. Some implications in the treatment of genetic disorders. *Biochem. J.*, **129**, 123–133 (1972).
16. Gregoriadis, G. and Ryman, B. E. Fate of protein-containing liposomes injected into rats. An approach to the treatment storage diseases. *Eur. J. Biochem.*, **24**, 485–491 (1972).
17. Heath, T. D., Edwards, D. C., and Ryman, B. E. The adjuvant properties of liposomes. *Biochem. Soc. Trans.*, **4**, 129–133 (1976).
18. Pagano, R. E. and Huang, L. Interaction of phospholipid vesicles with cultured mammalian cells. II. Studies of mechanism. *J. Cell Biol.*, **67**, 49–60 (1975).
19. Jaenicke, L. A rapid micromethod for the determination of nitrogen and phosphate in biological material. *Anal. Biochem.*, **61**, 623–627 (1974).
20. Johnson, S. M. and Buttress, N. The osmotic insensitivity of sonicated liposomes and the density of phospholipid-cholesterol mixtures. *Biochim. Biophys. Acta*, **307**, 20–26 (1973).

21. Kawaoi, A. and Nakane, P. K. An improved method of conjugation of peroxidase with proteins. *Fed. Proc.*, **32**, 840 (Abs. 3508) (1973).

22. Kimelberg, H. K. and Papahadjopoulos, D. Interactions of basic proteins with phospholipid membranes. Binding and changes in the sodium permeability of phosphatidyl-serine vesicels. *J. Biol. Chem.*, **246**, 1142–1148 (1971).

23. Kinsky, S. C. and Nicolotti, R. A. Immunological properties of model membranes. *Annu. Rev. Biochem.*, **46**, 49–67 (1977).

24. Lee, A. G. Local anesthesia: The interaction between phospholipids and chlorpromazine, propranolol, and practolol. *Mol. Pharmacol.*, **13**, 474–487 (1977).

25. Martin, F. J. and MacDonald, R. C. Lipid vesicle-cell interactions. III. Introduction of a new antigenic determinant into erythrocyte membranes. *J. Cell Biol.*, **70**, 515–526 (1976).

26. McDougall, I. R., Dunnick, J. K., Goris, M. L., and Kriss, J. P. *In vivo* distribution of vesicles loaded with radiopharmaceuticals: A study of different routes of administration. *J. Nucl. Med.*, **16**, 488–491 (1975).

27. Pagano, R. E. and Takeichi, M. Adhesion of phospholipid vesicles to Chinese hamster fibroblasts. Role of cell surface proteins. *J. Cell Biol.*, **74**, 531–546 (1977).

28. Papahadjopoulos, D., Hui, S., Vail, W. J., and Poste, G. Studies on membrane fusion. I. Interactions of pure phospholipid membranes and the effect of myristic acid, lysole-cithin, proteins and dimethylsulfoxide. *Biochim. Biophys. Acta*, **448**, 245–264 (1976).

29. Papahadjopoulos, D., Vail, W. J., Jacobsen, K., and Poste, G. Cochleate lipid cylinders: Formation by fusion of unilamellar vesicles. *Biochim. Biophys. Acta*, **394**, 483–491 (1975).

30. Poste, G., Papahadjopoulos, D., and Vail, W. J. Lipid vesicles as carriers for introducing biologically active materials into cells. *Methods Cell Biol.*, **14**, 33–71 (1976).

31. Poste, G. and Parahadjopoulos, D. Lipid vesicles as carriers for introducing materials into cultured cells: Influence of vesicle lipid composition on mechanism(s) of vesicle incorporation into cells. *Proc. Natl. Acad. Sci. U.S.*, **73**, 1603–1607 (1976).

32. Redwood, W. R., Jansons, V. K., and Patel, B. C. Lectin-receptor interactions in liposomes. *Biochim. Biophys. Acta*, **406**, 347–361 (1975).

33. Ryrie, I. J. and Blackmore, P. F. Energy-linked activities in reconstituted yeast adenosine triphosphatase proteoliposome. Adenosine triphosphate formation coupled with electron flow between ascorbate and ferricyanide. *Arch. Biochem. Biophys.*, **176**, 127–135 (1976).

34. Sessa, G., Freer, J. H., Celacico, G., and Weissmann, G. Interaction of a lytic poly-peptide, melittin, with lipid membrane systems. *J. Biol. Chem.*, **244**, 3575–3582 (1969).

35. Slack, J. R., Anderton, B. H., and Day, W. A. A new method for making phospholipid vesicles and the partial reconstitution of the (Na^+, K^+)-activated ATPase. *Biochim. Biophys. Acta*, **323**, 547–559 (1973).

36. Sone, N., Yoshida, M., Hirata, H., Okamoto, H., and Kagawa, Y. Electrochemical potential of protons in vesicles reconstituted from purified, proton-translocating adenosine triphosphatase. *J. Memb. Biol.*, **30**, 121–134 (1976).

37. Thorpe, P. E., Ross, W.C.J., Cumber, A. J., Hinson, C. A., Edwards, D. C., and Davies, A.J.S. Toxicity of diphtheria toxin for lymphoblastoid cells is increased by conjugation to antilymphocytic globulin. *Nature*, **271**, 752–755 (1977).

38. Tyrrell, D. A., Heath, T. D., Colley, C. M., and Ryman, B. E. New aspects of liposomes. *Biochim. Biophys. Acta*, **457**, 259–302 (1976).

39. Uemura, K., Nicolotti, R. A., Six, H. R., and Kinsky, S. C. Antibody formation in response to liposomal model membranes sensitized with N-substituted phosphatidyl-ethanolamine derivatives. *Biochemistry*, **13**, 1572–1578 (1974).

40. Weinstein, J. N., Yoshikami, S., Henkart, P., Blumenthal, R., and Hagins, W. A. Lipo-

some-cell interaction: Transfer and intracellular release of a trapped fluorescent marker. *Science*, **195**, 489–492 (1977).

41. Weissmann, G., Bloomgarden, D., Kaplan, R., Cohen, C., Hoffstein, S., Collins, T., Gottlieb, A., and Nagle, D. A general method for the introduction of enzymes, by means of immunoglobulin-coated liposomes, into lysosomes of deficient cells. *Proc. Natl. Acad. Sci. U.S.*, **72**, 88–92 (1975).

42. Weissmann, G., Cohen, C., and Hoffstein, S. Introduction of enzymes, by means of liposomes, into non-phagocytic human cells *in vitro*. *Biochim. Biophys. Acta*, **498**, 375–385 (1977).

43. Weissmann, G., Sessa, G., and Weissmann, S. The action of steroids and Triton X-100 upon phospholipid/cholesterol structures. *Biochem. Pharmacol.*, **15**, 1537–1551 (1966).

APPLICATION OF XENOGENIZATION
TO HUMAN CANCER

MELANOMA SKIN TEST ANTIGENS OF IMPROVED SENSITIVITY PREPARED FROM VESICULAR STOMATITIS VIRUS-INFECTED TUMOR CELLS

Charles W. Boone, Faye C. Austin, Mitchell Gail, Meera Paranjpe, and Edmund Klein

*Cell Biology Section, Laboratory of Viral Carcinogenesis, National Cancer Institute, National Institutes of Health[*1] and Dermatology Department, Roswell Park Memorial Institute[*2]*

Crude membrane (CM) extracts from three different cultured human melanoma lines that were "virus-augmented" (infected with vesicular stomatitis virus (VSV) and subsequently inactivated by ultraviolet ray) produced positive skin tests in 41/58 (71%) of trials in 20 melanoma patients. Identical CM extracts from the same melanoma lines that had not been infected with VSV gave positive skin tests in 8/58 (14%) of trials in the same 20 melanoma patients. In 18 control patients with other cancers or normal volunteers the virus-augmented extracts were positive in only 3/58 (5%) of trials. The "virus-augmented" CM extracts thus exhibited markedly greater sensitivity without significant loss of specificity as compared to nonvirus augmented extracts when used as tumor-specific melanoma skin test antigens. The isotopic footpad assay in mice proved to be a useful animal model for delayed hypersensitivity reactions to tumor cells and tumor cell extracts. Using the model, the kinetics of the antitumor delayed hypersensitivity response during progressive tumor growth could be followed, and the phase of specific immune suppression due to large tumor burdon analyzed.

It has been established that a significant proportion of cancer patients give positive skin test reactions to crude membranes (CM) or soluble extracts from their own tumors, including acute leukemia (4, 12), melanoma (5, 6, 9), and cancer of the colon (8, 11, 14), breast (1, 14, 15), lung (10, 11), and cervix (18). Some of these reports show that CM from allogeneic tumor cells also give positive cancer specific skin test reactions. The great advantage of using allogeneic CM is that a single preparation can be used to skin test a large number of cancer patients. Char *et al.* (4) compared the skin test reactions induced by allogeneic and autologous CM in patients with acute lymphocytic leukemia and acute myeolcytic leukemia and demonstrated that allogeneic CM were as reactive as autologous CM and gave tests which correlated with the clinical state in the same way as autologous CM.

[*1] Bethesda, Maryland 20014, U.S.A.
[*2] Buffalo, New York 14263, U.S.A.

Virus Augmented Skin Test Antigens in Melanoma Patients

In the course of studies on the phenomenon of "virus augmentation" of tumor rejection antigens in mice, we found that the delayed hypersensitivity reaction to tumor cell CM inoculated into the footpad of tumor-immune mice appeared to be substantially augmented of the CM were prepared from cells that had first been infected with influenza virus (2). We therefore turned to the evaluation of the use of virus-augmented allogeneic tumor cell CM as cancer specific skin test antigens in humans. We chose melanoma patients because the existence of a tumor tissue specific antigen has been documented in this disease (6). Since the preparation of CM from fresh tumors always entails the problem of variable antigenic potency resulting from the unknown proportion of tumor cells to stromal cells, we used three different established tissue culture lines of human melanoma as the starting material. The established melanoma lines also offered the advantage of reproducibly supporting a high titer of virus infection compared to primary explants of enzyme-disaggregated tumor tissue. We chose vesicular stomatitis virus (VSV) as the augmenting virus because of its relatively low pathogenicity in humans (mild flu-like syndrome) (7). CM from cultured melanoma cells infected with VSV and subsequently inactivated with ultraviolet ray did indeed give markedly heightened skin test reactivity in humans with little significant loss of speci-

TABLE I. Skin Test Response (mm of Induration at 48 hr) to Membrane Extracts from Cultured Melanoma Lines (Melanoma Patients)

Name	Sex	Age (year)	Recall antigen positive	Time disease free (months)	Melanoma		Melanoma		Melanoma	
					C101	V101	C375	V375	C875	V875
BuFr	M	55	P, V	6	5	20	10	20	5	20
BrJo	F	24	M	2	—[a]	2	—	—	—	—
DoFr	M	70	P, M, V, C	12	—	25	—	25	—	—
GaMa	F	51	M, V	0	5	15	8	20	10	8
GaWi	M	51	P, M, V, C	22	15	15	15	2	—	8
HoGa	M	42	M, V, T	13	—	10	—	10	—	18
HyWi	M	49	M, T	0	5	17	—	5	—	17
LeRu	M	29	P, M, V, C	13	—	11	—	—	ND	ND
LyRo	M	50	M, C	11	—	5	—	—	—	—
MeAn	F	72	P	0	—	10	—	—	ND	ND
MoNo	F	41	P, M, V	24	—	10	—	14	—	24
MoRi	M	46	P, M	4	2	10	5	—	—	10
NaAl	M	64	P, M, V	3	3	25	8	10	10	10
NeDo	M	60	P	0	—	15	—	15	5	10
RaDo	F	70	V, T	37	—	5	—	—	—	—
ReJa	M	55	V	33	—	8	—	10	—	10
RoJo	M	54	P, M, V, C	55	8	8	—	8	4	—
SiLe	M	63	P, M, V, C	10	—	45	5	20	—	15
SoJo	M	52	M, V, C	0	5	25	—	15	—	10
ViWi	M	34	P, V, C	13	—	8	—	—	—	10
					2/20	17/20	4/20	11/20	2/18	13/18

Proportion with positive skin tests (> 6 mm induration).

[a] Dashes indicate no visible skin test response.

ND, not done; M, male; F, female; P, PPD; V, Varidase; M, mumps; C, candida.

TABLE II. Skin Test Response (mm of Induration at 48 hr) to Membrane Extracts from Cultured Melanoma Lines (Patients with other Cancers and Normal Volunteers)

Name	Sex	Age (year)	Recall antigens positive	Time disease free (months)	Melanoma		Melanoma		Melanoma	
					C101	V101	C375	V375	C875	V875
Patients with other cancers										
AbMa	F	69	P, M, C	0	—a	—	—	5	—	—
AmCh	M	57	P, M, V	12	2	9	2	4	ND	ND
BiJa	M	66	P, M, C	0	—	—	—	—	—	5
DaEd	M	64	ND	0	—	—	—	—	—	—
DiVi	M	58	P	0	—	5	—	—	—	2
HuOt	M	65	P, C	0	—	2	—	2	—	4
KiWi	F	57	P, M, V, C	12	—	3	—	4	—	4
LiJo	M	73	M, V	0	—	2	—	—	—	—
PeCa	M	49	ND	0	—	—	—	—	—	—
ShMa	F	53	P	0	—	—	—	—	—	—
VaJa	M	75	M, V	0	—	2	—	—	—	—
YaMa	M	40	ND	0	—	5	—	5	—	5
Normal Volunteers										
CaCh	F	20	M, V, C	Vol	—	4	—	2	—	2
DoPh	F	33	M, V, C	Vol	—	2	—	—	—	17
FrGe	F	49	M, V	Vol	—	2	—	—	—	—
HeKa	F	26	V, C	Vol	—	3	—	—	—	2
PeGa	F	40	M, V, C	Vol	2	10	—	2	—	—
UzDe	F	25	V, C	Vol	—	2	—	—	—	—
					0/18	2/18		0/18	0/17	1/17

Proportion with positive skin tests ($> 6\,mm$ induration).
a Dashes indicate no visible skin test response visible.

ficity. The method for preparing the VSV-augmented melanoma skin test antigens has been recently published (3). Tables I and II give 48-hr induration responses for the 20 melanoma patients and for 18 control patients. It is easy to see that the virus-augmented skin test antigens gave reactions of markedly improved sensitivity without loss of specificity.

Mechanisms for Virus Augmentation of Skin Test Antigens

Possible mechanisms for the virus augmentation of skin test antigen reactivity can be broadly categorized into three groups. 1. *Improved antigen presentation.* Virus infection could bring about chemical stabilization of antigens in the tumor cell membrane or it could alter membrane conformation to give greater exposure of antigens to the immune system. 2. *Helper antigen effect.* This mechanism, discussed at length in another presentation of this workshop, does not appear too likely in this case because 48 hr may be too short a time to expect that a primary response to the virus would be intense enough to help the secondary response to the tumor antigen. 3. *Acute inflammatory helper effect.* The small but statistically significant inflammatory response to the virus-infected melanoma CM in control subjects suggests that cellular or soluble mediators generated during a mild acute inflammatory response to the virus might be sufficient to markedly intensify the secondary immune response to tumor antigen. This mechanism seems to be the easiest to accept as a possibility at this time.

We are now proceeding to test similarly prepared virus-augmented skin test antigens from cultured cell lines of human breast cancer and lung cancer. Studies on purified preparations derived from the virus-augmented melanoma CM are also in progress.

Utility of the Isotopic Footpad Assay in Mice as a Model for Studying Anti-tumor Delayed Hypersensitivity Reactions

Some years ago we developed a radioisotopic footpad assay in mice that has proven most useful in studying anti-tumor delayed hypersensitivity responses (*13*). At the time a tumor-immune animal is inoculated in the footpad with intact tumor cells or tumor cell extracts, ^{125}I-labeled mouse albumin is inoculated intraperitoneally. The labeled albumin enters the blood stream and remains there except at the site of inflammation in the footpad, where it leaks into the intracellular space because of the increased capillary permeability associated with the inflammatory reaction. Twenty-four hours after inoculation, the test foot and contralateral normal foot are cut off and counted in a γ-spectrometer. The results are recorded as the foot-count ratio, which is the counts-per-minute from the test foot divided by the counts-per-minute from the control foot. The isotopic footpad reaction is adoptively transferrable with immune spleen cells. For example, if the spleen cells from a tumor-immune mouse (*e.g.*, immunized with X-ray inactivated tumor cells) are mixed with intact tumor cells and inoculated into the footpad of a normal mouse, a positive foot-count ratio is produced (*16*). Interestingly, adoptive transfer of the footpad reaction can occur across allogeneic or even xenogeneic barriers. For example, spleen cells from a rat made immune to a syngeneic lymphoma, designated rat Gross lymphoma (FGT), when mixed with the FGT cells

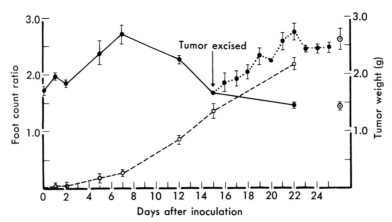

FIG. 1. Kinetics of cellular immunity in BALB/c mice injected with E4 tumors and subsequently challenged with E4 tumor cells.

●——● Average foot-count ratio in tumor-bearing mice; ●- - -● average foot-count ratio in tumor excised mice; ○- - -○ average tumor weight; ⊙ average foot-count ratio in E4 tumor immune mice; ⊗ average foot-count ratio in normal mice.

TABLE III. Reactivity of Spleen Cells from Unresponsive E4 Tumor-bearing
Mice after Local Adaptive Transfer to Normal Host

Group	Status of mice donating spleen cells	Status of recipient mice	Contents of challenge dose	Foot-count ratio	SE
1	—	E4 tumor immune	1×10^6 E4 tumor cells	2.23	±0.27
2	—	E4 tumor bearing	1×10^6 E4 tumor cells	1.59	±0.08
3	—	Normal	1×10^6 E4 tumor cells	1.40	±0.06
4	E4 tumor immune (same as group 1)	Normal	25×10^6 spleen cells $+1 \times 10^6$ E4 tumor cells	2.20[a]	±0.17
5	E4 tumor bearing (same as group 2)	Normal	25×10^6 spleen cells $+1 \times 10^6$ E4 tumor cells	2.61[a]	±0.19
6	Normal mice	Normal	25×10^6 spleen cells $+1 \times 10^6$ E4 tumor cells	1.63	±0.07

[a] Differences in groups 4 and 5 were not significant (by Student's t-test).

and inoculated into the footpad of a mouse, gave a positive footpad reaction (17).
Figure 1 is a graph of the kinetics of the isotopic footpad response at various intervals
during the growth of an SV40 induced transplantable tumor in BALB/c mice (E4
tumor). Note that as the tumor grows, the foot-count ratio rises for a time, but then
falls to normal levels as the tumor enlarges beyond a certain size. This decrease in
delayed hypersensitivity reactivity is specific for the tumor antigen (13). Most interestingly, when spleen cells from mice bearing large tumors and showing complete
suppression of footpad delayed hypersensitivity reactivity to the tumor cells were
removed, mixed with tumor cells of the same type as those producing the immune suppression, and inoculated into the footpads of normal mice, there was no suppression
of the footpad delayed hypersensitivity response compared to the reaction when
spleen cells from tumor-immune mice were used. Table III presents data illustrating
this effect (13). Note that there was no detectable suppressor cell activity. On the
contrary, even though the tumor-bearing animal from whom the spleen cells were
removed gave no footpad delayed hypersensitivity reaction to tumor cells due to
specific immune suppression produced by excess tumor burden, the adoptive transferred spleen cells mixed with tumor cells gave as strong a foot-count ratio in the normal
mice as did spleen cells from tumorimmune mice.

REFERENCES

1. Alford, C., Hollinshead, A. C., and Herberman, R. B. Delayed cutaneous hypersensitivity
   reactions to extracts of malignant and normal human breast cells. *Am. Surg.*, **178**, 20–24
   (1972).
2. Boone, C. W., Paranjpe, M., Orme, T., and Gillette, R. Virus augmented tumor transplantation antigens. Evidence for a helper antigen mechanism. *Int. J. Cancer*, **13**, 543–
   551 (1974).
3. Boone, C. W., Austin, F. C., Gail, M., Case, R., and Klein, E. Melanoma skin test
   antigens of improved sensitivity prepared from vesicular stomatitis virus-infected tumor
   cells. *Cancer*, **41**, 1781–1787 (1978).
4. Char, D. H., Lepourhiet, A., Leventhal, B. G., and Herberman, R. B. Cutaneous delayed hypersensitivity responses to tumor-associated and other antigens in acute leukemia. *Int. J. Cancer.*, **12**, 409–419 (1973).

5. Char, D. H., Hollinshead, A., Cogan, D. G., Ballentine, E. J., Hogan, M. J., and Herberman, R. B. Cutaneous delayed hypersensitivity reactions to soluble melanoma antigen in patients with ocular malignant melanoma. *N. Engl. J. Med.*, **291**, 274–277 (1974).

6. Fass, L., Herberman, R. B., Ziegler, J. L., and Kiryabuire, J.W.M. Cutaneous hypersensitivity reactions to autologous extracts of malignant melanoma cells. *Lancet*, **i**, 116–118 (1970).

7. Fields, B. N. and Hawkins, K. Human infection with the virus of vesicular stomatitis during an epizootic. *N. Engl. J. Med.*, **277**, 989–994 (1967).

8. Hollinshead, A. C., McWright, C. G., Alford, T. C., and Glew D. H. Separation of skin reactive intestinal cancer antigen from the carcinoembryonic antigen of Gold. *Science* **177**, 887–889 (1972).

9. Hollinshead, A. C., Herberman, R. B., Jaffurs, W. J., Alpent, L. K., Manton, J. P., and Harris, J. E. Soluble membrane antigens of human malignant melanoma cells. *Cancer*, **34**, 1235–1243 (1974).

10. Hollinshead, A. C., Stewart, T.H.M., and Herberman, R. B. Delayed hypersensitivity reactions to soluble membrane antigens of human malignant lung cells. *J. Natl. Cancer Inst.*, **52**, 327–338 (1974).

11. Hughes, L. E. and Lytton, B. Antigenic properties of human tumours: Delayed cutaneous hypersensitivity reactions. *Br. Med. J.*, **1**, 209–212 (1964).

12. Oren, M. E. and Herberman, R. E. Delayed cutaneous hypersensitivity reactions to membrane extracts of human tumour cells. *Clin. Exp. Immunol.*, **9**, 45–56, 1971.

13. Paranjpe, M. and Boone, C. W. Kinetics of the anti-tumor delayed hypersensitivity response in mice with progressively growing tumors: Stimulation followed by specific suppression. *Int. J. Cancer*, **13**, 179–186 (1974).

14. Stewart, T.H.M. The presence of delayed hypersensitivity reactions in patients toward cellular extracts of their malignant tumors. *Cancer*, **23**, 1368–1379 (1969).

15. Stewart, T.H.M. and Orizaga, M. The presence of delayed hypersensitivity reactions in patients toward cellular extracts of their malignant tumors. *Cancer*, **28**, 1472–1478, 1971.

16. Takeichi, N. and Boone, C. W. Local adoptive transfer of the anti-tumor cellular immune response in syngeneic and allogeneic mice studied with a rapid radioisotopic footpad assay. *J. Natl. Cancer Inst.*, **55**, 183–187 (1975).

17. Takeichi, N. and Boone, C. W. Local adoptive transfer of anti-tumor cellular immunity to xenogeneic animals studied with a radioisotopic footpad assay. *J. Natl. Cancer Inst.*, **57**, 131–134 (1976).

18. Wells, S. A., Jr., Burdick, J. S., Christiansen, C., Ketcham, A. S., and Adkins, P. C. Demonstration of tumor-associated delayed cutaneous hypersensitivity reactions in patients with lung cancer and in patients with carcinoma of the cervix. *Natl. Cancer Inst. Monogr.*, **37**, 197–203 (1973).

GANN Monograph on Cancer Research 23, 1979

VACCINIA VIRUS-AUGMENTED TUMOR VACCINES AS A NEW FORM OF IMMUNOTHERAPY

Marc K. Wallack

Section of Surgical Oncology, Barnes Hospital and Department of Surgery, Washington University School of Medicine*

A live vaccinia virus-augmented autochthonous tumor cell vaccine (vaccinia oncolysate) is used as a specific active immune mechanism stimulator in a syngeneic SV40 transformed mouse tumor system and against certain advanced human cancers. BALB/c mice pretreated with subcutaneous injections of vaccinia oncolysates prior to challenge with tumor cells failed to develop tumors at the injection sites. Cross immunization and immunotherapy experiments were also performed. Phase I human studies have shown that 29 patients with metastatic carcinoma who reacted to one or more common recall antigen skin tests have been treated with the vaccinia oncolysate intradermally in the thighs and upper arms until recurrence or exhaustion of the vaccine supply. The results of these trials show the vaccine to be safe, non-toxic, and potentially effective.

The fact that viruses are restricted to the cells in which they can replicate suggested the possibility of their use in the destruction of cancer cells. Since 1912, when the Italian physician, DePace, observed regression of cervical carcinoma in patients undergoing Pasteur's treatment for rabies, many viruses have been shown to exert an anti-neoplastic effect in either man or animals. All the reports included cases in which there had been at least some remission, effect, or cure in the tumors being treated (*21*). The striking oncolytic power of some viruses against transplantable mouse tumors (*15*) was unfortunately cytotoxic systemically for the tumor-bearing animal. The finding of strains of mice genetically unsusceptible to a particular virus, therefore, provided an opportunity to study viral oncolysis without killing the host. Koprowski *et al.* (*9*) found that West Nile virus could destroy ascites tumor in PRI mice without harm to the mice which were then able to resist rechallenge with the same tumor. This was the first suggestion that viral invasion of a tumor might lead to tumor immunity.

Similar and more extensive observations were made by Lindenmann (*10*), who performed a detailed immunological study in mice and established the value of a viral oncolysate, in contrast to a lysate prepared by other means. Lindenmann (*11*) used influenza A virus to lyse Erhlich ascites cells in the peritoneal cavities of A_2G mice and noted that mice which recovered from the influenza oncolysis had developed post-oncolytic immunity and resisted rechallenge with the same tumor (*10, 11*). Lindenmann (*12*) and Boone (*2*) showed that the product of the influenza virus-tumor cell interaction (the influenza oncolysate) was responsible for the post-viral oncolytic immunity.

---

* St. Louis, Missouri 63110, U.S.A.

Human application of this concept was difficult because most oncolytic viruses were harmful to man. We tested *in vitro* the vaccine strengths of six live viral vaccines (measles, mumps, smallpox, rubella, yellow fever, and rabies) against four human tumor lines (ovary, lung, melanoma, and colon) and noted that only the smallpox vaccine (vaccinia) duplicated the lytic action of the influenza virus on the Erhlich ascites cells. Since the safety of both lysed tumor cell vaccines (*6*) and the vaccinia vaccine has been established in both animals and man, an oncolysate prepared from vaccinia virus-lysed augmented tumor cells can logically be assumed to be benign.

This paper reports our results in using the live vaccinia virus-augmented tumor cell vaccine (vaccinia oncolysate) as a specific, active, immune stimulator in animals and as an immunotherapeutic agent in Phase I human trials.

Procedures for Animal Experiments

1) Animals

All experiments were conducted in BALB/c male mice, 8–10 weeks old at the time of implantation of the tumor isografts. Each treatment and control group consisted of 6–8 mice, randomly distributed.

2) Tumor cells

An SV 40-transformed peritoneal macrophage tumor from BALB/c male mice, designated GMMSV1, was used in all experiments. Tumor cells in doses ranging from 1×10^3 to 1×10^6 cells were injected subcutaneously in the left thigh of the mice.

3) Virus

For animal studies, The Wistar Institute's vaccinia virus is harvested from embryonic mouse fibroblasts (EMF) cells. Vaccine titers were determined on monolayers of EMF in Eagle's minimal essential medium (MEM), containing 3% fetal bovine serum (FBS). The vaccinia titer was approximately 1×10^7 $TCID_{50}$/ml.

4) Vaccine preparation

The vaccinia oncolysate was prepared by infecting monolayers of 1×10^6 $GMMSV_1$ tumor cells with 1 ml of live vaccinia virus (1×10^7 $TCID_{50}$/ml) and incubating for 96 hr. The oncolysate was then frozen and thawed three times and harvested by centrifugation of the virus-augmented cellular debris at 20,000 rpm for 45 min at 0°. The pellet was then resuspended in 10 ml of Eagle's MEM with FBS and further cell destruction accomplished by using a dounce homogenizer. This lysate was again centrifuged at 20,000 rpm and suspended in Eagle's MEM without FBS so as to effect a concentration of 1×10^6 vaccinia virus-augmented tumor cells/ml. This final concentration was the vaccinia oncolysate used in all the animal experiments. The vaccinia oncolysate was always injected subcutaneously into the right thigh. The quantity and number of treatments are described in the text and figures.

Patients and Procedures for Clinical Trials

The following cancer patients were selected for treatment with the vaccinia oncolysate in the Phase I study: 1) Cancer patients who had tumor resection and showed tumor metastases to local and/or regional lymph nodes; 2) patients submitted to radiation therapy for localized, unresectable disease; 3) patients with disseminated disease treated by chemotherapy but considered terminal; and 4) patients with disease so far advanced that they were deemed untreatable by surgery, chemotherapy, or radiotherapy. All patients involved in these therapeutic trials gave informed consent by signing authorization for the use of investigational therapy and showed a delayed hypersensitivity response to one or more of the common recall antigen skin tests used to gauge immunocompetence. An essential requirement was that cells from the tumor could be surgically obtained and grown in tissue cultures, either in suspension or monolayer.

1) Virus

The Wistar Institute's vaccinia virus is harvested from WI 38 cells. Vaccine titers were determined on monolayers of WI 38 cells in Eagle's MEM, containing 3% human serum. The vaccinia titer was approximately 1×10^7 $TCID_{50}$/ml.

2) Vaccine preparation

Tumor tissue removed from the patient in the operating room was processed as follows: 1) Those portions of the tumor which were not necrotic, fatty or hemorrhagic were finely minced by scalpels and placed in Eagle's MEM with 20% FBS plus penicillin and gentamicin; 2) the minced tissue was placed in an Erhlenmeyer flask with 30 ml of 0.25% trypsin, 1% versene solution, and stirred with a magnetic bar to effect a suspension of single cells; 3) approximately 1×10^7 $TCID_{50}$/ml of vaccinia virus was used to infect 1×10^6 ml of tumor cells in suspension; 4) the virus-tumor cell suspension was incubated for 96 hr at $37°$ in Spinner's media with 10% human serum while both tumor cell lysis and virus titer were monitored; 5) the live vaccinia virus-augmented tumor cell suspension was spun at 20,000 rpm for 60 min at $0°$, the supernatant was removed, and the pellet homogenized and suspended in enough Eagle's MEM to effect a concentration of 1×10^6 live vaccinia virus-augmented tumor cells/ml. These 1-ml aliquots were frozen at $-70°$ for use later.

3) Vaccine administration

The vaccinia oncolysate vaccine was injected in 1 ml doses intradermally into the anterior thigh, upper arm, and anterior thorax to stimulate regional lymph nodes. Oncolysate injections were given every 2 weeks for 3 months. Thereafter, 1 ml booster doses were given every month until recurrence or exhaustion of vaccine supply.

4) Patient monitoring

The following laboratory studies were done every 4 weeks during the course of immunotherapy:

1) complete blood count (CBC)
2) blood urea nitrogen (BUN)
3) glucose
4) serum glutamic pyruvic transaminase (SGPT)
5) serum glutamic oxalo-acetic transaminase (SGOT)
6) lactate dehydrogenase (LDH)
7) bilirubin
8) alkaline phosphatase
9) quantitative immunoglobulins
10) phytohemagglutinin (PHA)-induced blastogenesis (17)

11)   vaccinia antibody titer (22)
12)   anergy panel and DNCB (3)

5)   *Protocol design*

   This Phase I study had the following end points; 1) to establish the safety of the vaccine, 2) to establish the toxicity patterns and determine whether the toxicity was predictable and tolerable, and 3) to determine evidence of anti-tumor activity (4).

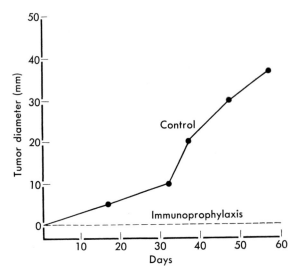

Fɪɢ. 1.   Immunization of GMMSVI$_2$ tumor with vaccinia oncolysate
Tumor burden, 1×10^3 cells; oncolysate given, day $-17, -12, -7, -3, 0$.

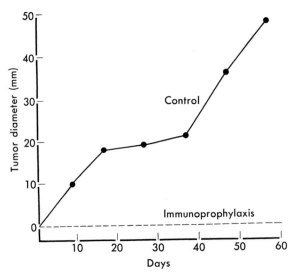

Fɪɢ. 2.   Immunization of GMMSVI$_2$ tumor with vaccinia oncolysate
Tumor burden, 1×10^4 cells; oncolysate given, day $-17, -12, -7, -3, 0$.

Tumor Growth in Mice Prevaccinated with Vaccine Oncolysate

Groups of 6–8 mice were injected subcutaneously into the right thigh with 0.5 ml of vaccinia oncolysate on day -17, -12, -7, -3, 0, and then received either 1×10^3 or 1×10^5 tumor cells subcutaneously into the left thigh on day 0. The mice were followed for 60 days.

Mice, prevaccinated with the vaccinia oncolysate before receiving the tumor cell challenge, failed to develop tumors at the injection site as compared to controls (see Figs. 1, 2, and 3).

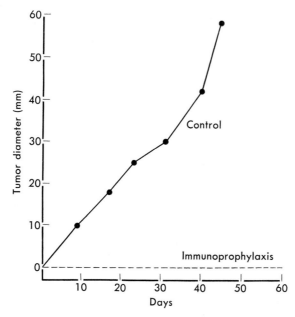

FIG. 3. Immunization of GMMSVI$_2$ Tumor with vaccinia oncolysate
Tumor burden, 1×10^5 cells; oncolysate given, day -17, -12, -7, -3, 0.

Groups of 8 mice which were preimmunized with 0.3 ml of vaccinia virus (diluted with phosphate buffered saline (PBS) to 1×10^5 TCID$_{50}$/ml) subcutaneously into the right thigh one week before pretreatment with the vaccinia oncolysates also failed to develop tumors in the left thigh injection site as compared to controls which received only the vaccinia virus and no oncolysate (Fig. 4).

Cross immunization studies performed with groups of 10 BALB/c male mice showed the GMMSV$_1$ oncolysates to provide specific, immunoprophylactic tumor protection only to the BALB/c mice receiving GMMSV$_1$ oncolysates as compared to groups of 10 BALB/c mice receiving either another BALB/c tumor oncolysate (BALB non-producer or BNP) or lysed GMMSV$_1$ tumor cells (Fig. 5). The lysed tumor cells alone were moderately immunogenic at lower challenge doses. However, when the tumor burden was increased to 1×10^6 cells the lysed cell vaccine failed.

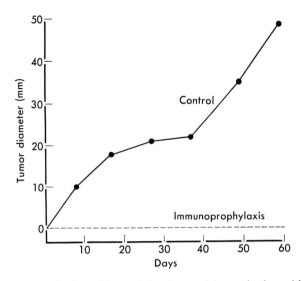

FIG. 4. Preimmunization with vaccinia virus and immunization with vaccinia oncolysate

Tumor burden, 1×10^4 cells; oncolysate given, day -17, -12, -7, -3, 0.

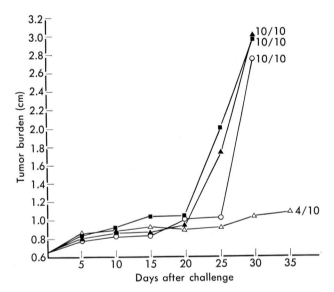

FIG. 5. Cross immunization of $GMMSVI_2$ tumors with vaccinia oncolysates

Tumor burden, 1×10^6 cells; oncolysate given, day -17, -12, -7, -3, 0.

○ BNP VT;   △ $GMMSVI_2$ VT;   ▲ lysed $GMMSVI_2$;   ■ saline.

Clinical Aspects of Effects of Vaccine Oncolysate

A total of 29 tumor patients have received the vaccinia oncolysate immunotherapy in this Phase I trial. These patients represent 10 cases of melanoma, 9 cases of colon carcinoma, 2 cases of gastric carcinoma, 1 case of cervical carcinoma, 1 case of lung

TABLE I. Side Effects of Vaccinia Oncolysates

Side effects	% of patents intradermal
Fever	20
Chills	7
Shaking	2
Malaise	7
Headache	5
Nausea	7
Vomiting	0
Increased blood pressure	0
Decreased blood pressure	0
Diarrhea	0
Pain at site of injection	45
Inflammation at site of injection	65

carcinoma, 1 case of hepatoma, 1 case of fibrosarcoma, 1 case of ovarian carcinoma, 1 case of renal carcinoma, 1 case of breast carcinoma, and 1 case of thyroid carcinoma.

Side effects of the immunotherapy were minimal except for pain and inflammation at the injection sites which seemed to correlate with the host's response to the tumor burden (Table I).

Patient response to the vaccinia oncolysate immunotherapy was as follows: 1) 0/29 patients had generalized vaccinia, allergy, anaphylaxis, and tumor growth at injection site; 2) 20/29 patients have died; 3) 9/29 patients died in the early part of the study; 4) 15/29 patients had delayed hypersensitivity reactions at vaccine injection sites; 5) 9/15 patients who had delayed hypersensitivity reactions at the vaccine injection sites, remain alive with control of tumor growth; and 6) 9/9 patients with control of tumor growth had elevated vaccinia antibody titers—a measure of non-specific immunostimulation.

The 9 patients who responded to the vaccine are summarized in Table II.

TABLE II. Nine Patients Surviving after Treatment with Vaccinia Oncolysates

Name	Age/Sex	Tumor	Clinical condition	Previous therapy	No. of injection	Results	Further clinical course in months
R.S.	46 M	Thyroid (undiff.)	Liver 8 neck	R	14	Regression	26
V.V.	47 M	Hypernephroma	Nodes L_1	O	20	Stable	22
E.O.	51 M	Melanoma	Level V	C	8	Stable	19
J.N.	53 M	Colon	Liver+ Duke's C	O	15	Stable	19
E.K.	61 F	Melanoma	Axillae+liver	O	14	Regression	19
E.N.	68 F	Colon	Duke's C	O	8	Stable	17
V.S.	59 F	Breast	14⊕Nodes	O	13	Stable	17
W.M.	71 M	Colon	Duke's C+ liver	O	16	Stable	17
M.M.	53 M	Melanoma	Level IV Stage II	O	11	Stable	10

R, radiotherapy; C, chemotherapy.

DISCUSSION

The phenomenon of viral oncolysis or the lysis of tumor cells by viruses with its resultant post-viral oncolytic immunity has been a subject of cancer research for approximately 30 years. Following initial observations of Koprowski et al. (9), Lindenmann (10) began a series of experiments to explore the phenomenon. He used a mouse-adapted strain of neurotropic influenza A virus against Erhlich ascites tumor growing in A_2G mice (10). The tumor became necrotic and disappeared, and survivors were resistant to rechallenge (11). Since post-oncolytic immunity was logically thought to be the result of neoantigens arising from the virus-tumor interaction, a viral oncolysate was prepared from the Erhlich ascites tumor cells exposed to influenza virus for 48–72 hr; the tumor homogenate was collected and four injections of this vaccine were given interperitonealy into A_2G mice at weekly intervals, enabling the majority of mice to resist challenge with both 1,000 and 100,000 tumor cells (13). This was evidence that the influenza oncolysate was a potent immunogen. Moreover, the fact that previous vaccination of mice against the influenza virus failed to hamper their ability to be immunized with an oncolysate in conjunction with the fact that the progress of active oncolysis could be prevented by the induction of anti-viral immunity, clearly shows that the immunogen must have been present in the lysing and that no active viral replication in the new host was required (13). Therefore, postviral oncolytic immunity could be explained as a viral adjuvant effect induced by the interaction of virus-specific and host-cell specific determinants, a situation very much like that in carrier-hapten systems (13) or helper antigen systems (14). Moreover, Webb (21) stated that in the treatment of cancer, infection with viruses may have a beneficial effect. One of the possible mechanisms of action include immunological cytolysis by both cell-mediated and humoral responses to viruses which incorporate cell membrane into their code and confer virus antigen determinants on the surface of the infected tumor cells. Lastly, Kobayashi (8) has revealed that transplantable tumors as well as primary tumors in rats failed to grow in susceptible rats after artifically infecting the tumors with Friend leukemia virus. It was proposed that the rat tumor cells infected with Friend virus acquired a new virus-induced specific transplantation antigen on the cell membrane which then would be recognized as foreign by the host and rejected. This phenomenon was called xenogenization of tumors.

Several investigators have decided to test the concept of post-viral oncolytic immunity in humans by using a live virus-augmented tumor cell vaccine. Sinkovics (20) treated metastatic soft tissue sarcomas with a PR8 influenza-augmented sarcoma oncolysate. Of 14 patients with metastatic sarcomas receiving comparable conventional modalities of treatment and immunotherapy with BCG and viral oncolysates, six had complete remission, six had partial remission, or are in stable disease status, and two have had disease progression. Green (7) reported that 12 patients, 11–20 years of age with recurrent osteosarcoma, were immunized with either autologous or allogeneic tumor cells infected with influenza virus. In all 12 cases, toxicity was negligible and immunizations boosted antibody titers to both tumor cell and influenza virus antigens. Although no clear-cut relationship or prognosis could be demonstrated, 3 of 6 patients with minimal disease have survived for 7–8 months after the first vaccination, without progression of the disease. Murray (16) reported that a melanoma cell oncolysate, prepared with Newcastle disease virus, was administered as an immunostimulant to 13 patients with metastatic melanoma. The oncolysate was well tolerated. Six treated patients evidenced a decrease in the size of skin nodules or diseased lymph nodes; visceral lesions were not favorably influenced. Finally, in a randomized prospective trial, Sauter (19) used influenza oncolysates in the treatment of acute myelogenous leukemia with poor results.

Instead of using influenza virus or Newcastle disease virus to augment tumor cells in the oncolysate, a live viral vaccine-augmented tumor cell oncolysate was used as a specific, active immunotherapeutic agent. The vaccine strength of six live viral vaccines (measles, mumps, vaccinia, rubella, yellow fever, and rabies) was tested *in vitro* against four human tumor lines and it was found that only vaccinia vaccine duplicated the lytic action of the influenza virus on Erhlich ascites cells. Vaccinia virus is known to inhibit the growth of malignant tumors directly because of its specific oncolytic activity (18). Also, the virus has been shown to act indirectly as an immunological adjuvant by increasing the cellular immune reaction against heterologous cell antigens in guinea pigs. This adjuvant effect seems to be due to a close association between host cell antigen and antigens produced by the virus (1). Finally, Chang and Metz (5) have reported that vaccinia virus entered HeLa cells by a process of direct fusion between the virus envelope and the plasma membrane of the cell. After fusion, components of the virus envelope become rapidly dispersed in the plasma membrane producing the juxtaposition of a strong viral antigen with a weak tumor specific transplantation antigen.

CONCLUSION

The vaccinia oncolysate was first tested in an SV 40 transformed BALB/c male mice peritoneal macrophage tumor system (GMMSV$_1$). These immunoprophylaxis experiments confirmed both the safety and potential efficacy of the vaccine in the animal model. There were no vaccine-associated mouse deaths; furthermore, tumors failed to grow in animals pretreated with the vaccinia oncolysate. Cross immunization studies showed that the GMMSV$_1$ oncolysate was specific for the GMMSV$_1$ tumor system.

Preliminary immunotherapy experiments using the same mouse tumor model produced moderate success. Because of the encouraging results in the mouse experiments, the vaccine was evaluated as an immunotherapeutic agent in Phase I trials in human cancer. All patients involved in this study had advanced metastatic disease, but showed delayed hypersensitivity reactions to one or more of the common recall antigen skin tests and had tumors that could be safely incised in the operating room. The Phase I trials have concluded. These trials have shown that the vaccine is safe (0/29 patients with untoward responses), non-toxic, and may even be effective in stimulating the patient's tumor immune response (9/29 patients with evidence of control of tumor growth). The heterogeneity of this early tumor group only reflects the type of patient available to the study during the early phase of testing vaccine safety. Obviously, positive responses to the vaccine in certain of these patients were interesting but difficult to evaluate. With completion of the Phase I trials, randomized prospective trials have begun in a more homogeneous tumor group so as to make analysis easier.

Acknowledgment
This work was supported by Cancer Research Institute Inc. and Schering Corporation.

REFERENCES

1. Bandlaw, G. and Koszinowski, V. Increased cellular immunity against host cell antigens induced by vaccinia virus. *Arch. Gesamte Virusforsch.*, **45**, 122–127 (1974).
2. Boone, C. and Blackman, K. Augmented immunogenicity of tumor cell homogenates infected with influenza virus. *Cancer Res.*, **32**, 1018–1022 (1972).
3. Brown, R. S., Haynes, H. A., Foley, H. T., Godwin, H. A., Berard, C. W., and Carbone, P. P. Hodgkin's disease: Immunologic clinical and histologic features of fifty untreated patients. *Ann. Intern. Med.*, **67**, 291–302 (1967).
4. Carter, S. K. Study design principles for the clinical evaluation of new drugs as developed by the chemotherapy program of the National Cancer Institute. *In* "The Design of Clinical Trials in Cancer Therapy," ed. M. Staguet, p. 242 (1972). Editions Scientifigues Europeanes, Brussels.
5. Chang, A. and Metz, D. H. Further investigation on the mode of entry of vaccinia virus into cells. *J. Gen. Virol.*, **32**, 275–282 (1976).
6. Currie, G. A. Effect of active immunization with irradiated tumor cells on specific serum inhibitors of cell-mediate immunity in patients with disseminated cancer. *Br. J. Cancer*, **28**, 25–35 (1973).
7. Green, A., Pratt, C., Webster, R., and Smith, K. Immunotherapy of osteosarcoma patients with virus-modified tumor cells. *Ann. N.Y. Acad. Sci.*, **277**, 396–411 (1976).
8. Kobayashi, H., Sendo, F., Kaji, H., Shirai, T., Saito, H., Takeichi, N., Hosokawa, M., and Kodama, T. Inhibition of transplanted rat tumors by immunization with identical tumor cells infected with Friend virus. *J. Natl. Cancer Inst.*, **44**, 11–19 (1970).
9. Koprowski, H., Love, R., and Koprowska, I. Enhancement of susceptibility to viruses in neoplastic tissues. *Tex. Rep. Biol. Med.*, **15**, 559–576 (1957).
10. Lindenmann, J. Resistance of mice to mouse-adapted influenza A virus. *Virology*, **16**, 203–204 (1962).
11. Lindenmann, J. Immunity to transplantable tumors following viral oncolysis I. Mechanism of immunity to Erhlich ascites tumor. *Immunology*, **94**, 461–466 (1965).
12. Lindenmann, J. Viruses as immunological adjuvants in cancer. *Biochem. Biophys. Acta*, **355**, 49–75 (1974).
13. Lindenmann, J. and Klein, P. Viral oncolysis: Increased immunogenicity of host cell antigen associated with influenza virus. *J. Exp. Med.*, **126**, 93–108 (1967).
14. Mitchison, N. A. Immunologic approach to cancer. *Transplant. Proc.*, **2**, 92–103 (1970).
15. Moore, A. E. The oncolytic viruses. *Prog. Exp. Tumor. Res.*, **1**, 411–439 (1960).
16. Murray, D., Cassel, W., Torbin, A., Olkowski, Z., and Moore, M. Viral oncolysate in the management of malignant melanoma. *Cancer*, **40**, 680–686 (1977).
17. Nowel, P. C. Phytohemagglutinin: An initiator of mitosis in cultures of normal human leukocytes. *Cancer Res.*, **20**, 462–466 (1960).
18. Roenigk, H. H., Jr., Deodhar, S., St. Jacques, R., and Burdick, K. Immunotherapy of malignant melanoma with vaccinia virus. *Arch. Dermatol.*, **109**, 668–673 (1974).
19. Sauter, C., Cavalli, F., Lindenmann, J., Gmur, J. P., Berchtold, W., Alberto, P., Obrecht, P., and Senn, H. J. Viral oncolysis: Its application in maintenance treatment of acute myelogenous leukemia. *In* "Immunotherapy of Cancer: Present Status of Trials in Man," ed. W. D. Terry and D. Windhorst, p. 355 (1978). Raven Press, New York.

20. Sinkovics, J. Immunotherapy with viral oncolysates for sarcoma. *J. Am. Med. Assoc.*, **237**, 869 (1977).

21. Webb, H. E. and Gordon Smith, C. E. Viruses in the treatment of cancer. Lancet, **i**, 1206–1208 (1970).

22. Weir, D. M. Hemagglutination inhibition. *In* "Handbook of Experimental Immunology," pp. 781–786 (1967). Blackwell Scientific Publications, Oxford.

ATTEMPTS AT VIRUS-ASSISTED IMMUNOTHERAPY IN HUMAN CANCER

J. Lindenmann

*Institute of Medical Microbiology, Division of Experimental Microbiology, University of Zürich**

Patients with acute myelogenous leukemia received injections of virus-infected, allogeneic myeloblasts in an attempt at virus-assisted maintenance immunotherapy. The virus in the cell homogenate was inactivated. This randomised trial showed no effect, beneficial or otherwise, of the procedure.

Two terminal cancer patients with carcinomatous pleural effusions, in whose cells avian influenza A virus replicated *in vitro*, were injected with the virus by the intra-pleural route, the virus being given live. Viral replication could be demonstrated *in vivo*, with effects on the tumor both locally and at distant sites. No conclusions as to the possible benefits of this procedure could be drawn.

Controlled Trial of Maintenance Chemotherapy versus Maintenance Chemotherapy plus Virus-assisted Immunotherapy in Acute Myelogenous Leukemia

Details of this collaborative study have been reported (*4*). Briefly, patients diagnosed as suffering from acute myelogenous leukemia were subjected to initial chemotherapy. Those entering remission were randomised into two groups, the first receiving, at monthly intervals, a standard regimen of maintenance chemotherapy. The second group was treated, in addition to exactly the same maintenance chemotherapy, with injections of allogeneic, virus-infected, homogenized, formalin-treated myeloblasts 2 weeks after each preceding chemotherapy course. The allogeneic myeloblasts were obtained from patients with acute myelogenous leukemia before the start of treatment and were infected *in vitro* with a strain of avian influenza virus which had been serially passed through myeloblasts from several patients (*3*). The material injected consisted of a high speed pellet of culture supernatant plus the disrupted cells. Formalin was added to inactivate the virus. Each monthly injection contained the equivalent of 10^9 infected cells.

1) Results

As judged by overall survival, actuarial survival curves, and length of remission, both groups followed the same course. Thus neither beneficial nor adverse effects of the immunotherapeutic maneuvre could be detected.

---

* CH-8006 Zürich, Switzerland.

2) *Critique*

The protocol was intended as a pilot study for testing logistic problems under conditions of minimal risk both to the patient and to his surroundings. This was the reason for inactivating the virus with Formalin. Although in animal models with allogeneic tumors Formalin treatment had not greatly impaired immunogenicity of viral oncolysates, it is doubtful whether this can be extrapolated to the human situation where the relevant tumor-associated antigen, if indeed there is one, might be destroyed by Formalin. Inactivation of the virus was deemed necessary to avoid the possibility of producing recombinants between our strain of avian influenza virus adapted to human cells and human influenza virus strains that patients might accidentally pick up while under treatment. Such recombinants might conceivably give rise to new pandemic variants, a risk we did not want to run. However, on second thought we may have exaggerated this danger. In influenza virus laboratories all over the world laboratory personnel routinely work with influenza strains from animal and human sources, and are at the same time exposed to the normal risks of acquiring influenza. Particular precautions are not taken, and laboratory-centered influenza outbreaks have not been reported.

There are several other weak points in this pilot experiments: The supposed immunotherapy was given to immunologically compromised hosts, since we did not want to deprive one group of patients from the benefits of chemotherapy. The use of allogeneic cells, although it greatly facilitated certain practical aspects of the trial, may have left out the very antigens that could be important. Furthermore, the total amount of antigen injected may have been insufficient.

Individual Attempts at Producing Oncolysis in Terminal Cancer Patients

With the strain of avian influenza virus adapted to grow in myeloblasts and used in the trial mentioned above, we have also inoculated a patient suffering from acute myelogenous leukemia. The virus was injected live, and the number of myeloblasts decreased, suggesting some effect of the virus. This case has been reported in detail (2). In parallel with the controlled trial of acute myelogenous leukemia mentioned before, we have used live avian influenza virus in two terminal cancer patients. The main purpose was to test for replication *in vivo* of a strain which had been adapted *in vitro* to the particular cancer cell type involved. In addition, we wanted to get an impression of possible side reactions under the extreme condition of tumor-adapted virus brought in immediate contact with a large tumor mass. The first case concerned a 54-year old woman with bronchiogenic carcinoma, with an extended carcinomatous pleural effusion and palpable lymph node metastases. Tumor cells could be cultivated from the pleural effusion. An avian strain of influenza A virus serially adapted to grow in carcinoma cells BT20 readily grew to high titers in the *in vitro*-held tumor cells of this patient. Virus having replicated in the patient's cells *in vitro* was injected into the carcinomatous pleural effusion. It replicated to high titers within the pleural cavity. Fever developed, and later the pleural effusion regressed. High antiviral titers became detectable in the serum. Palpable lymph nodes regressed distinctly. Intrapleural virus inoculations were repeated after 6 and 10 months without much further improvement. The patient died 2 years after the first virus injection. There was no evidence that "viral oncolysis" had in any way shortened her life. On the contrary, both subjective and objective improvement, although insufficient to influence the inevitable fatal outcome, was noticeable.

The second case, which will be reported in full details elsewhere (Ch. Mayer, in preparation), was that of a 56-year old nurse with disseminated mammary cancer, again with carcinomatous pleural effusion. The same strain of avian influenza virus as above, but now adapted to grow in mammary tumor cell lines obtained from a number of patients with carcinomatous effusions (*1*), was shown to grow in the patient's cells *in vitro*, and in the patient's pleural cavity *in vivo*. There was high fever 2 and 3 days after virus instillation, and the virus could be recovered repeatedly from the pleural cavity and once from the blood. Tumorous infiltrates around the neck became softer with evidence of local inflammation. The pleural exudate changed from one containing an almost pure suspension of tumor cells to one dominated by macrophages. High antiviral antibody titers developed. The patient survived for another 5 months after oncolysis. There was again no evidence for a deleterious effect of the procedure. Subjectively both patients, who had been fully informed and had consented to be subjected to a novel therapeutic attempt, felt transiently much improved. This was probably due in a large extent to psychological factors, since these hopeless cases were surrounded with much attention, and since obvious effects on distant foci were unmistakable. It is questionable whether life was prolonged, but it does not seem to have been shortened.

Critique

These two cases show that properly adapted avian influenza A virus can grow in tumor cells *in vivo*, at least in cells floating in the pleural cavity. The virus did not seem to be excreted in an epidemiologically significant way: Throat washings remained free of virus in both cases. Our attempt suffered from the drawback inherent in many similar applications of therapeutic measures to patients who are definitely beyond the point of no return: Objective improvement was not lasting, and subjective improvement may have been due more to the effects of a psychological than of an immunological adjuvant.

Nevertheless, it is felt that the successful adaptation of avian influenza virus to human tumor cells and its capacity to replicate *in vivo* form important steps towards application of the principles of viral xenogenization in human cancer.

REFERENCES

1. Illiger, H-J., Sauter, Chr., and Lindenmann, J. Replication of an avian myxovirus in tumor cell cultures obtained from effusions of mammary carcinoma patients. *Cancer Res.*, **35**, 3623–3627 (1975).
2. Sauter, Chr., Gerber, A., Lindenmann, J., and Martz, G. Akute myeloische Leukämie: Behandlungsversuch mit einem Myeloblasten adaptierten Myxovirus. *Schweiz. Med. Wochenschr.*, **102**, 285–290 (1972).
3. Sauter, Chr., Baumberger, U., Ekenbark, S., and Lindenmann, J. Replication of an avian myxovirus in primary cultures of human leukemic cells. *Cancer Res.*, **33**, 3002–3007 (1973).

4. Sauter, Chr. and Lindenmann, J. Virusassistierte Immunotherapie bei der akuten myeloischen Leukämie. *In* "Erkrankungen der Myelopoese," ed. A. Stacher and P. Höcker, pp. 280–281 (1976). Urban & Schwarzenberg, München-Berlin-Wien.

SUBJECT INDEX